PRACTICAL DEMENTIA CARE

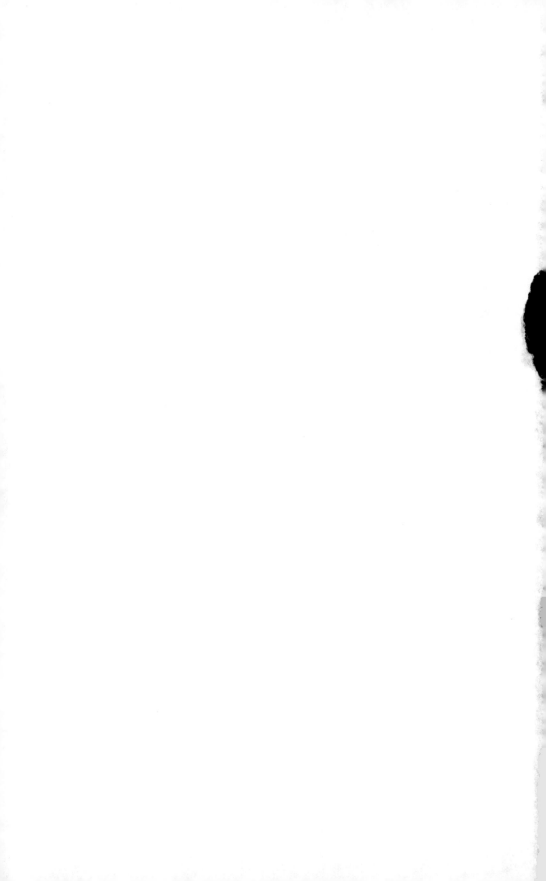

PRACTICAL DEMENTIA CARE

Second Edition

Peter V. Rabins, M.D., M.P.H.
Constantine G. Lyketsos, M.D., M.H.S.
Cynthia D. Steele, R.N., MP.H.

*Johns Hopkins School of Medicine
and Bloomberg School of Public Health
The Johns Hopkins University
Baltimore, Maryland*

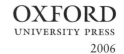

OXFORD
UNIVERSITY PRESS
2006

OXFORD
UNIVERSITY PRESS

Oxford University Press, Inc., publishes works that further
Oxford University's objective of excellence
in research, scholarship, and education.

Oxford   New York
Auckland   Cape Town   Dar es Salaam   Hong Kong   Karachi
Kuala Lumpur   Madrid   Melbourne   Mexico   City Nairobi
New Delhi   Shanghai   Taipei   Toronto

With offices in
Argentina   Austria   Brazil   Chile   Czech Republic   France   Greece
Guatemala   Hungary   Italy   Japan   Poland   Portugal   Singapore
South Korea   Switzerland   Thailand   Turkey   Ukraine   Vietnam

Published by Oxford University Press, Inc.
198 Madison Avenue, New York, New York 10016
www.oup.com

Oxford is a registered trademark of Oxford University Press

Library of Congress Cataloging-in-Publication Data
Rabins, Peter V.
Practical dementia care / Peter V. Rabins, Constantine G. Lyketsos, Cynthia D. Steele.—2nd ed.
p. cm.
Includes bibliographical references and index.
ISBN-13: 978-0-19-516978-2
ISBN 0-19-516978-6
1. Dementia—Patients—Care.   I. Lyketsos, Constantine G.   II. Steele, Cynthia, 1947–   III. Title.
RC521.R33 2005
616.8'3—dc22   2005040670

The science of medicine is a rapidly changing field. As new research and clinical experience broaden our knowledge, changes in treatment and drug therapy do occur. The author and publisher of this work have checked
with sources believed to be reliable in their efforts to provide information that is accurate and complete, and
in accordance with the standards accepted at the time of publication. However, in light of the possibility of
human error or changes in the practice of medicine, neither the author, nor the publisher, nor any other party
who has been involved in the preparation or publication of this work warrants that the information contained herein is in every respect accurate or complete. Readers are encouraged to confirm the information
contained herein with other reliable sources, and are strongly advised to check the product information sheet
provided by the pharmaceutical company for each drug they plan to administer.

9   8   7   6   5   4   3   2   1

Printed in the United States of America
on acid-free paper

FOREWORD

Alzheimer's disease and other dementing disorders are becoming so prevalent in aging global societies that they represent a major threat to the public health and public purse. The frequency of dementia increases markedly among the old-old, and this population is among the fastest-growing segments of societies around the world. Cognitive, functional, and behavioral compromises associated with dementia syndromes reduce the quality of life for patient and caregiver, increase the costs and distress associated with care, may precipitate institutionalization, and eventually lead to the death of the affected individual.

The growing population of persons afflicted with cognitive impairment demands clinicians with expertise in dementia management. There are few volumes that comprehensively address the wide range of strategies potentially useful in limiting the progression and treating the symptoms of patients with dementia. *Practical Dementia Care,* second edition, helps fill this information gap. Building on the success of the first edition, this revised volume provides scientifically based yet practical information useful to the clinician faced with the multifaceted challenges of working with patients suffering from dementia and their caregivers. This volume addresses dementia assessment; cortical, subcortical, and mixed dementia syndromes; dementia care management; pharmacotherapy of dementing disorders; supporting the family and the care provider of dementia patients; normal aging; care of the advanced dementia patient; and legal and ethical issues relevant to dementia care. When the complex issues of management of behavioral disturbances are discussed, both pharmacologic and nonpharmacologic interventions are described. Adopting a disease-state management approach, the authors provide care pathways for the major diagnostic and therapeutic challenges encountered while providing humane care to patients with cognitive disorders.

Practical Dementia Care is a resource to which dementia care providers can refer for guidance in the increasingly complex area of dementia management.

Jeffrey L. Cummings, M.D.
Los Angeles, California

PREFACE

The recognition in the 1970s and 1980s that the dementias are prevalent sources of morbidity for patients, families, and society, the demonstration that the dementias are brain diseases and not the expected outcomes of normal aging, and dramatic advances in our understanding of brain function have all fueled a dramatic increase in knowledge about the causes and treatments of this group of illnesses.

This second edition of *Practical Dementia Care* updates the first edition by describing the advances in our understanding of the biology of Alzheimer disease, a reorganization of how the fronto-temporal dementias are organized and diagnosed, and new information about several other diseases known to cause dementia. The treatment sections present new information about medication therapies, while the problem management sections expand approaches to specific neuropsychiatric and behavioral problems.

The section on competency assessment has also been expanded and a new chapter on early diagnosis and prevention has been added. The latter signals an appreciation that the best opportunities for reversing symptoms lie in starting treatment at the very earliest possible time, perhaps even before symptoms start.

Knowledge about dementia is advancing a rapid pace. We believe this second edition will help clinicians improve their practice and experience the excitement that new gains in knowledge bring to a field.

Contents

Foreword, *Jeffrey L. Cummings, M.D.*   vii

Introduction   xiii

CHAPTER 1   Definitions and Overview of the Book   1

CHAPTER 2   The Evaluation and Formulation of Dementia   15

CHAPTER 3   Diseases Causing a Cortical Pattern of Dementia   43

CHAPTER 4   Diseases Typically Causing Subcortical
            or Mixed Pattern Dementias   57

CHAPTER 5   Overview of Dementia Care   75

CHAPTER 6   Supportive Care for the Patient with Dementia   89

CHAPTER 7   Supporting the Family and Care Provider   109

CHAPTER 8   Noncognitive Behavioral and Neuropsychiatric
            Disorders   131

CHAPTER 9   Noncognitive Functional Disorders and
            Disturbances in Sleeping, Eating, and Sexuality   169

CHAPTER 10 Pharmacologic and Other Biologic Treatments
            in Dementia   201

CHAPTER 11 Prevention, Early Detection, and Mild Cognitive
            Impairment   231

CHAPTER 12 Terminal Care   241

CHAPTER 13 Ethical and Legal Issues   251

CHAPTER 14 Clinical Genetics and Dementia   269

            Appendices   277

            Glossary   301

            Bibliography   311

            Index   319

INTRODUCTION

This book is meant to be used by professionals involved in the evaluation and treatment of people who suffer from one of the many disorders that cause dementia. This includes primary care and specialist physicians, nurses, psychologists, social workers, activity therapists, occupational therapists, physical therapists, and gerontologists. The book takes a broad, holistic approach to dementia and should be useful to professionals treating patients in settings varying from the community to the hospital. It may be of particular interest to professionals caring for people with dementia who reside in long-term care facilities such as retirement communities, assisted living facilities, and nursing homes. We hope that the book will also be useful to policy makers, health administrators, and others who want to understand the skills involved in providing care for people with dementia.

The care of people with dementia carries with it many challenges. Among the most difficult is the need to consider the disorder and the ill person from several different viewpoints. Paul McHugh and Phillip Slavney have suggested that four perspectives guide the clinician approach. All will agree that the cardinal disturbance of dementia, the cognitive disorder, results from an impairment of brain function. This approach must be the starting point and is called the *disease perspective*. In addition, the disease afflicts a person who has attributes that she or he has carried throughout life—personality traits, innate cognitive abilities, likes and dislikes, skills and interests. These are universal characteristics of human beings and are best considered as graded *dimensions* because people differ in the amount or extent of these characteristics. Dimensional characteristics of people with dementia are important to consider since they shape the persons' symptoms, reactions, and behaviors. In addition, these essential characteristics of a person are sometimes changed by the disease. For example, a person who has been suspicious and irritable may become pleasant and trusting. Helping the family describe a patient's characteristics prior to the development of the illness can help the clinician appreciate how the patient is responding to the illness and how the family is reacting to its manifestations.

A very different viewpoint shapes a third aspect of dementia care. At the level of *behavior,* we become less interested in the cause of a problem and focus more on helping the person adapt more comfortably to the problems imposed by the disease. Problems in behavior are common in persons with dementia and will be extensively discussed in Chapter 10. The ability to take a behavioral approach is one of the most important requirements of the professional providing care for individuals with dementia. It requires a set of skills that can be learned and taught.

The fourth perspective, the *life story* approach, requires the professional caregiver to appreciate the uniqueness of each individual who is suffering from dementia and to appreciate the many meanings that these illnesses carry with them. The ability to understand the fear and sense of loss experienced by many patients with dementia and by their loved ones complements the other three viewpoints (or perspectives) and is as necessary as they are for providing good care.

The challenge is clear. Professionals who dedicate themselves to caring for individuals with dementia must be willing to think at multiple levels. The artificial boundaries imposed by the profession (nurse, doctor, social worker, activity therapist) and models of care (medical model, social model, holistic model) break down in the face of complex diseases like the dementias. A major challenge faced by students, practitioners, policy makers, and planners is that each approach and each profession makes unique contributions to the care of people with dementia. The skillful provider is the person who can move from one mode of thinking to another, the choice depending on the circumstances.

The difficulties and challenges of caring for individuals with dementia should not be underestimated or exaggerated. The rewards of providing care are many. They are based on the improved quality of life that good professional care brings to the ill, their family members, their loved ones, and society as a whole. This book is based upon the belief that the best care is provided by individuals who are well trained, who have developed a variety of techniques, who can treat each patient as an individual, and who are able to identify, within themselves, the rewards and frustrations of caring for people with chronic and usually progressive, debilitating diseases.

PRACTICAL DEMENTIA CARE

1

Definitions and Overview
of the Book

Dementia is a clinical syndrome caused by a wide range of diseases that affect the brain. Its core feature is a decline in cognition. Dementia has multiple causes and presentations. It can be stable or progressive. It can afflict the young or the old. Dementia is also associated with a wide range of mental and behavioral disturbances, many of which are reminiscent of other psychiatric disorders. Dementia causes functional impairments that derive from the impairments in cognition, but it can also be the result of behavioral disturbances. Dementia renders individuals more vulnerable to the effects of coexisting medical conditions and medications. Finally, dementia occurs in a family context and affects the lives of many others. The care of the dementia patient is a complex endeavor. It requires multiple skills and the involvement of the patient, family, care providers, and health professionals.

This chapter will introduce definitions that professionals caring for patients with dementia need to keep in mind. It will discuss the magnitude, burdens, and costs of dementia. This will be followed by a detailed discussion of the complexities of dementia care. Finally, the organization of this book and how it might help professionals in providing dementia care will be reviewed.

DEFINITIONS

Dementia

The word *dementia* derives from the Latin *de mens* and means "from the mind" and is mentioned in the Bible and early Egyptian, Greek, and Roman writings. This suggests that it has affected humankind since the dawn of time. To many, the word *dementia* implies craziness, irrationality, and hopelessness, but none of these meanings is accurate. While many terms have been proposed to replace *dementia,* all have taken on the same undesirable connotations. This suggests that it is not the word that is frightening but rather the disorder it describes. Dementia is best defined as a *syndrome,* a pattern of clinical symptoms and signs that meets the definition presented in Table 1.1. The first element of the definition is a decline or deterioration in the cognitive or thinking capacities. This decline from a previous level of ability distinguishes dementia from disorders of cognition that have been present since birth, such as mental retardation and learning disabilities. The severity of this decline must be such that there is some effect on day-to-day functioning. This differentiates dementia from milder forms of cognitve decline dicussed in Chapter 11.

The second element of the definition requires that more than one area of cognition be impaired. Memory is affected in almost every disease that causes dementia, while the other cognitive impairments in judgment, perception, language, abstraction, persistence, and calculation depend on the specific disease and the stage of the illness. This criterion distinguishes dementia from disorders in which only a single cognitive ability is impaired, for example aphasia, in which language disorder is present, and the amnestic syndrome, in which only memory is impaired (see also Chapter 11).

Even though dementia requires multiple impairments, not all cognitive functions are necessarily affected. In addition, the functions that are impaired often vary in the degree to which they are affected. Thus, there is variation from patient to patient in the type and severity of cognitive processes that are impaired. The identification of retained capacities is an important component of treatment planning that can help the ill person remain as functional as possible.

Based on the pattern of cognitive impairment (phenomenology), two types of dementia syndromes are recognized, cortical and subcortical. In the cortical type, the brain pathology predominantly affects cognitive functions that are located in the outside layers of the brain, that is, the cortex, such as memory, language, gnosis, and praxis. Loss of memory capacity is called *amnesia;* language impairment is referred to as *aphasia;* impairment in the ability to do learned motor tasks is called *apraxia;* and impairment in recognition is called *agnosia.* Thus, the cortical dementias are characterized by amnesia, aphasia, apraxia, and agnosia (the *four A's*). Alzheimer disease is the best-known example. In subcortical dementia the pathology involves primarily deeper brain structures. Patients lose the ability to coordinate cognition and have difficulties with memory (forgetfulness), slowed thinking and moving, and decision making, and have reduced complexity of thought

TABLE 1.1. Definition of Dementia

1. Decline of cognitive capacity (memory, language, judgment, etc.), with some effect on day-to-day functioning

2. Impairment in multiple areas of cognition (global)

3. Normal level of consciousness (absence of delirium)

(dysmnesia, delay, dysexecutive function, and depletion—the *four D's*). Of note, cortical and subcortical disturbances can coexist, in which case patients are said to have *mixed* dementia.

Table 1.2 summarizes the differences between cortical and subcortical dementia. Patients with cortical dementia lose cognitive capacities, the ability to do things. In contrast, patients with subcortical dementia lose the ability to coordinate cognition but retain the ability to use it. A parallel with motor disturbances is apt: patients with a stroke in the motor area lose the ability to do movement (cortical), while patients with Parkinson disease can move but are unable to coordinate movement properly so that their actions are delayed, slowed, imprecise, and lack dexterity (subcortical).

The third element of the definition of dementia is that alertness and awakeness are not impaired. This criterion is sometimes stated as having a normal level of consciousness. It distinguishes dementia from delirium. *Delirium* is a condition in which the patient is drowsy, inattentive, or unable to sustain concentration and in which multiple impairments in thinking are present. Delirium usually begins suddenly and is often associated with disordered sleep, visual hallucinations, and behavior change.

Delirium is most commonly caused by a metabolic abnormality (such as abnormal electrolytes), an infectious process, or medication toxicity. Dementia and delirium often occur together because dementia is a risk factor for the development of delirium. Since delirium is often reversible, its recognition should lead to an intensive search for a cause.

It can be difficult to distinguish between delirium and dementia when memory or language is so severely impaired that the patient is unable to sustain a conversation, or when perceptual dysfunction is so marked that the patient seems not to pay attention to other people or to the environment. If patients are fully alert, they do not meet the altered level of consciousness criterion of delirium.

The frequent occurrence of delirium and dementia was illustrated by a large Finnish study in which 2000 individuals were examined on admission to a general hospital. Fifteen percent of the patients over age 55 suffered from delirium. Twenty-five percent of this group were later found to be suffering from an underlying dementia, twice the rate of dementia in nondelirious ad-

TABLE 1.2. Cortical versus Subcortical Dementia

	Cortical	Subcortical
Key feature	Loss of core ability (capacity) to cognate	Loss of ability to coordinate cognition
Mneumonic	The four A's	The four D's
Features	Amnesia	Dysmnesia
	Apraxia	Delay
	Aphasia	Dysexecutive
	Agnosia	Depletion
Typical Symptoms	Cannot recall or recognize	Benefits from cues to remember
	Repeats questions or statements	Thinking and movement are slowed
	Cannot do things	Trouble planning and executing
	Does not know things	Inflexible
	Trouble with language	Poor initiative

missions. Among those who developed delirium while hospitalized, 22% suffered from dementia.

Dementia is caused by a disease of the brain. By *disease* we mean a process that causes something to be broken in the structure or function of the brain. This might be due to a direct mechanical injury such as trauma, degeneration or death of brain cells, or a factor that temporarily disrupts brain cell function such as an abnormal level of thyroid hormones. These pathologic changes can have one or several causes. Ultimately, every dementia syndrome will be associated with a specific pathologic change due to a specific disease. The location and extent of the damage to the brain will explain the symptom profile (the syndrome). Table 1.3 lists the most common diseases that cause dementia.

Noncognitive neuropsychiatric symptoms

The term *noncognitive neuropsychiatric symptoms* refers to a wide range of disturbances in mental life and behavior that afflict almost all patients with dementia. These are defined descriptively, sometimes as individual symptoms and at other times as syndromes. They are sometimes referred to as the *behavioral and psychological symptoms of dementia* (BPSD). They are distinguished from *cognitive neuropsychiatric symptoms* such as amnesia and agnosia for several reasons. Cognitive and noncognitive neuropsychiatric

TABLE 1.3. Dementia-Causing Diseases

Degenerative brain diseases	*Traumatic brain injuries*
Alzheimer disease	Closed head injury
Parkinson disease	Open head injury
Frontotemporal degeneration	Subdural hematoma
Huntington disease	
Progressive supranuclear palsy	*Vitamin deficiencies*
Spinocerebellar degeneration	Vitamin B_{12} deficiency (subacute
Multiple sclerosis	combined sclerosis, pernicious
	anemia)
Cerebrovascular diseases	Vitamin B_6 deficiency (pellagra)
Multiple infarct disease	Vitamin B_1 (thiamine) deficiency
Binswanger disease	
Subcortical leukoareosis	*Endocrine diseases*
Thalamic infarct	Hyperthyroidism
	Hypothyroidism
Cerebral vasculitides	Growth hormone deficiency
Lupus erythematosus	Hyperparathyroidism
Temporal arteritis	Cushing disease (hyperadrenalism)
Giant cell arteritis	Conn disease (hypoadrenalism)
Infectious diseases	*Cerebral tumors*
Syphilis (general paresis of the insane)	Intrinsic brain tumor
Tuberculosis	Metastatic cancer
HIV disease (AIDS dementia	
complex)	*Toxin exposure*
Prion diseases (Creutzfeld-Jakob	Alcohol
disease)	Heavy metals (lead, arsenic, mercury)
Fungal encephalitides	Volatile hydrocarbons
Viral encephalitides	Medications
Psychiatric disorders	*Other*
Major depressive disorder	Normal pressure (communicating)
Schizophrenia	hydrocephalus

AIDS, acquired immune deficiency syndrome; HIV, human immunodeficiency virus.

symptoms are caused by damage to different parts of the brain from the dementing disease. The noncognitive are more often affected by environmental circumstances and at times are a consequence of the cognitive symptoms (e.g., becoming upset when confronted with forgetfulness). In addition, the noncognitive neuropsychiatric symptoms are more responsive to currently available treatments.

The most common noncognitive neuropsychiatric disturbances are listed in Table 1.4 (for definitions see the Glossary). In this book, at times we use the terms *behavioral disturbances* and *noncognitive symptoms* interchange-

TABLE 1.4. Hierarchical Grouping of Noncognitive Neuropsychiatric Disturbances in Dementia

Delirium	*Disturbance of basic drives*
Affective cluster	Sleep disorders
	Feeding disorders
Major depression	Sexual disorders
Depression of Alzheimer disease	
Alzheimer-associated affective disorder	*Miscellaneous problem behaviors*
Anxiety disorder	Rummaging and hoarding
	Aggression-agitation
Psychotic cluster	Wandering and pacing
	Social withdrawal and apathy
Psychosis of Alzheimer disease	Catastrophic reactions
Isolated hallucinosis	Uncooperativeness with care
Delusions, suspiciousness, paranoia	

ably to refer to these symptoms. Table 1.4 groups these disturbances into specific areas using a hierarchic approach. By a *hierarchic approach* we mean that conditions listed earlier in the table take precedence over conditions listed later for purposes of classification and treatment. Thus, for example, a diagnosis of an affective cluster disturbance will not be made if a diagnosis of delirium can be made. Smilalry, a diagnosis of a sleep disturbance will not be made if a diagnosis of an affective disturbance can be made.

The etiopathogenesis of these noncognitive neuropsychiatric symptoms is complex. In some instances, the disease causing the dementia also injures brain areas important to the regulation of mood, perception, and behavior. In other cases, these symptoms are a consequence of the cognitive disorder itself. Additionally, they may be the consequence of preexisting psychiatric disorders, or may be due to comorbid medical problems or medications, that dementia patients are receiving. This is discussed in greater detail in Chapter 9.

The importance of noncognitive neuropsychiatric disturbances in dementia is underscored by their high prevalence and high morbidity. From 25% to 40% of patients with mild dementia and as many as 75% to 80% of patients with severe dementia, particularly those who are institutionalized or in nursing homes, suffer from experience such symptoms. Over a lifetime of suffering from dementia, 90% of individuals experience a noncognitive neuropsychiatric symptom. In addition, these disturbances contribute to the disability experienced by dementia patients. For example, problems as diverse as depression, hallucinations, and irritability can prevent participation in day-care programs even when the cognitive and physical capacities to do so are present. Furthermore, behavioral disturbances contribute to the burnout of those who care for dementia patients and are a primary reason for the placement of patients with dementia in long-term care facilities.

Impairment and disability

The word *impairment* refers to loss of function directly due to the illness causing a disease. The word *disability* is defined as the loss of function that results from this impairment. The disabilities associated with dementia range from the very mild to the very severe. Mild disabilities include the inability to do instrumental activities of daily living (IADLs). These include the ability to work, maintain a living space, shop, clean house, handle money, use the telephone, get from place to place, drive, and so forth. Almost all patients with dementia have impairments in some of these instrumental activities, and most are dependent on others for all of these activities. As the dementia progresses (or in more severe cases of dementia), patients lose the ability to perform more basic activities of daily living (ADLs) such as dressing, bathing, personal care, toileting, navigating in their homes, and eating. An additional source of disability for some patients is a loss of the capacity for self-regulation. This results in doing things that are inappropriate, socially objectionable, or dangerous, for example wandering and getting lost, hitting others who try to help them with daily activities, or sitting in one place all day, becoming deconditioned and being at high risk for falling. Table 1.5 provides one approach to staging functional impairment, the Functional Assessment Staging of Alzheimer Disease (FAST) system of Reisberg and collaborators. This was developed in Alzheimer disease but is applicable to other dementias as well.

Co-morbidity

Many patients with dementia suffer from other medical and psychiatric illnesses. Rates of medical co-morbidity and medication treatment for co-morbidity are similar to those of age-comparable people without dementia. In addition, dementia patients are very vulnerable to illness. The more co-morbidities they have, the greater their impairments in cognition and functioning. The explanation for this is not clear but may have to do with the fact that dementia reflects widespread disease of the brain. In part, this is due to the association between old age and chronic illnesses such as arthritis and diabetes, but it also probably results from the fact that brain dysfunction lowers the threshold for developing symptoms. For example, an elderly patient without dementia is better able to handle the flu than an elderly person with dementia. Dementia also makes patients more likely to develop side effects from medications.

TABLE 1.5. FAST Stages

FAST Stage	Characteristics	Clinical Diagnosis
1	No objective or subjective functional decrement.	Normal Adult
2	Subjective deficit in recalling names or other word-finding and/or subjective deficit in recalling location of objects and/or subjectively decreased ability to recall appointments. No objectively manifest functional deficits.	Normal Aged Adult
3	*Deficits noted in demanding occupational and social settings* (e.g., the individual may begin to forget important appointments for the first time; work productivity may decline); problems may be noted in traveling to unfamiliar locations (e.g., may get lost traveling by automobile and/or public transportation to a new location or spot).	Compatible with Incipient AD
4	*Deficits in performance of complex tasks of daily life* (e.g., paying bills and/or balancing checkbook; decreased capacity in planning and/or preparing an elaborate meal; decreased capacity in marketing, such as in the correct purchase of grocery items).	Mild AD
5	*Deficient performance in choosing proper attire, and assistance is required for independent community functioning*—the spouse or other caregiver frequently must help the individual choose the appropriate clothing for the occasion and/or season (e.g., the individual will wear incongruous clothing); over the course of this stage, some patients may also begin to forget to bathe regularly (unless reminded), and automobile driving capability becomes compromised (e.g., carelessness in driving and violations of driving rules).	Moderate AD
6a	*Requires physical assistance in putting on clothing properly*—the caregiver must provide increasing assistance with the mechanics of helping the individual clothe himself properly (e.g., putting on clothing in the proper sequence, tying shoelaces, putting shoes on proper feet, buttoning and/or zipping clothing, putting on blouse, shirt, pants, skirt, etc., correctly).	Moderately Severe AD
6b	*Requires assistance in bathing properly*—the patient's ability to adjust bathwater temperature diminishes; the patient may have difficulty entering and leaving the bath; there may be problems with washing properly and completely drying the body.	Moderately Severe AD
6c	*Requires assistance with mechanics of toileting*—patients at this stage may forget to flush the toilet and may begin to wipe themselves improperly or less fastidiously when toileting.	Moderately Severe AD

Fast Stage	Characteristics	Clinical Diagnosis
6d	*Urinary incontinence*—this occurs in the absence of infection or other genitourinary tract pathology; the patient has episodes of urinary incontinence. Frequency of toileting may somewhat mitigate the occurrence of incontinence.	Moderately Severe AD
6e	*Fecal incontinence*—in the absence of gastrointestinal pathology, the patient has episodes of fecal incontinence. Frequency of toileting may somewhat mitigate the occurrence of incontinence.	Moderately Severe AD
7a	*Speech limited to about six words in the course of an average day*—during the course of an average day the patient's speech is restricted to single words (e.g., "Yes," "No," "Please") or short phrases (e.g., "please don't hurt me," "get away," "get out of here," "I like you").	Severe AD
7b	*Intelligible vocabulary generally limited to a single word in the course of an average day*—as the illness progresses the ability to utter even short phrases on a regular basis is lost, so that the spoken vocabulary becomes limited to generally one or two single words as an indicator for all things and needs (e.g., "Yes," "No," "okay" for all verbalization-provoking phenomena).	Severe AD
7c	*Ambulatory ability lost*—patients gradually lose the ability to ambulate independently; in the early part of this substage, they may require actual support (e.g., being physically supported by a caregiver) and physical assistance to walk, but as the substage progresses, the ability to ambulate even with assistance is lost; the onset is somewhat varied, with some patients simply taking progressively smaller and slower steps; other patients begin to tilt forward, backward, or laterally when ambulating; twisted gaits have also been noted as antecedents of ambulatory loss.	Severe AD
7d	*Ability to sit up lost*—the patients lose the ability to sit up without assistance (e.g., they need some form of physical brace—an arm rest, a belt, or other special devices to keep them from sliding down in the chair).	Severe AD
7e	*Ability to smile lost*—patients are no longer observed to smile, although they do manifest other facial movements and sometimes grimace.	Severe AD
7f	*Ability to hold head up lost*—patients can no longer hold up their head unless the head is supported.	Severe AD

Source: Adapted from Reisberg, B. Functional assessment staging (FAST). Psychpharm Bull 1998; 24:629–36.

AD, Alzheimer disease.

The presence of co-morbid medical illness and the use of medications to treat other diseases often result in a worsening of the cognitive symptoms of dementia, the development of delirium, the onset of noncognitive neuro-psychiatric symptoms, or accelerated cognitive decline. The provision of good medical, surgical, dental, gynecologic, and psychiatric care to dementia patients is critical in minimizing the effects of co-morbidity.

Caregivers

Given the disabilities associated with dementia, all patients with dementia need some assistance. The degree of caregiver involvement is usually proportional to the patient's level of impairment and disability. The majority of caregivers are family members, usually women, who are spouses, adult children, or siblings. Chapter 7 discusses their needs and the needs of professional caregivers.

THE SCOPE OF THE PROBLEM

Epidemiology is the study of the occurrence of a disorder in the population. It is an information science that seeks to discover the cause or causes of disease by studying how the condition is distributed in the population, identifying protective and causative factors, and studying treatment and prevention strategies.

Prevalence refers to how common a condition is in the community. Below age 65, the prevalence of dementia is low, on the order of 5–10 per 1000 people (0.5% to 1%). In this younger age group, dementia is most commonly caused by trauma to the brain. Brain diseases such as multiple sclerosis and Alzheimer disease, toxins such as lead, metabolic diseases such as Metachromatic Leukodystrophy or infections such as encephalitis can cause dementia in the young and others.

Over age 65, the prevalence of dementia increases dramatically (Fig. 1.1). Among all people 65 years of age and older, 70–100 per 1000 (7%–10%) suffer from dementia. This number increases to 180–200 per 1000 (18%–20%) for those 75 and older and to 350–400 per 1000 (35%–40%) for individuals 85 years of age and older. Over age 65, Alzheimer disease is the cause of 60%–70% of dementia.

The prevalence of dementia depends on the age distribution of the population. Currently in the United States, there are 4 to 5 million people with dementia, most of whom are elderly. This number will increase dramatically over the next few decades because the number of people living to old age is increasing. As a result, the number of people with dementia will double by

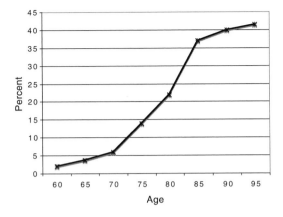

FIGURE 1.1 The prevalence of dementia at different ages.

the year 2020 unless a prevention or cure is developed for at least one of the common causes. The most rapidly growing age group is those 85 years old or older, the very old group, in which Alzheimer disease is most prevalent. This is the primary reason that the number of people with dementia will increase so dramatically.

The incidence rate of dementia also increases with age. *Incidence* is defined as the number of *new* cases of a disorder in a given period of time. At age 65, an individual who does not have dementia has a 25 per 1000 (0.25%) chance of developing dementia during the next year. This rate then doubles every 5 years (Fig. 1.2) so that by age 70, an individual who does not have dementia has a 50 per 1000 (0.5%) chance of developing dementia in the next year. By age 85, the annual incidence rate is 4%. Thus, the longer one lives, the greater the chance becomes of developing dementia. Furthermore, as average life expectancy increases, the risk of developing dementia increases, since living longer means living to an age at which the incidence rate is higher.

Valid data on incidence beyond age 90 are sparse because we know little of what happens to people who live into their 90s and 100s. Several possibilities can be imagined. In one scenario, the trend will continue with the incidence of dementia doubling every 5 years. If this in fact is true and the incidence continues to rise throughout the life span, then almost every individual will develop dementia by age 112. This conclusion has been supported by recent epidemiologic data from the Framingham Study in Massachussetts. An alternative possibility is that the incidence rate of dementia peaks at age 90 or 95 and then stabilizes or begins to decline. Recent data from the Cache County Memory Study in Utah suggest stabilization fol-

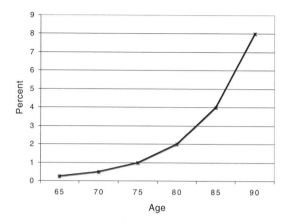

FIGURE 1.2 The incidence of dementia at different ages.

lowed by a reduction in the incidence of dementia after age 90, but other studies will need to confirm this before any conclusion can be drawn.

Another way of looking at the scope of dementia is to examine its costs to society. Direct costs, estimated at $80 billion per year in the United States, relate to the direct care provided for people with dementia. Indirect costs, which result from nonmedical expenses, are an additional $20 to $30 billion per year. They include the health care costs of caregivers, the years of productive life lost by the patient, and the loss of productivity of caregivers caaused, for example, by missing work or retiring early.

THE COMPLEXITIES OF DEMENTIA CARE

Professionals who care for patients with dementia need to be aware of the diverse presentations of dementia, the multiplicity of treatments that are available, and the importance of social, environmental, medical, and psychological issues. Dementia care can be provided at a variety of geographic locations, but the care needs to be coordinated among these sites.

Patients with progressive dementia require structure in their day, protection from victimization, and good medical care. As the dementia progresses, patients lose their capacity for independent decision making, so others have to make decisions for them. They also lose the ability to drive and live alone. Each of these losses adds a layer of complexity to their care.

Dementia care involves providing support to family members and other care providers, including helping them understand the patient's symptoms and condition, helping them care for the patient, and helping them access resources. Additionally, family care providers require considerable emotional support, because day-to-day caregiving is taxing and emotionally devastating.

Families, particularly children of dementia patients, also have another major concern. They live with the question "Is this likely to happen to me?" This arises from the recognition that they will grow old and may suffer a similar dementing illness, and from evolving knowledge reported in the mass media that certain dementias are heritable. Having a parent or another relative with dementia clearly affects a child's risk of getting it, perhaps at a younger age than expected.

Professional care providers are confronted with caring for patients with a complex, multifaceted, relentless disease, often terminal in nature. Cognitive, behavioral, and functional impairments all occur, and incapacitate patients and families. Care providers need to understand the various diseases that cause dementia, be prepared to detect it early, keep up with new scientific information about dementia, and maintain stamina and hope in the face of the cruelty of the disease. These needs make the task of dementia care a challenging one for the professional.

How to Use This Book

While the discussion above illustrates how dementia care is challenging, we believe that it is possible to go about it systematically, in a way that maximizes benefits to patients and families, and that continues to retain the interest and warmth of the professional care provider, thus preventing burnout. This book is intended to be a practical source of information and reference for the professional providing day-to-day care to patients. It is not intended to be a comprehensive reference book. We have forgone systematic referencing in order to keep the book more user-friendly. We suggest that beginners read the entire book and then refer to it periodically to brush up. Experts can refer to specific segments of the book as necessary. We have included many tables and figures, as well as practical aids to clinical practice, such as checklists, for use in day-to-day care of dementia patients.

The organization of this book is as follows: This chapter provides an overview of dementia focusing on a description and scope of the conditions. It is complemented by the Glossary. Chapter 2 presents in detail the process of evaluating and formulating a case of suspected dementia. Chapters 3 and 4 provide an overview of basic facts about the most common dementia-causing diseases. Many of these facts will change over time as new knowledge develops about dementia and the different diseases that cause it. However, some basic issues, such as definitions and complexities of care, are unlikely to change. The same is true of the practical approaches to evaluation and treatment that are presented throughout the book.

Chapter 5 provides a systematic overview of dementia care, and is organized to include principles, goals, and the development of treatment plans. The next two chapters (6 and 7) discuss in detail the supportive care that must be provided to both patients and caregivers. Chapters 8 and 9 focus on problem solving and discuss a long list of clinical problems frequently encountered in dementia care. For each of these problems, the chapters provide a definition of the problem and specific approaches to addressing it. Chapter 8 focuses on dealing with problems that arise directly out of noncognitive neuropsychiatric symptoms (behavioral and psychological symptoms). Chapter 9 deals with problems that arise out functional decline and disturbances in the basic drives of eating, sleeping, and sexuality. Chapter 10 provides an overview of currently available medications that may be used in the care of dementia patients. Chapter 11 is an overview of milder cognitive impairments, such as *cognitive impairment, not dementia* and *mild cognitive impairment.* These terms are used to refer to the cognitive decline that occurs in older people but is not severe enough to meet the criteria for a diagnosis of dementia. Chapter 12 discusses care for patients in the late stages of dementia. Chapter 13 presents practical approaches to legal and ethical issues that arise in dementia care. Chapter 14 includes a genetics primer and an approach to providing genetic counseling for patients with dementia. Following is a glossary of common terms in dementia care that should be consulted while reading the book if unfamiliar or unclear words are encountered. A bibliography is provided for professionals to give to patients and their caregivers. Finally, appendicies containing materials that can be copied and distributed to others are provided.

Professionals who read this book are strongly encouraged to augment their day-to-day practice and use of this book with ongoing education about dementia care, such as by subscribing to professional newsletters related to dementia and by participating in groups that advocate better care of patients and research of dementia, such as the Alzheimer's Association and The Brain Injury Association.

2

THE EVALUATION AND FORMULATION OF DEMENTIA

This chapter will discuss the evaluation of a patient with memory complaints or suspected dementia. The first part of the chapter addresses the following questions: (1) When should a comprehensive dementia evaluation be performed? (2) What is the purpose of such an evaluation? (3) Who is involved in performing such an evaluation? (4) What is the process of this evaluation?

The second part of the chapter discusses how to perform an assessment of a person with suspected dementia. Chapter 5 discusses how to use the information from the assessment in the differential diagnosis and workup of dementia.

BACKGROUND

When should a comprehensive dementia evaluation be performed?

In most cases, the recognition that an evaluation is needed does not come from the patient. Typically, a family member, such as a spouse or a child, notices forgetfulness, communication difficulty, problems in functioning, or a personality change and persuades the patient to be evaluated. Primary care physicians, neurologists, psychiatrists, geriatricians, and specialists in dementia are often the first professionals to see patients with such complaints.

This reliance on family members and patients to recognize dementia often leads to delays in diagnosis. Of the patients seen for an initial evaluation at the Johns Hopkins Comprehensive Alzheimer Program, only 15%–20% are in the early stages of the disease and one-third are in the late stages of dementia. More often than not, evaluations are sought when crises occur such as dangerous behavior, forgetting to pay bills, having a car accident, withdrawing from social activities, or stopping activities such as cooking and yard work.

There are several benefits of early diagnosis. First, the functional decline due to dementia and its consequences can be better managed if anticipated and addressed early. For example, financial catastrophes and injuries from car accidents or falls can be prevented by the knowledge that the patient is impaired. Second, early identification helps the family and patient understand changes in behavior and judgment that are often early symptoms. Behavioral disorders such as depression, delusions, and aggression are more likely to respond to treatment if caught early and treated appropriately. Third, early diagnosis allows patients and families more time for long-range planning to manage the consequences of dementia. This includes the ability to do estate planning, appoint power of attorney (Chapter 13), and so forth. Fourth, early diagnosis may improve the response to treatment for the cognitive symptoms and delay progression in some diseases.

Despite this, we do not believe that widespread screening of asymptomatic individuals can be justified at present. In the future, when more effective therapies are available and preventive treatments are developed, screening evaluations of at-risk individuals will be warranted.

To improve recognition and early diagnosis of dementia, we recommend that an evaluation be considered for elderly persons and other persons with neurologic disease or head injury who develop any of the signs or symptoms listed in Table 2.1.

Of the problems listed in this table, memory impairment and impaired functioning are most likely to be ascribed to normal aging and to be explained away or ignored. Since there are slight declines in cognition and functioning associated with aging, awareness of the usual changes associated with aging is necessary. For example, difficulty remembering names or coming up with the right word without any of the other symptoms in Table 2.1 is unlikely to be due to dementia. One piece of information that is especially useful in the primary care setting is a standardized cognitive assessment done during routine medical checkups. Tests such as the Mini-Mental State Examination (MMSE) can be administered annually or biannually in less than 10 minutes by a physician or an allied health professional. A decline of more than 3 points on the MMSE from a stable baseline should trigger an evaluation.

TABLE 2.1. Signs and Symptoms That Should Trigger Consideration of a Dementia Evaluation

1. *Cognitive changes*
   Worsening new forgetfulness
   Excessive repetition of questions and
     statements
   Trouble understanding spoken and
     written communication
   Difficulty finding words
   Not knowing previously known
     information
   Disorientation as to time, place, or
     person

2. *Psychiatric symptoms*
   Withdrawal or apathy
   Depression
   Suspiciousness
   Anxiety
   Insomnia
   Fearfulness
   Paranoia
   Abnormal beliefs
   Hallucinations

3. *Personality change*
   Inappropriate friendliness
   Blunting and disinterest
   Social withdrawal
   Excessive flirtatiousness
   Easy frustration
   Explosive spells

4. *Problem behaviors*
   Wandering
   Agitation
   Noisiness
   Restlessness
   Being out of bed at night

5. *Changes in day-to-day functioning*
   Difficulty driving
   Getting lost
   Forgetting recipes in cooking
   Neglecting self-care
   Neglecting household chores
   Difficulty handling money
   Making mistakes at work
   Trouble with shopping

What are the purposes of a dementia evaluation?

The primary purpose of the dementia evaluation is to determine whether dementia is present or absent. Dementia is a clinical diagnosis that depends on the demonstration of multiple declines in cognitive capacity and clear consciousness. The evaluation may demonstrate that dementia is not present and that the complaints or concerns that initiated the evaluation can be attributed to some other cause, such as usual aging, depression, a previously unrecognized neurologic or medical condition such as Parkinson disease or hypothyroidism, or an offending factor in the environment such as alcohol or medication.

Another purpose of the dementia evaluation is to ascertain the cause of the dementia syndrome. This is a necessary step in determining the most appropriate treatment and the prognosis, that is, the likely course over time. An important aspect of assessment is the identification of both disabilities that result from the dementia and remaining abilities, as both should be addressed in the treatment plan. Finally, the evaluation lays the groundwork for developing a family support plan. It determines the kinds of information, guidance, and emotional support that the patient and family require to deal with a chronic and usually progressive illness.

Who is involved in performing a dementia evaluation?

Most dementia assessments can be accomplished in the community in primary care settings. Specialists are best used when the diagnosis is in question, the case is atypical, the symptoms are complex, or initial management strategies here failed. Specific examples of when specialist input should be sought include the following: the diagnosis of dementia is uncertain, the patient is young (<65), the dementia is rapidly progressive, motor symptoms are prominent, behavioral disorder is pronounced, the dementia is potentially reversible, or the care needs are beyond those usually required.

The assessment of dementia uses medical skills that are within the capabilities of all physicians. Some elements of the evaluation, such as history taking, simple cognitive testing, and psychosocial assessment, can be performed by allied professionals (nurses, psychologists, or social workers) who are specially trained.

In many settings, an interdisciplinary team can carry out such an evaluation. In this model, an allied health professional takes the history from the family and caregiver and performs a mental status exam; a neuropsychologist performs the neuropsychological assessment; and a physician performs a physical examination and a comprehensive mental status exam and reviews the case with the other professionals. We believe such a model can be applied to any practice setting with the appropriate training and experience.

The physician who does not have such a team available should take the history, perform a physical examination and mental status examination of cognitive and noncognitive realms, and order appropriate laboratory studies. Indications for laboratory studies and referrals to a neuropsychologist and other professionals are discussed later in this chapter.

What processes are involved in a dementia assessment?

A comprehensive assessment is typically done in stages (Table 2.2). The first stage involves the patient and one or several informants, requires 1–2 hours, and consists of a complete neuropsychiatric assessment (discussed below). The second stage consists of a family evaluation and is done only if the initial assessment confirms the diagnosis of dementia. It can be performed by a social worker or nurse and requires approximately 1 hour to complete. This, too, will be discussed below. A series of diagnostic tests described later in

TABLE 2.2. Stages of a Comprehensive Dementia Evaluation

Stage 1: Neuropsychiatric assessment (directed by any trained physician)

Stage 2: Family assessment

Stage 3: Diagnostic tests

Stage 4: Conference discussion, diagnosis and recommendations to patient, family, and others as appropriate

this chapter should be obtained. These include laboratory studies, brain imaging studies, and neuropsychological tests. They are almost always done on an outpatient basis, but an inpatient assessment may be necessary if severe medical or behavioral problems are present. Finally, the whole picture is pulled together at a Diagnostic and Recommendation Conference where the interdisciplinary team meets with the patient and care providers to review the history and the results of the assessment, to explain the diagnosis, and to develop a treatment plan.

Each of these stages, including the initial assessment, has several purposes. The involvement of family members and/or other informants is crucial at several points, but the patient and family should be evaluated separately to diminish patient embarrassment and allow family members to answer freely questions about the patient's history and current symptoms. Performing the entire assessment with the patient and family together can be awkward and uncomfortable since the patient is being talked about as if he or she were not there. On rare occasions, patients will refuse to be seen alone. We sometimes call the family by telephone at another time to collect information and address concerns.

We typically start an assessment by meeting briefly with the patient and all family members who are present. We begin by stating that we will first meet briefly with everyone, then talk with the patient and family separately, and conclude by meeting together to discuss the findings. Before separating the patient and family, we ask whether there are particular issues that should be discussed with everyone present. We specifically ask whether there are questions that the patient and family want addressed by the end of the evaluation. Occasionally, the family will begin to give a full history at this point. If this happens, we ask them to wait until later. The purpose of this brief joint meeting is to raise general issues that can be explored separately with both care provider and patient. Sometimes patients will say that they do not know why they are coming for an evaluation and do not want to be there. In this case, they can often be reassured that the evaluation will be relatively brief and that they will be returning home in an hour or two.

THE EVALUATION

The history

The cornerstone of a comprehensive dementia evaluation is the neuropsychiatric assessment, which is outlined in Table 2.3. The goal of this assessment is to obtain information that will enable the clinician to determine an initial impression, develop a differential diagnosis, and plan treatment. Selected sections of this evaluation are highlighted here.

Family history

A detailed family history of the grandparents, parents, siblings, and children is taken. This is best recorded as a pedigree on a genogram. An example is provided in Figure 2.1. A genogram helps the clinician and family ask questions about each relative and increases accuracy. This helps the clinician focus on the family's health history, which will aid in the differential diagnosis, and on the current status of the family, which will identify potential and actual human resources available for the patient's care.

Personal history

The patient's personal background provides the data by which the whole case can be understood. Specifically, information should be obtained about early life cognitive and behavioral difficulties, educational achievement, work history, marital history, quality of relationships among family members, and religious background. In addition to allowing an estimation of premorbid functioning and cognitive reserve, the personal history illustrates the patient's life in a way that allows a clearer understanding of this individual and his or her response to illness. It also identifies interests and wishes, which in turn guide treatment planning. A sexual history should be obtained to assess for possible exposure to human immunodeficiency virus (HIV) risk factors.

Substance abuse history

It is important to be complete here because several dependency-producing substances, including alcohol and benzodiazepines, impair cognition even at low doses.

Medical history and review of systems

This is essential. All patients should be asked about hypertension, diabetes, heart disease, cancer, lung disease, surgery, and blood transfusions. Careful attention should be given to determining all medications taken in the prior

TABLE 2.3. Outline of a Neuropsychiatric Assessment

1. *Identifying Data:* age, marital status, race, sex, referral source

2. *Chief Complaint:* including the reason for referral and questions to be answered

3. *Family History:* vital status of parents, grandparents, siblings, and children; if deceased, age at death and cause; any members with psychiatric or neurologic illness; pedigree

4. *Personal and Social History:* where born, summary of early life experience, education, work history, marital state, living situation, leisure practices, religious faith, typical daily activities

5. *Substance Abuse:* use of cigarettes, alcohol, prescription and over-the-counter medications; history of abuse or dependency on any of these substances

6. *Medical History:* medical and surgical problems, active problems and their severity, review of systems, current medications, physicians and other health care providers involved in providing medical care

7. *Premorbid Personality:* traits, predispositions, affect, activity, reactivity

8. *Neuropsychiatric History:* psychiatric symptoms or disorders, psychiatric assessments or treatments, seizures, head trauma, stroke, other neurologic disorders

9. *History of Present Illness:* onset date, course, features, rapidity, and pattern of change; systematic review of systems to include information on cognitive capacity, mental syndromes, unusual experiences, functional status, and behaviors

10. *Current Psychosocial Environment:* living environment at present, care providers, financial issues, legal issues, use of community resources

11. *Examinations:* physical, neurologic, cognitive, and mental status exams

12. *Laboratory Evaluations:* brain imaging, laboratory studies, and other tests

6 months. Over-the-counter drugs such as aspirin, vitamins, nutraceuticals, and sleeping potions are important to note. Possible exposure, including occupational exposure, to toxins such as heavy metals (lead), organic solvents, and other chemicals should be determined.

Premorbid personality

This will provide a good picture of the patient's predispositions, character, temperament, and interests. It is important in understanding symptoms and in planning treatment and supportive care.

Past neuropsychiatric history

Special attention is paid to a history suggestive of brain injury including trauma, transient ischemic attacks, stroke, paralysis, sensory loss, speech or

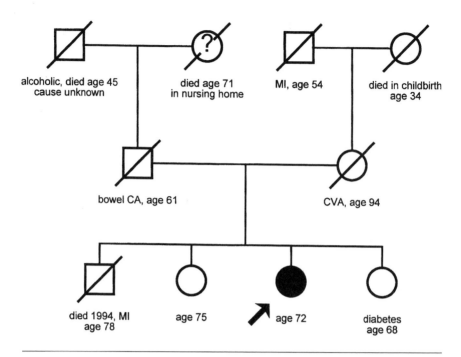

FIGURE 2.1 Example of a pedigree drawing. CA, cancer; CVA, cerebrovascular accident; MI, myocardial infarction. Box, male; circle, female; arrow, patient (proband).

language impairment, and tremor. A full psychiatric history is also taken, including a history of mental symptoms such as depression, prior evaluation, prior treatment, or hospitalization.

History of present illness

The examiner should identify the earliest symptoms and provide a chronological history up to the present using a detailed symptom checklist (Table 2.4). Family members and other informants play a major role in obtaining this part of the history. They should be asked specific questions about the functions and impairment listed in Table 2.4. In addition to helping with the differential diagnosis, this symptom checklist aids in the identification of target symptoms requiring treatment.

The mental status examination

Since the primary symptoms of dementia are impairments in cognition, behavior, and function, a thorough mental status examination is a necessary part of the evaluation. Some clinicians believe that the mental status examination is intrusive, while others are concerned that it is insulting or too

TABLE 2.4. Symptom Checklist in the Evaluation of Dementia

Impaired Cognition		*Problem Behaviors*	
Memory	Concentration	Verbal abuse	Catastrophic
Language	Planning and	Uncooperative	reactions
Orientation	organization	Physically aggressive	Noisy
Writing	Personality	Sundowning	Wandering
Reading	change	Demands	Hoarding/
Calculating	Executing	interaction	rummaging
Recognizing	Loss of social	Outbursts	Intrusive
Attention	rules		
		Disturbances in Drives	
Abnormal Mental Phenomena		Poor appetite	Sleeps a lot
		Weight loss	Out of bed
Depression	Death,	Poor Sleep	at night
Self-deprecating	suicidal	Hypersexual	Sexual
Somatic complaint	Disinterested	Excessive	aggression
Crying spells	Anhedonic	appetite	Hyposexual
Diurnal variation	low energy		
Socially	level	*Impaired Function*	
withdrawn	Apathetic	Cooking	Mobility im-
Anxiety	Panicky	Finances	pairments
Irritability	Labile	Housekeeping	or falls
Euphoria	Rapid speech	Driving	Bathing/
Delusions	Hallucinations	Shopping	grooming
Illusions	Acute	Dressing	Feeding
Fatigue	confusion	Hearing/sight	Continence

medical. Similar reluctance was reported years ago about taking a sexual history. Refusal is rare if the examiner believes it is an important part of the examination and so informs the patient. It is helpful to assure the patient that this is a routine part of the assessment for every person. In our experience, those who resist are almost always impaired. When individuals refuse to answer questions by saying "That's a silly thing to ask" or "Of course I can do that," it is best to turn temporarily to another area of questioning such as the medical history and to ask the questions again later.

It is not uncommon for cognitively impaired patients to be reluctant to answer direct questions. Individuals who will not or cannot answer direct questions about cognition are more likely to answer questions asked in the course of a general conversation. For example, orientation to year can be determined during the life history review. "Where were you born? What year was that? Do you know what year it is now? How old does that make you?"

Resistance to the mental status examination can sometimes be overcome by the examiner's emphasizing that the assessment is being carried out to identify remaining abilities as well as impairments ("Let's see how well you do with this one") and by acknowledging that some questions are difficult ("I'm going to ask you a more difficult one now. Let's see how good you are at math. Take 7 away from 100"). Sometimes it is useful to say that the information is being gathered for the benefit of the patient ("I know this is hard, but if I know what you have problems with, I'll be better able to help you"). There is a fine line between being supportive and being condescending, but helping a person over a difficult question is often reassuring. For example, if a person answers the question "Do you know where we are now?" with "I can't remember" and is upset, the examiner can be supportive by responding, "Well, let me help you. Do you know what city we are in?" Even in the best of hands, however, some individuals (perhaps 1%–2%) are unwilling to undergo this part of the assessment.

The mental status examination we recommend has seven major headings. An outline is presented in Table 2.5. It is not necessary to ask all the questions together. For example, some aspects of the mental status examination can be assessed during the general patient interview. Examples include appearance and behavior, talk, and mood. However, focused questions pertaining to these and other areas are usually necessary, and we believe it is useful for the examiner to have a specific outline in mind. This allows the clinician to check at the end of the evaluation and determine if all appropriate questions have been asked. It is also helpful to record the information obtained in a specific order because this allows the clinician to check for completeness and, more importantly, put the information together in a meaningful fashion. In addition, having the data in a specific order enables the clinician to present them to others in a comprehensive fashion.

Elements of the mental status and cognitive examinations

Appearance and behavior

First and foremost, practitioners are nonjudgmental observers. Training and experience guide what the clinician considers relevant. Issues of note include whether patients recognize the clinician as a professional, whether they act in a manner consonant with their background, and whether they are neat in appearance. In general, how patients approach the examination reflects how they react to situations that are unusual or stressful.

The predominant demeanor of patients during the assessment should be noted. Are they relaxed and calm, tense, or distressed? Does the examiner have to work hard to put them at ease? Are they restless, slow-moving, fidgety, or tremulous? Are there frequent, easily induced changes in mood or behavior? None of these actions is necessarily abnormal, but each can be relevant for diagnosis and treatment.

TABLE 2.5. Parts of the Mental Status Examination

1. *Appearance/Behavior*	5. *Content of Thought* Delusions
2. *Talk* Rate Rhythm Fluidity Spontaneity Latency Thought disorder	Obsessions Compulsions Phobias 6. *Insight and Judgment* 7. *Cognition* Consciousness
3. *Mood and Affect* Observed and reported stability, reactivity, and appropriateness Vital sense Self-attitude Thoughts of death, suicide, homicide	Orientation Memory Praxis Language Abstraction Gnosis Knowledge
4. *Perception* Hallucinations Illusions	Attention Calculation Executive function

Observing how patients are dressed is important. Are their clothes neat or do they seem disheveled, mismatched, misbuttoned, or dirty? Are they appropriate for the weather? Individuals who are reported to have always been neat and who come in with messy or stained clothes are probably having significant trouble not only with dressing but also with other complex activities such as preparing meals and keeping house. These clues should raise concern about safety.

The description of behavior should also state whether patients are able to walk into the room unaided, require a wheelchair, use a cane, or are lying in bed. Do they have the stooped posture and flexed body habitus of a person with parkinsonism? Is there obvious weakness or does the person seem to neglect one side of the body? Do they have a tremor or rapid, jerking movements? Do they appear fearful—for example, glancing around the room as if hearing someone talking? Do they seem uninterested, sad, or resistant? Do they become more or less cooperative as the assessment evolves?

Talk

Several aspects of the patients' talk (speech) should be assessed. First, speech should flow naturally (*fluency*) and spontaneously, that is, its speed should follow the examiner's. Speech should demonstrate an appropriate rate, rhythm, and prosody (smoothness). The pragmatics of speech (appropriate use of facial expression and gestures in conversation) should be assessed.

Hesitant speech, in which word-finding difficulty is prominent, speech is telegraphic or without the usual connecting words, and talking is frustrating to the patient suggests a nonfluent (Broca) aphasia. Speaking a great deal but saying little that makes sense indicates a fluent (Wernicke) aphasia. Substituting one word for another—for example, calling a watch a tie, saying words that are combinations of other words (time teller for watch), or saying words that are not in the lexicon (walm for watch)—all called *paraphasic errors*—also indicate a language disorder. Occasional difficulty finding words in the course of a conversation can be normal but repeated instances are not. Therefore, it is important to notice that such difficulties are occurring and to keep track of their frequency.

Second, the patient should be able to *comprehend* questions and *follow instructions*. An inability to do so in response to normally spoken statement or question might be due to a hearing deficit but often indicates difficulty in comprehending spoken language (receptive aphasia). Problems in this realm should be suspected if patients ask for questions and instructions to be repeated, or if they seem to understand simple and straightforward questions but have difficulty with more complicated ones, even if the examiner asks them with the same loudness of voice.

If words are *slurred* or incomprehensible, a disorder of the motor or production aspects of speech is likely. This points to damage of the neurologic or oropharyngeal control mechanisms responsible for producing speech. In contrast, word-finding problems are indicative of an impairment of language processing.

The ability to control speech can be impaired. Hesitancy before answering questions and speaking very softly, slowly, and deliberately can indicate depression. Rapid speech that dominates the conversation and prevents the examiner from interrupting (push of speech) suggests hypomania or mania. If the content of speech does not flow logically, there might be evidence of tangentiality (answering questions well off the mark), circumstantiality (giving excessive detail), or derailment (having no clear *string* or line of thought). *Pallilalic* speech, consisting of repetitive sounds (e.g., *la la la*) or words (e.g., *go go go*), or frequent perseveration (repetition) of words or phrases indicates a severe language disorder.

Mood and affect

Clinicians sometimes distinguish between the terms *mood* and *affect,* although there is not universal agreement on their definition. It is best to describe both how patients feel in their own words (subjective mood) and how the examiner perceives their predominant mood to be (observed mood). It is always helpful to use quotation marks specifying patients' exact words. Variations in mood during the course of the interview and examination should be described if they occur. The examiner should note if patients cry or laugh easily and if they are emotionally labile. The sudden starting and stopping of crying or laugher following a minor stimulus or no stimulus, referred to as *emotional incontinence,* indicates damage to specific neural fiber tracts and can aid in diagnosis. Mood should reflect what the conversation is about; for example, when patients talk about someone's death, they should appear sad. A lack of reactivity and evidence of unresponsiveness in mood should be noted. Irritability, anxiety, and emotional explosiveness or anger when confronted with a difficult task (a catastrophic reaction) is also important to report.

Vital sense

This refers to patients' assessment of their energy level and whether it differs from their usual self-perception. Patients should be asked if they feel interested and energetic in performing their usual activities, whether they derive enjoyment and pleasure from usually enjoyed activities, whether their body feels well or sick, and whether they feel they will be able to sustain activity over time.

Self-attitude

This is a complicated construct that assesses how patients perceive their own capabilities, and whether they believe these are different from their usual self-concept. Self-attitudes can be elevated, with better than usual self-confidence and self-esteem, or lower than usual, with guilt, remorse, self-deprecation, self-blame, and feelings of incompetence and failure. Low self-attitude is often accompanied by hopelessness, while elevated self-attitude often coexists with an inappropriately elated mood and grandiosity. Fluctuations in self-attitude, especially those not linked to environmental events, may be indicative of a mood disorder. Even when dementia is present, the identification of a *change* in self-attitude is a particularly important indicator of the presence of a mood disorder.

Assessment for thoughts of death, suicide, or homicide

Patients who can understand should be asked if they have thoughts about death, catastrophe, or disaster. Do they wish death upon themselves and, if so, why? Do they think they would be better off dead? Would they consider hurting themselves? If they would rather be dead but are not thinking of hurting themselves, what is stopping them? Are they angry with someone else? Are they thinking of hurting someone? What is the reason for this? What has prevented them from doing it thus far?

Perception

The examiner should investigate the presence of both hallucinations and illusions. *Hallucinations* are sensory perceptions without actual stimuli. They can occur in any of the five sensory modalities (hearing, sight, smell, taste, and touch). The examiner should ask patients if they hear sounds or people, or see things when nobody else is around or that others do not hear or see, whether they smell peculiar or odd odors that others cannot, or if there has been a specific repetitive taste or sensation that has been upsetting. Hallucinations are distinguished from *illusions*. In the latter, there is an actual stimulus that is misinterpreted or distorted—for example, seeing a face in the folds of curtains, believing a lamp is an animal, or looking into a mirror and seeing the face of a stranger.

Thought content

This refers to ideas, beliefs, and explanations a person reports. Included under this heading is the presence of *delusions*. These are defined as ideas that appear to the examiner to be false, fixed (unshakable), and idiosyncratic (unique to the specific patient). Delusions are common in persons with dementia, are often a source of distress to them and others, and can lead to behavior problems. Common delusions in dementia include the belief that someone is coming into the house and stealing, that family members are taking money, or that a spouse is unfaithful. It is important to distinguish between delusions and ideas based on culture and background. One helpful way is to ask family, friends, and acquaintances whether they also believe what the patient believes. For example, the patient may have a religious belief that the examiner does not share. If relatives have the same belief, then it is unlikely to be a delusion and the most appropriate conclusion is that the difference between the examiner's and patient's perspective rests on culture rather than disordered content of thought.

Obsessions, compulsions, and phobias are also surveyed. *Obsessions* are recurrent, intrusive *thoughts* that the patient perceives as his or her own and attempts to resist. They often concern matters described by the patient as trivial or foolish. Over time, resistance may fade. Typical obsessions include preoccupation with cleanliness, orderliness, infestation, and disaster. *Compulsions* are repetitive *behaviors* that the person feels driven to perform, such as handwashing or touching the wall, but that the person perceives as unreasonable and attempts to resist. Compulsions often occur in response to obsessions and are followed by a reduction in anxiety. *Phobias* are disproportionate fears of specific objects or situations. They should be distinguished from the fearfulness that arises in response to a delusion or depression. Although obsessions, compulsions, and phobias occur in patients with dementia, they are usually manifestations of a psychiatric disorder that preceded the dementia.

Insight and judgment

Insight refers to a patient's awareness of cognitive or other deficits or of certain abnormal mental states. Insight is often impaired or lacking in dementia patients, especially those with one of the cortical dementias. This lack of awareness is a consequence of the underlying dementia rather than a psychological denial since it is uncommon in the subcortical dementias. The inability to perceive a deficit is called an *anosagnosia*. Insight is assessed by asking questions such as "Do you think there is something wrong?" or specific questions relating to the individual's function such as "Is your memory functioning well or are you having difficulty with it?" Lack of insight can explain what seem to be foolish, dangerous, or unusual behaviors and, more importantly, can determine how clinicians and caregivers should best relate to the patient. For example, a severely impaired patient with poor insight should not be confronted with a diagnosis of a degenerative disorder such as Alzheimer disease because this could lead to brief distress without a clear benefit (since the patient cannot become aware that there is a deficit).

Judgment refers to a person's ability to assess a situation, consider the facts and issues and draw an appropriate conclusion. It can be assessed by asking questions about a health-related situation, for example, "If you had a serious health problem, who would you talk to?" Judgment is also assessed from the history provided by the family and throughout the course of the interview by observing the way the patient approaches the examiner.

The cognitive examination

Since cognitive impairment is the core feature of all dementias, every patient should undergo a thorough assessment of cognition. The extent of the cognitive assessment can vary, however, depending upon the purposes of the examiner and the setting in which the examination is being carried out. A neuropsychologist would be expected to carry out an in-depth, extensive inventory of a patient's cognitive abilities that would take several hours. A social worker, nurse, or physician reassessing a person with Alzheimer disease might use a brief global assessment to monitor the patient's course.

The cognitive assessment should also vary based on the patient's background. Individuals who have always been very bright or have depended on intellectual functions for their livelihood often need to be asked more complex questions to identify and assess cognitive deficits. For example, a bookkeeper should be able to do more complex math. Patients with other strengths should be tested in areas about which they are especially knowledgeable. Given the wide variability in premorbid ability and exposure, there is no single assessment instrument that is appropriate for all situations or all patients.

Nonetheless, it is useful to have a standard method of cognitive examination with which one starts and then modifies as appropriate, for an individual patient. The most widely used standard cognitive examination is the The Mini Mental State Examination (MMSE) developed by Folstein, Folstein, and McHugh. The major strengths of this examination are its brevity and its broad coverage of cognitive functions. The chief limitations are its inability to identify very early dementia (called the *ceiling effect*), its dependence on language (resulting in very low scores in persons who have primary aphasia), and its inability to discriminate the degree of impairment in severely impaired individuals (called the *basement effect*). As with all cognitive tests, persons with little education do less well. Despite these limitations, the MMSE is a useful tool for assessing and following most individuals with dementia. It can also be used by the individual practitioner to follow normal individuals over time since a *sustained* drop of 3–4 points indicates a high likelihood of dementia. An occasional patient will remember items from previous testing, but this is rarely a problem in clinical settings. Several methods are used to score the MMSE. What is presented below is the version we most often use. Consistency of scoring is important because it allows an individual's performances to be compared over time and the comparison of the capacities of different individuals.

The Mini Mental State Examination. The first half of the MMSE consists of items related to memory, attention, and concentration. The second half measures cortical functions. Items 1 and 2 measure *orientation* to time and place. Questions include "Can you tell me where we are now?" and "What city and state are we in?" One point is given for each correct answer. When testing orientation to time (knowledge of the year, month, season, day of the week, and date), the first question asked may depend on whether the person appears, based on the initial conversation, to have a significant impairment. If disorientation is likely, we often first ask if the person knows the month and introduce the questioning in a nonthreatening fashion, for example, "Have you been keeping up with the date? Do you know what month it is?" When a person is doing well, every question should be asked, even the year, since mildly impaired patients sometimes know the day and date but not the year.

Item 3 tests *registration*, that is, the ability to immediately repeat back items being committed to memory. This is the first part of *memory testing*. Three words are given to remember in the following manner: "I'd like to test your memory by asking you to remember three words. Please listen carefully and repeat these three words after me." We always choose the same three words for new patients. This not only has the benefit of preventing embarrassment should the examiner forget the words (or forget to write them down) but also teaches the examiner that normal individuals are able to repeat that words without difficulty unless they have a marked hearing deficit. This item is scored by counting the number of words the person is able to repeat correctly the *first* time. If a person misstates a word, he or she does not receive a point for it. If the person asks for the words to be repeated, the examiner should first ask him or her to repeat as many words as are remembered since the score for registration measures how many words an individual reports on the first try. The three words are repeated until the patient is able to say all three or it is clear that they cannot be said all at once.

Difficulty in registering the words can indicate a hearing problem or a language problem. If not previously alerted to the possibility of a hearing problem, the examiner should note this as a possibility and perform a hearing assessment at some point. Sometimes the examiner can raise his or her voice and find that the patient is still unable to respond to a command or question appropriately. Whispering words or commands in the patient's ear and having the patient listen to a watch or tuning fork are other forms of brief auditory testing.

The next item serves two functions. First, it distracts the patient from reciting the three words just asked; second, it is a test of *attention* and *concentration*. An individual with an eighth-grade or higher education is asked to subtract 7 from 100 and then to continue subtracting 7 from the answer. This is called *serial sevens*. If it is clear that respondents have memorized answers from prior examinations, the subtraction is altered and they are asked instead to subtract beginning from 101 or 103. This is one item that many practitioners do not expect older persons to perform correctly. It is a good example of why it is important to have experience testing the normal elderly. Experience and research demonstrate that individuals with an eighth-grade education or better can perform serial sevens. The speed of performance may slow down with age, so the examiner should be patient. An individual who is able to subtract 7 from 100 correctly should be able to do all the subtractions. One point is scored for each correct subtraction even if the previous subtraction was incorrect (so that "93, 87, 80, 73, 66" is given 4 points).

When individuals do not attempt the first subtraction (note: we do not say whether they *cannot* or *will* not) or when they have less than an eighth-grade education, they are asked to spell backwards a five-letter word with three consonants in a row (usually with *world* or *spray* as a backup). To determine whether persons have the ability to spell the word, it is best to ask them to spell *world* or *spray* forward and then, when they are finished, to

spell it backward. For the occasional person who misspells the word forward, the incorrect spelling in reverse is used as the correct sequence. When
scoring backward spelling, a point is given for each response that matches
the correct position in the sequence *d-l-r-o-w*. For example, *d-l-o-r-w* would
score 3 points, while *d-r-o-l-w* and *l-r-d-o-w* would score 2.

After the distraction task, patients are asked if they can remember any of
the three words that they were asked to remember (this tests recall or working memory). It is important to give individuals adequate time. Those in
their eighties may take 30 seconds to recall all three words. One point is
given for each word correctly recalled. The words must be *spontaneously* remembered to receive a point. For words that cannot be recalled (and thus
scored as no points), the examiner may want to determine whether giving a
cue or hint or asking the patient to chose the correct word from a list of
words, some of which were not in the original three, improves performance.
These questions can provide useful information but are *not* scored on the
MMSE. For example, persons who cannot benefit from cues will need more
direct help in remembering than individuals whose memory benefits from
cuing. In giving cues, the clinician might start with a category. For example,
"One was an animal." Persons who are still unable to remember can then be
given a choice such as "Was it a puppy, pony, or kitten?" Because the MMSE
does not have a set time interval after which items are recalled, it is sometimes best to attempt a recall task with a 5-minute interval, particularly if
the patient seems to have memory difficulty but recalls the items correctly
the first time.

Several aspects of language are assessed in the MMSE. *Naming* is tested
by asking the person to name two simple objects, such as a pen and a watch.
A point is given for each correct response. Visually impaired individuals can
be asked to name a pencil and a key placed in their palm. Examiners may
also want to assess naming in more depth by asking the patient to name less
common objects, for example, a button, an eraser, a lapel, the stem of a
watch, shoelaces, or the buckle of a belt. Points are not given on the examination for these words, but repeated failures suggest a naming deficit. *Repetition* is assessed by testing the ability to repeat a specific phrase. The suggested MMSE phrase is "No ifs, ands, or buts." The phrase must be repeated
exactly, including all the *s*'s at the end of the words. The patient is allowed
only one attempt. One point is given for a correct repetition. An alternate
phrase is "Methodist, Protestant, Episcopal." These phrases are difficult for
individuals of some ethnic backgrounds or for these for whom English is not
native. If there is a question about this being a problem, the sentence "Today
is a (sunny) day in the month of (April—substituting the current weather
and month)" can be used in its place. It is necessary that the patient say every
word correctly. Repetition is an excellent screen for determining whether a

person has any language problem. It requires intact comprehension, intact registration, and intact expression of language. Repetition can be adversely affected by a hearing impairment. If this is present it should be noted, since this can have important clinical and therapeutic implications, but the item is still sscored as not performed correctly. The next item addresses the ability to *read* a sentence *and carry out* the action. Reading the sentence "Close your eyes" is included in the MMSE. Patients are asked to read the sentence to themselves and then carry out the action. The print should be large so that it can be easily read by those with visual problems. Some patients are able to say the sentence but not carry out the action. A point is not given in this case.

Following a *three-step command* requires that people comprehend that the examiner wants them to do something, that they can hear what is said, and that they are able to carry out the three distinct steps. This tests several cognitive abilities but is most indicative of *praxis,* defined as the ability to carry out learned motor movements. The three-step command on the MMSE asks the subject to take a piece of paper in the right hand, fold it in half, and then place it on the floor. A point is given for each step done correctly. The reliability of this item is surprising to some people. Patients who are able to do only one or two steps when first asked will usually be able to do only the same number of steps when asked to do them a second time.

Next, a person is asked to *write* a sentence spontaneously. One point is given if it is a complete sentence (with a subject and a verb), if it is grammatically correct, and if it does not contain language errors. Some patients say that they do not know what to write. In this instance, we encourage them to "write anything that comes to mind." When an individual is still not able to write a simple sentence, the examiner might suggest one, for example, "Today is a (warm or cold) day," changing the adjective depending on the temperature. However, a point is given only if the patient *spontaneously* writes a complete, grammatically correct sentence. Finally, the patient is asked to *copy* a design with 2 five-sided interlocking shapes. A point is given if each figure has five sides and five angles and if the overlap is a four-sided figure. This assesses *visuospatial function and praxis.*

The interpretation of an MMSE total score depends on the presence or absence of non-cognitive impairments (e.g., blindness, dominant arm weakness) that might account for the loss of certain points, as well as on the person's estimated premorbid cognitive abilities, based among other things on his or her education and occupation. An MMSE score below 24 is indicative of significant impairment. For blind individuals, a score of 27 is probably normal, as they would be unable to complete three items due to blindness. In contrast, a score of 25 might be abnormal for a person with a high premorbid ability, such as an attorney or a nuclear physicist.

The expanded cognitive examination. The MMSE adequately tests orientation, memory, praxis, language, attention, and calculation. However, there are other aspects of cognition (see Table 4.5) such as consciousness, fund of knowledge, and executive function that are not assessed well by the MMSE. Since successful performance on the MMSE does not necessarily indicate the absence of a dementia, particularly in persons who premorbidly were quite high-functioning intellectually, a more in-depth cognitive examination is sometimes indicated. For these reasons, more sophisticated clinicians may choose to use in their day-to-day practice the Modified MMSE (3MS), which quantifies cognitive functioning on a broader 100-point scale and overcomes many of the limitations of the MMSE, such as the ceiling effect. The 3MS was developed by Teng and Chui in California and has been used in many studies that provide norms against which to compare the performance of specific patients. The scale can be obtained from the original publication (Teng EL, Chui HC. The Modified Mini-Mental State (3MS) examination. J Clin Psychiatry 1987; 48(8):314–18).

Alternatively, clinicians may choose to conduct an in-depth assessment of a particular aspect of cognition. The discussion below gives examples of other important parts of the examination.

Level of consciousness is assessed by evaluating the patient's ability to engage in and focus on the examination without fluctuation or *waxing and waning*. The presence of any limitation or fluctuation in attention might be indicative of delirium. Attention can be tested by having the patient repeat a sequence of numbers. Normally, seven numbers can be repeated forward and five backward at a minimum.

A more in-depth examination of recent *memory* (or memorizing or memory for newly learned material) includes determining whether the patient can recall lists of more than three words or recall the second of a pair of words when given the first word of the pair. Testing for current events (e.g., what is in the news) is also a memory test. Almost every intact individual knows who the current president is, and the ability to name the previous four presidents also suggests intact memory. An inability to name previous presidents or to name the current vice-president should be interpreted in light of the patient's estimated premorbid abilities. *Remote memory* (or memory for previously learned material) refers to previously learned material such as events from one's personal life, important dates, names of prior acquaintances, historical events, or personalities. It is tested by asking patients about dates, people, and places they would be expected to know. Failure to know the names and ages of grandchildren is a likely indication of impairment, for example.

A more detailed assessment of *praxis, planning,* and *visuospatial* function includes asking the patient to draw a flower pot or to draw a clock with the numbers in the correct place and the hands pointing at "10 minutes past 11." Assessments of ideomotor (cannot pretend that they are using a tool or instrument) and ideational (can imitate an action only if they copy someone else) praxis include asking patients to demonstrate how people brush their teeth, comb their hair, button a button, or salute.

Testing the patient's *fund of knowledge* provides information about premorbid intellectual ability and current intellectual ability. Questions asked include knowledge of recent news events or the functioning of certain equipment such as a barometer, the color of a ruby, or the capitals of certain states or countries.

Abstraction is an element of cognitive function that can be tested through proverb interpretation and the ability to identify similarities and differences. The interpretation of proverbs requires intact language skills but is primarily a measure of abstraction. Abstraction is strongly influenced by cultural factors. Thus, proverbs must be in the cultural repertoire of the patient to be appropriate. When testing this, it is common to start with an easily interpretable proverb such as "Don't cry over spilled milk" ("What's done is done"). A second, more difficult proverb is "People who live in glass houses shouldn't throw stones" ("Don't criticize others if you also have faults"). Another often used proverb is "A stitch in time saves nine" ("Don't put things off"). A difficult proverb that is unfamiliar to most individuals but that usually can be interpreted by individuals with intact normal intelligence is "The tongue is the enemy of the neck" ("Don't talk too much").

The ability to abstract can also be tested by asking individuals how an apple and an orange are alike. The correct response is "fruit." If an incorrect answer such as "They are both round" is given, the examiner should say, "And they're both fruit. Now try . . ." Subsequently, more difficult pairs of items are given, such a hammer and a saw (tools), a table and a chair (furniture), a bicycle and an airplane (means of transportation), or a bird and a tree (both alive). The ability to abstract is also tested by asking the difference between a river and a canal (natural vs. man-made) or a dwarf and a child (a child will grow tall).

Tests that require the ability to focus attention and switch sets (concepts) in rapid succession, sometimes referred to as *executive function,* should be considered, particularly when frontal lobe impairment is possible. Three tests are commonly used in this regard. The first is a verbal form of the Trail Making Test. The test is introduced by saying, "I'm going to ask you to alternate numbers with letters. Please complete the sequence. 1-A, 2-B; keep going." This requires the ability to recite the alphabet and to count to 15. The examiner keeps track of the patient's responses and corrects them as needed. For example, the patient might say "1-A, 2-B, 3-C, 4-D, 5-F," in which case the examiner would say, "5E; keep going." If the patient reverses the sequence, as in "1-A, 2-B, C-3, 4-D," no correction or penalty is applied. Two minutes are allowed for the patient to go all the way to 13-M. The examiner keeps track of time. Taking more than 60 seconds or making three or more errors indicates impairment.

A second test of executive ability is the Luria Hand-Sequencing Test, in which the patient is asked to mimic or copy a sequence of hand movements done by the examiner. The examiner demonstrates a series of three hand positions, which might be an open palm, a fist, or scissor fingers. After each set of three hand positions the patient is asked to copy the exact sequence. Five sets of three positions are given. Most well elderly patients are able to successfully copy four of five sets in the absence of impairment. Younger persons can do better.

The final test is referred to as the Go-No Go Test, in which the examiner gives the instruction, "I am going to tap on the table with my fist. If I tap once, I want you to respond by tapping twice. If I tap twice, I want you to respond by not tapping at all." Ten trials are given. Most well elderly respondents can successfully complete 6 or 7 of 10; younger persons can do better, often a perfect 10.

Use of standardized scales to supplement assessment

The process of assessment is often complemented by the use of a limited number of standardized scales that assess different domains. The rating of these scales allows the clinician to summarize and organize a complex case by reference to a set of numbers. This is useful in communicating information about severity to other caregivers, provides an objective means of charting the course of illness over time, and helps assess the response to interventions.

Many scales have been developed for rating different features of dementia. We favor the use of scales that are simple to administer, have been shown to be reliable, and have broad coverage. The domains that are important to consider are cognition, mood, behavioral disturbances, and ADLs (both instrumental and basic).

To rate cognition in early and moderately advanced stages, we recommend the MMSE or the 3MS. For late-stage patients we recommend the Severe Impairment Rating Scale (SIRS). To rate depression, we recommend the Cornell Scale for Depression in Dementia (CSDD). To rate dependency on caregivers and to assist in making level-of-care decisions, the Psychogeriatric Dependency Rating Scale-Behavior subscale is preferred (PGDRS). To rate IaDLs we recommend the IADL, and to rate ADLs we recommend the PGDRS-physical subscale. These scales can be copied for individual use and can be obtained from the original references. To rate noncognitive neuropsychiatric disturbances we favor the Neuropsychiatric Inventory (NPI) or its derivative caregiver questionnaire. Both can be obtained by writing to Jeffrey L. Cummings, M.D., Department of Neurology, Reed Neurology Center, UCLA. School of Medicine, 710 Westwood Plaza, Box 951769, Los Angeles, CA 90095–1769.

The family assessment

The importance of evaluating the patient's family and personal environment cannot be overemphasized. The family has been described as "the lifeline of the patient." Their well-being is essential to the patient's status, and the family is appropriately considered a partner in care. As professionals embark on the care of the patient and family, it must be remembered that the provision of a diagnosis and treatment recommendations will aid the family in the years ahead but must be supplemented by the many other approaches discussed in this book. Data on the family that are collected at around the time of the initial contact can be crucial for understanding the family's needs.

Table 2.6 lists the elements important to the family and their assessment. The family's well-being is best monitored over time by revisiting these areas at intervals of no longer than 6 months. Although family assessment is frequently provided by social workers, it can be accomplished by other health care providers as long as the information is systematically collected. Construction of a family genogram is one effective way to gather these data. An example is in Figure 2.1.

The assessment of the patient's functioning within the family should cover the following topics: knowledge of how the patient's needs and wants are provided for; the way in which the patient spends his or her time; the extent to which family and/or care providers have insight into the patient's condition and its prognosis; the extent to which care providers require help in caring for the patient; and the resources family caregivers have available to provide help.

Through the psychosocial assessment, the clinician will develop an understanding of the patient's immediate environment, day-to-day functioning, and resources. This will add to the intervention problem list and will lay the groundwork for developing appropriate long-term supportive care for the patient and family (see Chapters 7, 8 and 9).

DIFFERENTIAL DIAGNOSIS AND WORKUP OF DEMENTIA

After completing the assessment discussed at the beginning of this chapter, the clinician is faced with the task of making sense of the information. Doing so has two purposes: diagnosing the cause of the dementia and developing a

TABLE 2.6. Assessment Domains for the Family Evaluation

1. Family members, their roles, frequency of interaction
2. Health status of care providers
3. Financial status of care providers
4. Spiritual beliefs
5. Knowledge about dementing illnesses
6. Other responsibilities, including work and other dependents, such as children or other ill relatives

care plan. A list of possible diagnoses, called the *differential diagnosis,* is made, and this clarifies what other information is needed.

The goals of the differential diagnosis are the formulation, classification, and determination of the cause. This process is best understood in a series of sequential steps (outlined in Fig. 2.2) to which we refer throughout this chapter.

In the *formulation,* the clinician organizes the history, physical examination, mental status examination, and laboratory studies in a coherent and systematic fashion. The first step is to decide whether dementia is present or absent. If cognitive impairment is absent (in which case dementia is absent), then the differential diagnosis typically involves disorders such as depression, schizophrenia, factitious disorder, or a neurologic disorder that spares cognition. If cognitive impairment is present, then the clinician must decide if the *clinical* definition of dementia is met (i.e., a decline in multiple cognitive capacities occurring in clear consciousness). If cognitive impairment is present but does not represent a decline, then a diagnosis of mental retardation, borderline intellectual functioning, or development delay (DD) is appropriate. If cognitive decline is evident but is either not global or not sufficiently severe to affect functioning (i.e., does not meet criteria for dementia presented in Table 1.1), then then another diagnosis such as cognitive impairment, no dementia (CIND), mild cognitive impairment (MCI), amnestic disorder, aphasia, mild cognitive disorder, or age-associated memory impairment should be considered (see also Chapter 11). If the clinician is still uncertain about the presence or absence of dementia after the initial assessment, then long-term follow-up will be necessary to determine whether dementia is present. Uncertainty is most common when the patient was highly functioning premorbidly and is only mildly impaired, when the clinician is not persuaded that the patient's current functioning represents a decline, or when the patient is very old. Neuropsychological testing, a series of standardized and normed tests of cognitive function performed by a specially trained clinician, can be an invaluable tool in the evaluation of dementia. Referral for testing is indicated

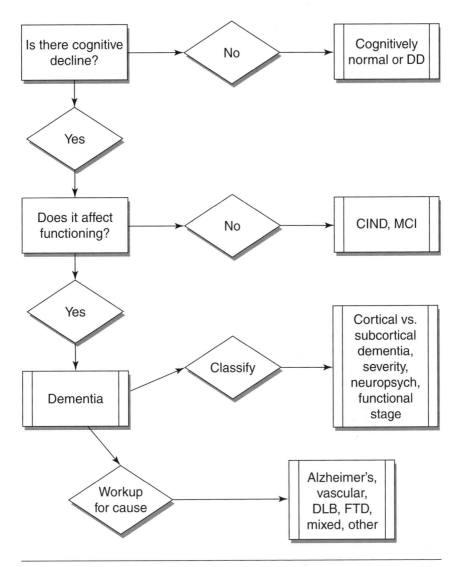

FIGURE 2.2 Differential diagnosis of dementia. CIND, cognitive impairment, no dementia; DD, development delay; DLB, dementia with Lewy bodies; FTD, frontotemporal dementia; MCI, mild cognitive impairment.

when there is cognitive impairment but it is not clear if it is severe enough to be a dementia, when the impairment could be accounted for by advanced age, when there is dementia but there is uncertainty about its cause, or when there is a need to differentiate dementia from depression or schizophrenia.

If the clinician decides that dementia is present, the next step is the *classification* of the syndrome according to its cognitive features (cortical,

TABLE 2.7. Laboratory Investigations for the
Evaluation of Dementia Syndromes

Urinalysis and microscopy
Blood tests
   Complete blood count
   Serum electrolytes, including magnesium
   Serum chemistries, including liver tests
   Thyroid testing
   Vitamin B_{12}
   *Erythrocyte sedimentation rate
*Serologic tests for syphilis (or similar conditions)
*Chest X-rays
*Electrocardiogram
*Toxicology screens
   Urine toxicology
   Serum toxicology (alcohol, salicylates, other)

---

*Consider; not universally needed.

subcortical, mixed), noncognitive features (behavior, mood, function, motor), and functional impairments. This classification lays the foundation for determining etiology and directing treatment. Tables 1.2, 1.4, and 1.5 will assist in this classification.

The *differential diagnosis* is a list of potential causes (Table 1.3). It is constructed by matching the patient's history, signs, and symptoms with known disorders. Ideally, further clinical and historical data, as well as laboratory testing, imaging, or neuropsychological testing, will identify a single likely cause.

Table 2.7 lists laboratory evaluations for all patients with dementia. The recommendations here are consistent with those developed by the relevant guidelines of the American Psychiatric Association and the American Academy of Neurology. As noted in the table, certain laboratory studies should be ordered in all cases mostly to rule out rare causes of dementia. Note that the table does not include laboratory studies that are being marketed for the diagnosis of Alzheimer disease, such as apolipoprotein E genotyping, presenilin-1 genotyping, or cerebrospinal fluid testing for neutropil protein or different forms of tau protein. At this point, there is not sufficient evidence to support the use of the latter in the differential diagnosis of dementia.

Brain imaging should be considered in all cases but is not always necessary, so clinical judgment should be exercised. If the dementia is long-standing (more than 3 years) or very advanced, we sometimes forgo imaging because a treatable cause is very unlikely and the identification of less common dementias is unlikely to affect care. While a brain computed tomogram (CT)

TABLE 2.8. Second-Stage Laboratory Investigations

Test	Indication
Electroencephalogram (EEG)	Possible seizures; Creutzfeld-Jakob disease
Lumbar puncture	Onset of dementia of <6 months to rule out rare infectious causes
	Obtain cerebrospinal fluid to assess for Creutzfeld-Jakob disease proteins (G-14) or Whipple disease proteins
	High-volume "tap" or continuous pressure monitoring to assess for normal pressure hydrocephalus
Heavy metal screen for mercury, arsenic, and lead (urine or serum)	History of potential exposure
Human immunodeficiency virus (HIV) test	History of potential exposure
Lyme disease titer	History of exposure and compatible clinical picture
Ceruloplasmin, arylsulfatase electrophoresis, Slit lamp exam	History and exam suggest Wilson disease
Apolipoprotein E testing	Need to increase the likelihood that the diagnosis of Alzheimer disease is correct
Genetic testing for presenillin-1 Alzheimer gene, CAG repeat determination in Huntington gene or other dementia genes	Family history is strong and confirmation is clinically necessary

is sometimes adequate, we usually order a brain magnetic resonance imaging (MRI) scan because it offers more information. Single photon emission tomography (SPECT) or positron emission tomography (PET) should be ordered to rule specific causes in or out. For example, SPECT/PET can identify specific patterns of blood flow or metabolic abnormality and confirm or rule out specific disorders, such as frontotemporal dementia or Alzheimer disease.

When the clinical circumstances, history, or examination indicate that a *specific* cause might be present for which a specific diagnostic test is available (Table 2.8), it should be ordered. Table 2.8 also contains genetic testing for Alzheimer-associated genes that may be of value in specific clinical circumstances.

Differential diagnosis is a top-down process in which the clinical phenomena, both signs and symptoms, first indicate the presence or absence of the syndrome of dementia and then direct the classification of the syndrome into recognizable patterns. Because it is assumed that in all cases of dementia there is an underlying disease of the brain, and since in most cases the clinical pattern correlates well with findings at autopsy, knowledge and understanding of the clinical syndrome is important. However, clinicians should not lose sight of the fact that in a sizable number of cases, perhaps 15%–20%, the clinical presentation of dementia is atypical—that is, it does not follow a recognizable pattern and therefore the pathologic cause is less certain.

We do not favor classifying dementia as reversible or irreversible, however. Even when a dementia for which there is a specific treatment is diagnosed, it often does not fully respond to treatment, particularly if it has been present for more than several months. Also, many of the treatments that are available now and others that will become available in the near future will lead to partial or transient improvement but not full recovery.

3

DISEASES CAUSING A CORTICAL PATTERN OF DEMENTIA

One of the major themes of this book is that making a specific diagnosis of the cause of dementia is important because it conveys important knowledge about prognosis and treatment. Many disease processes lead to dementia and they differ substantially, depending on what parts of the brain they affect and their symptoms. For many of the diseases discussed, dementia is an inevitable and defining characteristic. However, for some, such as multiple sclerosis and Parkinson disease, dementia is not inevitable. Table 1.3 lists some of the 100 or so diseases associated with the clinical syndrome of dementia. Only the more common conditions and those that make important teaching points will be discussed in detail.

Diseases associated with typically cortical syndromes will be discussed in this chapter. Disease causing typically subcortical or mixed dementia syndromes will be discussed in Chapter 4. For each disease, three areas will be reviewed:

1. The *clinical picture* of the dementia syndrome associated with that disease, including prominent cognitive abnormalities, the associated noncognitive behavioral disorders, other common neurologic features, course, and prognosis of the disease.
2. *Epidemiology,* including population prevalence (number of cases in the population), incidence (number of *new* cases in a given time period), and known risk factors.
3. *Pathology* (structural brain abnormalities) and *etiology* (cause) of the

disease process. The focus will be on the mechanism of brain injury associated with each disease process and how this mechanism leads to a specific dementia syndrome.

OVERVIEW OF THE CORTICAL DEMENTIAS

Alzheimer disease

Clinical picture

Alzheimer disease (AD) is defined clinically by the criteria listed in Table 3.1. Its earliest symptoms are often recognized only in retrospect because it has an insidious onset and is slowly progressive. The dementia of AD is a classic cortical dementia with impairments in memory (amnesia), coordination/ dexterity (apraxia), language (aphasia), and perception (agnosia). Roughly speaking, the progression of the AD dementia is broken down into three clinical stages, each lasting 3 years on average. In the first stage, memory impairment predominates. In some individuals, personality changes occur in this stage as well. Impairments in IADLs are present, but ADL impairment is absent or minimal. In the second stage, patients develop significant impairments in language, in the ability to perform everyday activities, and in recognition of people, places, and situations. Functioning becomes impaired to the point that instrumental daily activities such as shopping, paying bills, or cooking must be supervised. In the third stage, the impairments in memory, communication, and praxis and recognizing become severe. Impairments in basic capacities, such as walking and toileting, develop. As a result, patients need considerable help with basic daily activities such as bathing, dressing, and mobility. Most patients in the third stage are fully dependent on others for all basic daily activities.

Patients with AD frequently suffer from a variety of noncognitive behavioral disorders. Delusions, hallucinations, sleep disturbance, overactivity/ aggression/agitation, and depression are most common. Delusions and misinterpretations occur in 30%–40% of patients with AD at some point in the illness. From 10% to 25% experience a hallucination. These are most often visual, but auditory hallucinations also occur and can be distressing. The delusions and the hallucinations differ from those seen in schizophrenia. In AD the delusions are fairly circumscribed, that is, not very elaborate—for example, the belief that someone is stealing one's money. It is rare for patients to offer complex explanations for how they know this and why it is occurring. Delusions and hallucinations can lead to troubling behaviors such as striking out at others, barricading oneself in a room, hiding things, or refusing to eat.

TABLE 3.1. Criteria for Probable Alzheimer Disease

1. Dementia
   Decline on examination and objective testing
   Deficits in two or more areas of cognition

2. Gradual progression

3. Intact level of consciousness

4. Onset after age 40
5. No other cause after workup

The reported rates of depression in AD vary widely. In several studies in which patients have been evaluated thoroughly, 20%–25% were found to have depressive symptoms. Depression can lead to mental suffering, striking out, weight loss, and social uninterest.

A variety of problem behaviors develop in the middle and late stages of AD, but no widely accepted classification system has been developed. We group them according to their phenomenology (symptomatology) and by assumptions about the mechanisms that cause them. Altogether, noncognitive symptoms afflict as many as 60% of patients with AD at any one time and 90% over the course of the illness.

In the early stages of AD, neurologic symptoms are limited to the cognitive abnormalities. In the third stage, hyperreflexia, apractic gait, and frontal release signs (grasp and snout reflexes) develop. Some patients develop parkinsonian symptoms, that is, become slowed and rigid. Sudden jerking movements of the limbs, trunk, or head, called *myoclonus,* occur in 15% of patients and seizures occur in 10%. Difficulty walking due to gait apraxia and poor balance is common, and fine motor coordination becomes progressively impaired. In the very late stages, patients often become incontinent and immobile and develop problems with swallowing. In the preterminal stages, many patients become bed-bound. Marked rigidity (stiffness) is common, as are diffuse hyperreflexia, spasticity, and inability to swallow.

Alzheimer disease lasts for 8–10 years on average, but durations as brief as 2 years and as long as 22 years have been reported and confirmed pathologically. For many patients the diagnosis is not made until symptoms have existed for 2–3 years. The confidence in the clinical diagnosis based on the criteria in Table 3.2 is high. Over 90% of patients who meet these criteria are found to have the characteristic brain changes of the disease at autopsy. Decline is usually steady, and for most individuals the rate seems to stay consistent, but the rate of progression can vary. Some studies suggest an acceleration of the decline in the middle stage and slower declines early and late, but this may be due to the way decline is measured and the fact that certain symptoms such as language disorder are more impairing.

Epidemiology

The prevalence of AD is age-dependent. In the United States, 5%–7% of persons 65 years of age or older are estimated to suffer from the disease. The prevalence increases with age and is 8%–10% for persons 75 years of age or older, 20%–25% for persons 85 years of age or older, and 40%–50% in those older than 90. The estimates are consistent across almost all racial and cultural groups. The incidence (rate of new cases per year) of AD at age 65 is around 0.25% per year. This doubles every 5 years, so that the incidence is 1% per year at age 75 and approaches 4% per year at age 85.

Alzheimer disease is always associated with a dementia if one requires both the clinical syndrome and the brain pathology to make the diagnosis. However, some individuals are found at autopsy to have the pathology of AD without having manifested symptoms of a dementia syndrome. Since the pathology precedes the clinical syndrome, it is likely that all individuals who develop the pathology and live long enough will develop dementia, but this hypothesis cannot be tested at present.

Pathology and etiology

The pathology of AD has two prominent features, both described by Dr. Alois Alzheimer in 1906–7. First are extracellular accumulations called *neuritic* or *senile plaques*. These contain a protein predominantly consisting of beta-amyloid, a breakdown product of a protein present in all nerve cell (neuron) membranes known as the *amyloid precursor protein* (APP). The way in which APP becomes beta-amyloid has now been characterized and may lead to treatments or prevention. Under the microscope, this protein can be visualized because it stains in a characteristic pattern.

The second element of the brain pathology is the intracellular *neurofibrillary tangle*. This, too, is a protein, made up predominantly of hyperphosphorylated tau protein. Normally, this protein links together pieces of the microtubule, structures that make up the cytoskeleton or skeleton of each cell. The precise ways in which neuritic tangles develop is also not known.

Another important finding in the pathology of AD is widespread loss of neurons. In the early stages of the disease, this is most prominent in the entorhinal and hippocampal areas of the temporal lobes. As the disease progresses, it spreads throughout the temporal region and into the parietal regions. Cell loss is also found to varying degrees in the frontal lobes, subcortical structures such as the nucleus basalis of Meynert (the main source of brain acetylcholine), and deeper structures such as the locus ceruleus (the source of most brain norepinephrine) and the raphe nuclei (the source of most brain serotonin). This widespread loss of neurons accounts for the atrophied or shrunken appearance of the brain at autopsy.

The distribution of neuropathology helps explain the clinical syndrome. Neuritic plaques and neurofibrillary tangles in the hippocampus and entorhinal cortex are responsible for impaired memory. Temporal lobe pathology explains the prominence of language disorder, while cell loss in the parietal lobes leads to visuoperceptual impairments. Loss of neurons occurring in subcortical nuclei such as the locus ceruleus and raphe nuclei may lead to hallucinations, delusions, and impaired regulation of mood.

The cause of the neuropathology and the mechanism by which it spreads are not yet known. Heredity plays an important role in the causation of the disease. About 2% of cases are transmitted as an autosomal dominant trait, with 50% of people in each subsequent generation affected. Genes on chromosomes 21 (the APP gene), 1 (the presenilin-2 gene), and 14 (the presenilin-1 gene) have been implicated in the causation of AD in these familial cases. In addition, a gene on chromosome 19, the apolopoprotein E gene, increases the risk of developing AD, likely by causing it to begin 5 years earlier on average. Clearly, other genes are involved in the development of AD that remain to be discovered.

In terms of the ways in which the pathology of AD develops, there are probably primary and secondary processes. It now appears that the disease process occurs for many years (10 or more) before the first symptoms develop. Thus, it is likely that some process initiates a cascade that leads secondarily to cell death. The death of neurons leads to the loss of neurotransmitter release, and this in turn may lead to the development of specific symptoms. For example, the loss of acetylcholine is hypothesized to lead to memory loss and perhaps other cognitive impairments. Loss of the neurotransmitters norepinephrine, dopamine, somatostatin, and serotonin is probably linked to the development of other specific cognitive and noncognitive symptoms, while an increase in the neurotransmitter glutamate, which may occur in response to the diminishing function of neurons, may lead to overstimulation and death of remaining neurons. Figure 3.1 provides a simplified summary of our current undestanding of the etiopathogenetic cascade involved in AD.

Fronto-temporal degeneration

A group of dementias in which there is variable degeneration of the frontal and temporal lobes is now referred to as the *fronto-temporal dementias* (FTDs). These have been referred to by a variety of different names, including *dementia lacking distinctive histologic features*, *dementia of the frontal lobe type*, *frontal lobe dementia*, *frontal lobe degeneration*, *lobar atrophy*, and *Pick's disease*. These conditions are now grouped together because, over time, they become similar clinically and because similarities in their neuropathology are increasingly being recognized.

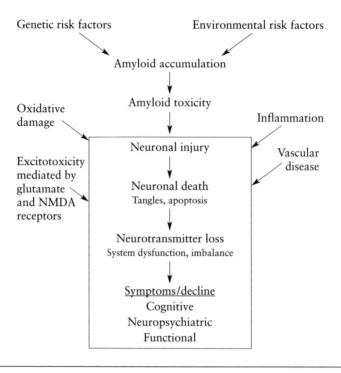

FIGURE 3.1 The Alzheimer disease cascade. NMDA, *N*-methyl-D-aspartase.

Clinical syndrome

Fronto-temporal dementia most commonly begins with changes in personality and behavior, language, and executive function. *Executive function* refers to a set of capacities required to abstract, follow social rules, be mentally flexible, and initiate, sustain, and stop behavior. Apathy, disinhibition, intrusiveness, explosiveness, irritability, and assaultiveness are common early manifestations of FTD. Depression, delusions, and hallucinations are relatively infrequent. In some individuals, language disorder is the only symptom for years because the temporal lobes are the predominant site of pathology. Apraxia and agnosia can develop within several years but are often less prominent than in AD. The motor dysfunction generally develops later in the disease and consists of slowness and rigidity, but gait disorder is an occasional early manifestation, as is an unusual symptom called *alien hand syndrome*, in which a person does not recognize a hand as his or her own or cannot make the hand move in response to a command, even though there is no weakness. The average age of onset is 54 and the average age of death is 64, that is, younger than in AD, but FTD can begin in the 70s.

Diagnostic criteria for FTD are found in Table 3.2. These clinical criteria are just now being linked to autopsy diagnosis, so their sensitivity and specificity are not yet known. Five subtypes of FTD have been proposed, and several diseases that were once thought to be distinct illness are now being included under the rubric of FTD because they are associated with abnormalities of the tau protein, because the diseases become clinically similar as they progress, and because at autopsy a disease with the clinical picture of one of these illnesses sometimes is found to have the neuropathology of another.

In the *frontal lobe type,* disinhibition and poor insight are the earliest manifestations. Memory loss, rigidity, and dysarthria develop in the middle stage, followed by withdrawal, apathy, aphasia, and amimia (lack of spontaneity). The average duration is 5–7 years.

In the *thalamostriatal type,* personality changes and extrapyramidal motor symptoms such as rigidity and slowness occur early. Disinhibition is less common. The thalamostriatal type progresses more slowly, typically lasting for 7–10 years. Visuospatial impairment is sometimes present early. Progressive supranuclear palsy (PSP), a disease in which truncal rigidity, opisthotonus (head thrust back), loss of voluntary eye movements (loss of up-gaze initially), and falls are prominent, and cortico-basalganglionic degeneration (CBD), in which the alien hand syndrome, slowness, and clumsiness occur early, are now included in this group

Patients with the *motor neuron type* develop the spinal cord pathology and clinical symptoms of amyotrophic lateral sclerosis (ALS), or Lou Gehrig's disease, and also have these inclusion bodies in brain neurons in addition to the characteristic brain pathology of FTD. Language and memory disorder occur early along with the frontal lobe symptoms. The duration is typically 2–4 years.

The *asymmetric type* resembles the frontal lobe type except that the condition localizes to the dominant temporo-parietal area. Language disorder predominates if the dominant (almost always left) hemisphere is involved and visuospatial symptoms predominate if the nondominant hemisphere is involved. The duration is 2–4 years.

The *amnestic type* is characterized by slowly developing impairment in memory and relative sparing of other cognitive symptoms. Pathology is often limited to the hippocampus. This condition has been referred to as *hippocampal sclerosis* for this reason.

Epidemiology

The population prevalence of FTD is equal to that of AD before age 65. Autopsy studies report its prevalence at 3%–5% for all patients with dementia

TABLE 3.2. Criteria for Fronto-Temporal Degeneration

1. Progressive personality change and breakdown in social conduct
   Restless, distractible, disinhibited, or apathetic, slowed, amotivated
   Hypochondriasis with bizarre complaints
   Stereotyped behavior
   Echolalia and perseveration
   Variable memory disturbance

2. Normal neurologic examination
   May have frontal release signs

3. Supportive features
   Family history of dementia
   Reduced frontal lobe blood flow on functional imaging
   Normal electroencephalogram

and 10% for patients with dementia who die before age 70. The disease has been reported throughout the world. Evidenece now suggests that about one-third of cases have a genetic etiology, but this figure may increase over time. An autosomal dominant form of inheritance is seen with mutations in the tau gene on chromosome 17.

Pathology

Neuronal loss, astrocytosis (increased numbers of brain cells called *astrocytes*), and vacuolization (development of balloon-like holes) of the superficial layers of the frontal and temporal cortices are common to all forms of FTD. The subtypes are distinguished pathologically by variable involvement of subcortical and limbic structures. The frontal lobe subtype has less subcortical involvement, whereas in the thalamostriatal subtype there is prominent loss of neurons in multiple subcortical nuclei. In the motor neuron type there is loss of brain stem and spinal cord hypoglossal nucleus cells and anterior motor neurons, and intraneuronal inclusions appear. The asymmetric type has pathologic features similar to those of the frontal lobe type, but the dominant hemisphere (usually the left) is most affected. In some cases, characteristic abnormal inclusions called *Pick bodies* are found in the nuclei of dying neurons. In such instances, the pathologic diagnosis of Pick's disease is made. In the amnestic type, cell loss and gliosis are limited to the hippocampus.

There are molecular differences among these subtypes that do not always parallel the clinical subtypes. When Pick bodies are present, the inclusions have three microtubule binding repeats. Four microtubule binding repeats are usually associated with PSP and CBD, the thalamostriatal subtype. Some cases have both three and four microtubule binding repeats, while the motor neuron type has distinctive inclusions seen in motor neurons.

DISSEMINATED LEWY BODY DISEASE

Clinical presentation

Dementia with Lewy Bodies (DLB) has been described in recent years, although it is certainly not a new disease. In addition to the impairments of memory, language, and praxis that are seen in cortical dementia, mild parkinsonism (resulting in falls), hallucinations, and delusions are present early in the course. Cognitive impairment can fluctuate over time so that days of moderate impairment alternate with periods of nearly normal functioning. This fluctuation, in conjunction with falls and the noncognitive psychopathology, is central to making the diagnosis. At least 70% of patients have complex visual hallucinations and/or paranoid delusions. Auditory hallucinations occur in 15%. Depression is present in 40% of individuals.

Motor disorder is prevalent early in LBD, primarily manifested as parkinsonism (rigidity, slowed movements, and poor balance). Tremor is rare. Whenever parkinsonian symptoms and cognitive impairments characteristic of cortical dementia are present at the onset of a dementia, LBD should be strongly considered. Up to 40% of patients experience unexplained falls by the time they present to clinicians. As the disease progresses, the parkinsonian signs become more prevalent, occurring in more than 50% of patients. Neuroleptic drugs can worsen parkinsonism and lead to marked rigidity, tremor, postural instability, and gait disturbance even at low doses.

Dementia with Lewy bodies, also referred to as Lewy body dementia, appears to evolve in stages, but good data are lacking. The earliest period consists of episodes of forgetfulness, lapses of concentration, periods of gait instability, and depression. Functional impairments are uncommon at this stage, but careful testing will often reveal visuospatial deficits.

In the second stage, which often coincides with presentation for evaluation, the cognitive impairments continue to fluctuate but problems become frequent at night, perhaps due to distressing visual hallucinations, auditory hallucinations, and paranoid delusions. Extrapyramidal symptomatology leads to frequent falls. Electroencephalographic abnormalities consisting of anterior temporal lobe theta and delta activity, often with sharp components and occasionally with marked lateral asymmetry, can be seen.

The third stage of DLB is characterized by a rather sudden acceleration of cognitive decline, delusions, hallucinations, and behavioral disturbance.

The decline of the patient is fairly dramatic. Death may occur within months, typically due to aspiration. During this terminal phase, patients can remain behaviorally disturbed, with shouting, aggression, and delirious-like spells.

Lewy body dementia shares similarities with both Parkinson disease and AD, but it can be distinguished both clinically and pathologically. Several sets of operational criteria have been proposed. Those of the group at Newcastle-Upon-Tyne in England are presented in Table 3.3. These have good sensitivity (95%) and adequate specificity (82%) based on pathologic confirmation.

The age of onset of DLB is similar to that of AD, with the median age being in the early to mid-70s. Noncognitive symptoms occur earlier in the course of DLB than in AD. The duration of illness is shorter than for AD, ranging from 3 to 8 years.

Epidemiology

Since DLB has only recently been recognized as a distinct entity, precise epidemiologic data are not available. Between 5% and 18% of patients coming to autopsy suffer from DLB. Extrapolating from population estimates of dementia, perhaps 0.5%–1% of persons over 65 suffer from this disease. Although men predominantly suffer from this condition, this finding is controversial.

Pathology

The hallmark pathology of the DLB is the Lewy (pronounced *loo'-ee* in the United States and *le'-vee* in Europe) body, an intracellular inclusion body. Lewy bodies were first described early in the twentieth century by a student of Alois Alzheimer, and for much of the twentieth century were believed to occur primarily in Parkinson disease in the substantia nigra. In DLB, Lewy bodies are seen outside the substantia nigra in the cortex. Lewy bodies are relatively dense in the brain stem, and in the entorhinal cortex and other areas of the temporal lobes. The parietal and frontal cortices exhibit lower levels of Lewy bodies. Lewy bodies are less common in the occipital cortices.

In some cases of DLB, senile plaques are common and reach levels similar to those seen in AD. However, few cases have sufficient numbers of neurofibrillary tangles to meet that criterion for AD. This has led some authors to suggest that there are two types of DLB, one called the *Lewy body variant* of AD and the other DLB, a distinct disease. Further studies are needed to clarify this.

Cholinergic activity is reduced in DLB, especially in the temporal, frontal, and parietal cortices. Loss of cholinergic function in the parietal cortex par-

TABLE 3.3. Criteria for Disseminated Lewy-Body Disease

1. Fluctuating cognitive impairment
   Memory and one other area affected
   Episodic confusion followed by lucid intervals
2. One of the following:
   Visual or auditory hallucinations, paranoid delusions
   Mild extrapyramidal symptoms or neuroleptic sensitivity
   Unexplained falls, transient clouding or loss of consciousness
3. AA and AB sustained over a period of months
4. No other evidence after workup
5. No evidence of vascular dementia

allels impairments on mental tests of cognition. Cholinergic neuron counts have been found to be lower in hallucinating than nonhallucinating patients with DLB. This suggests that the cholinergic deficiency system may play a role in the development of hallucinations.

Neuronal cell loss parallels the distribution of Lewy bodies, just as the presence of plaques and tangles parallels cell loss in AD. Direct neuropathologic comparisons between AD, Parkinson disease, and senile dementia of the Lewy body type suggest that the qualitative aspects of the DLB pathology (i.e., the Lewy bodies) mostly resemble those of Parkinson disease, although the distribution of this pathology resembles that of AD (i.e., it is widely distributed in the brain).

The risk of developing a dementing disorder in the context of DLB is unknown, although it is likely to be very high. No autopsy series have documented the presence of disseminated LDB pathology in the absence of the clinical syndrome of dementia.

There is a correlation between the pathology in the temporal lobes and the hallucinatory syndrome, as well as an association between the pathology in the parietal lobes and the severity of cognitive impairment. Thus, the unique clinical picture can be partly understood by the distribution of neuropathology, but much more work is needed to prove this.

The prion dementias

Clinical syndrome

This is a group of rare brain diseases first described in 1921. Presently, two forms of the disease have been associated with dementia: a sporadic (nonfamilial) form, referred to as *Creutzfeldt-Jakob disease* (CJD), and a familial (heritable) type referred to as *Gerstmant-Straussler-Scheinker syndrome* (GSS), which follows an autosomal dominant pattern of transmission.

Early symptoms of prion dementias include executive dysfunction, aphasia, apraxia, and amnesia. Progression is rapid, and change can be observed over a period of several weeks. Motor disorders also occur early. These include myoclonus (brief, quick muscle jerks), spasticity, and ataxia.

The age of onset of the prion dementias is usually after age 55. Both sexes appear to be affected equally. There is some evidence that brain trauma might advance the age of onset of the disease. In nonfamilial cases the disease has a rapid onset and course, leading to death within 12–18 months, although longer durations of up to 5–6 years have been reported. The genetic forms of prion dementias are less malignant and run a more protracted course, particularly in women. The onset is usually characterized by personality change and disinhibition, gradually followed by the four A's of cortical dementia.

A new form of CJD has emerged in Europe that typically begins between ages 20 and 40, presents with psychiatric symptoms and ataxia, and progresses in a fashion similar to that of the nonfamilial disorder. This is now referred to as *variant CJD* (vCJD) and is thought to be a human form of bovine spongiform encephalitis (BSE) or "mad cow disease." Individuals who develop this condition have a genetic variation in the prion gene; at codon 129 they have a methionine in both genes (this is call being *homozygous*). How this makes them vulnerable is not known.

Although systematic study is limited, noncognitive behavioral disorders such as depression, mania, delusions, and hallucinations are relatively rare in the nonfamilial form but are common in the familial younger-onset form. Problem behaviors such as agitation and irritability may be more frequent, but their prevalence is unknown.

At onset the diagnosis of prion dementias can be difficult, but the rapid progression and early myoclonus are suggestive. The electroencephalogram (EEG) often shows generalized, repetitive triphasic complexes with virtual abolition of background rhythms. However, this is absent in 20% of cases. Brain imaging can be normal or show focal frontal atrophy. Recent studies suggest that a characteristic protein, the 14-3-3 protein, is present in the spinal fluid of many individuals with CJD. This has high specificity but limited sensitivity for CJD; that is, when found, it likely indicates CJD, but its absence does not rule out the disease

Epidemiology

The population prevalence of CJD is approximately 1 per million. The disease has a population incidence of 0.5 per million per year worldwide, although there may be a higher incidence in Israel. It is thought to be due to either spontaneous mutations of the human prion protein or infection with mutated prion proteins, such as occurred with a disease known as *Kuru* that was associated with cannibalism in New Guinea. Gerstman-Straussler-Scheinker syndrome is even less prevalent than CJD. Its population prevalence is unknown.

Pathology

The predominant pathologic features of prion disease are a characteristic spongy appearance of the brain and cell loss that has given rise to the term *spongiform encephalopathy*. In early-onset familial cases, protein plaques are found within the spongiform degeneration.

The etiology of prion disease is thought to be an altered form of a normal brain protein known as the *protease resistant protein* (PRP) or *prion* (*pro*teinous *in*fectious particle) protein. Prion proteins are encoded by a gene on chromosome 20 and are thought to cause the disease by acting like an infectious agent (although they do not contain DNA). Because this disease is transmissible through the transfer of the prion proteins, it was thought for many years to be due to a "slow" virus. However, no virus particle and no immunologic response have been found. Several families with GSS have been described, with each family carrying specific mutations in the human prion protein on chromosome 20.

The pathophysiology of the disease is not known. It is presumed that prion protein becomes widely distributed in the brain and leads to neuronal injury and death with the formation of characteristic spongiform patterns. It is very likely that 100% of patients with CJD and GSS develop dementia. The presence of spongiform encephalopathy in the cortex likely explains the predominance of cortical symptoms. Ataxia and cranial nerve signs are explained by cerebellar and brain stem involvement.

4

DISEASES TYPICALLY CAUSING SUBCORTICAL OR MIXED PATTERN DEMENTIAS

OVERVIEW OF THE SUBCORTICAL DEMENTIAS

Parkinson disease

Clinical syndrome

Parkinson disease (PD) is a degenerative neurologic illness characterized by four features: (1) a coarse "pill-rolling" tremor of several beats per second, usually worse at rest, (2) rigidity or stiffness, (3) bradykinesia or motor slowness, and (4) poor balance.

Not all persons with PD develop dementia. In fact, until the 1980s, many researchers and clinicians believed that PD did not cause dementia. While there is now universal agreement that it can, there is still debate about the criteria that should be used to diagnose dementia in PD, so we prefer to use the broad definition in Table 1.1. Fewer than one-third of patients with PD suffer from dementia at any one time. However, an additional 50% have mild cognitive impairments, most often in mental speed and flexibility. The significance of these mild cognitive changes is unknown, but their recognition is important because they may adversely affect function and well-being. Over the course of an individual case of PD, the prevalence of dementia is at least 60%.

The clinical profile of the dementia of PD is typical of the subcortical dementias. The memory disorder is characterized by impaired free recall, with relative preservation of recognition memory; that is, patients have difficulty spontaneously recalling information but can pick the correct response when given a right and a wrong choice. Impairments in attention, verbal output (mostly with deficits in the motor aspects of speech—rate, loudness, prosody, and flow), and selection, anticipation, planning, and monitoring of goals are common. One feature atypical of subcortical dementia is impairment in visuospatial function. In the late stages of PD, a pronounced anomia can be seen.

Patients with PD exhibit high rates of apathy and social withdrawal that can be misinterpreted as dementia. The differentiation between apathy or slowness and dementia can be made by finding intact performance on a thorough cognitive mental status exam.

As many as 30% of patients with PD experience visual hallucinations. Dementia is a risk factor for these hallucinations, but they occur in many patients who do not have dementia. The most common hallucinations are of groups of humans or animals. Visual hallucinations are associated with the anti-Parkinson medicine levodopa (L-dopa) and occur more commonly at night. Hallucinations in nonvisual modalities have also been reported in up to 12% of patients.

From 30% to 60% of patients with PD develop a major depressive syndrome. This prevalence is higher than that reported in most other chronic neurologic disorders. The relationship between dementia and depression in PD is unclear.

Delusions, particularly paranoid or persecutory delusions, are uncommon in untreated patients but are frequent complications of pharmacotherapy. Frequencies of 3% to 8% have been reported in untreated patients. The presence of dementia predisposes to delusions, as do dopaminergic agents such as bromocriptine and L-dopa.

Epidemiology

Parkinson disease affects 100 per 100,000 population. This prevalence is age dependent, rising from approximately 50 per 100,000 at age 60 to approximately 130 per 100,000 at age 75. Estimates of the incidence of dementia in PD range from 8% to 84%. The only prospective study found an incidence of 29%. The most significant risk factor for developing dementia is age of onset. Parkinson disease beginning after age 60 is more likely to lead to dementia. Early-onset PD that is unresponsive to L-dopa may also be a risk factor for developing dementia, although this lack of response usually indicates a related disorder such as DLB (Chapter 3), PSP (Chapter 4), or multisystem atrophy (previously called *Shy-Drager syndrome*).

Pathology and etiology

Loss of dopamine-producing cells in the subcortically located substantia nigra is the basic pathologic change in PD. Loss of 80% or more of these neurons is necessary before the clinical syndrome occurs. The degree of dopamine loss in the substantia nigra correlates with the degree of the motor disorder, but its association with dementia is less clear. There is some loss of cells in the frontal lobes and other basal ganglia nuclei besides the substantia nigra.

The importance of the dopamine system in this disease is further supported by the fact that the clinical syndrome responds to drugs that increase levels of brain dopamine. Treatment with dopamine agonist medications (i.e., drugs that increase brain dopamine activity in some way), such as L-dopa and bromocriptine, have greatly benefited the motor disorder. Performance on cognitive tests improves in patients treated with L-dopa, but it is not clear whether this benefit occurs in individuals with moderate or severe dementia.

Cells in the substantia nigra of patients with PD also contain intracellular inclusions called *Lewy bodies*. Lewy bodies may also be found in other areas of the brain, especially the nucleus basalis, the locus ceruleus, the raphe nuclei, and occasionally the cortex. Some individuals with PD dementia are found to have the pathologic findings of both AD and PD at autopsy. It is not known whether this is due to the coincident occurrence of the two diseases, whether one disorder is caused by the other, or whether there is a common trigger to both. It is possible that some of the clinical variability seen in PD results from this pathologic variability.

The etiology of PD is unknown in most cases. A small percentage of cases are genetic, and abnormalities in several genes have been found in familial cases. In addition, the proteins produced by these genes are present in Lewy bodies, the pathologic hallmark of PD, in more typical later-onset non-familial cases. The genesis of these proteins is under extensive scrutiny but has not yet been determined.

Toxins such as the metal manganese and the drug MPTP cause a parkinsonian syndrome. Parkinsonism is also induced by neuroleptic medications such as haloperidol, risperidone, olanzapine, and others (see Chapter 10). Cerebrovascular disease with stroke in the basal ganglia is an uncommon etiology. The fact that PD was not described until the industrial age has led to the suggestion that environmental toxins may be etiologic agents, but this has not yet been substantiated. Cigarette smoking has been shown to be protective.

Progressive supranuclear palsy

Clinical syndrome

Progressive supranuclear palsy (PSP) is an uncommon disorder that resembles PD in causing rigidity, bradykinesia (slowness), and poor balance but in which tremor does not occur. Eye movement disorder, initially presenting as a diminished or absent ability to look upward, is almost always present. The head is often thrust back due to trapezius muscle overactivity in a position referred to as *opisthotonos*.

Progressive supranuclear palsy was one of the first subcortical dementias to be described. Marked cognitive slowness is usually present and may precede the development of frank dementia. The distinction between slowness and true dementia can be made by a careful cognitive mental status exam. For example, patients with PSP may take 10–20 seconds or longer to recall the words given in a free recall task and may take 10 seconds or more for each serial seven subtraction. However, they ultimately come up with the correct answer, where as patients with dementia do not. Many patients with PSP are *both* slow and unable to answer cognitive questions and have a subcortical form of dementia. While PSP is now included as one of the FTDs, the pattern of difficulty in accessing memory and marked slowness make it most similar to the subcortical dementias. However, as in PD dementia and DLB, visuospatial impairment is present as well.

Visual hallucinations are common. These can be frightening and sometime cause secondary delusions, that is, delusions that arise from interpretation of the hallucinatory experience.

Epidemiology

The prevalence and incidence rates of PSP are unknown. The rate of dementia in PSP is controversial because some studies have not distinguished between slowness to respond and true inability to respond correctly.

Pathology and etiology

Cell loss in the serotonin-producing cells of the raphe nuclei is characteristic. However, immunostaining techniques also demonstrate abnormalities in microtubule-associated proteins, as described in Chapter 3 under the frontotemporal dementias.

Huntington disease

Clinical syndrome

Huntington disease (HD) is an inherited, chronic, progressive dementia characterized by the presence of a choreiform motor disorder and dementia. The family history follows the pattern of a dominantly inherited disease (approximately 50% of each generation is affected). A core feature of HD is the motor disorder, which has two components: (1) dyskinesias (excess movements) in the form of choreic, brief, dance-like, nonrepetitive, involuntary movements, athetoid (writhing) movements of the face, limbs and trunk, and, later in the disease, dystonic (sustained), rigid postures and (2) impairments of voluntary movement leading to poor coordination of fine motor skills such as buttoning. The earliest evidence of incoordination is an eye movement disorder characterized by impaired saccade and jerky pursuit movements, that is, an inability to move the eyes smoothly when looking sideways. The motor disorders of HD cause gait instability and lead to frequent falls in the middle stage of the disease.

The clinical features of the dementia of HD are consistent with a subcortical dementia and include apathy, bradyphrenia (slowness of thinking), impaired mental flexibility, slowed thought processing, executive dysfunction, and impaired recall. Recognition memory is relatively spared. As the disease progresses the impairments become more global, so that what begins as a subcortical dementia broadens throughout the course of the illness to impair all cognitive capacities. The disease usually begins in midlife, although it can begin as early as the teenage years or as late as the 70s. When it begins in adolesence or early adulthood, rigidity is usually prominent early in the course of the disease.

Huntington disease is associated with high rates of depression. As many as 30% of patients suffer from depression, occasionally as the initial symptom. The depression in HD appears to run in families. Up to 10% of patients with HD develop episodes of mania in which irritability and elation are prominent. Other common noncognitive symptoms include irritability, explosiveness, and agitation. Delusions, hallucinations, and personality disturbances are less common but occur in up to 10% of patients. These noncognitive symptoms can worsen the motor and cognitive impairments and may respond to symptomatic treatment with medications (see Chapter 10).

Epidemiology

Huntington disease is inherited as an autosomal dominant trait. The population prevalence is 1 per 10,000 live births. The prevalence is similar in men and women. The average age of onset of the clinical syndrome is the late 30s to early 40s, but it can begin in adolescence or old age. The average patient lives 10–12 years after the development of symptoms.

Pathology and etiology

Major strides have been made in understanding the genetics and pathophysiology of HD in recent years. It is caused by a specific mutation in a gene located on the short arm of chromosome 4. This gene contains a region in which the three amino acids cytosine (C), adenosine (A), and guanine (G) are repeated multiple times. This is called a *CAG triplet repeat.* In normal individuals, this sequence is repeated fewer than 30 times. In persons who develop HD, the number of repeats is greater than 36. Earlier age of onset is associated with a higher number of repeats. Thus, individuals with 80 or more triplet repeats tend to have the earliest age of onset, often in adolescence. Patients with greater numbers of repeats also appear to suffer from more severe disease. Additionally, when the disease is transmitted through a male proband, that is, from father to child, there are usually more triplet repeats in the child's genome than in the father's. This process is referred to as *anticipation.*

The earliest pathologic change in HD is progressive shrinkage of the caudate nucleus bilaterally. In at-risk patients who carry the mutated gene, caudate atrophy can be seen on brain imaging before the clinical syndrome develops, suggesting that the brain has substantial reserve and that the clinical syndrome does not develop until a significant portion of this reserve is depleted. Several groups have reported intraneuronal intranuclear inclusion bodies in several triplet repeat diseases including HD. Their sensitivity and specificity are not yet established.

The gene product of the HD gene has been identified and is a protein called *huntingtin.* Its function is not yet known. It appears to cause a *gain of function;* that is, the protein may cause something to occur that does not usually occur. If this is true, a preventive therapy is possible, since blocking the action of this gene product might prevent brain damage from occurring.

Normal pressure hydrocephalus

Clinical Syndrome

Normal pressure hydrocephalus (NPH) is a rare syndrome defined clinically by the triad of dementia, gait ataxia, and urinary incontinence. The median age of onset is in the early 70s. Prevalence is equal in men and women. It was first described in 1964 by McHugh based on autopsy findings of a normal cortical mantle, enlarged ventricles suggesting hydrocephalus, absence of an obstruction causing the hydrocephalus, and absence of specific pathology suggesting another cause.

The clinical features of the dementia reflect the periventricular subcortical locus of the pathology, with impairments in executive function, memory (recall), apathy, and mental inflexibility being prominent. Rates of depression are reported to be high. Rates of mania, delusions, hallucinations, problem behaviors, and personality change are unknown.

The motor disorder of NPH is an ataxic gait disturbance with a broad-based, "magnetic" (feet seem to stick to the ground), short-stepped walk and multistep turning. Weakness and spasticity of the legs occur late. The progression of the syndrome is fairly rapid unless it is treated, but natural history data on large numbers of patients are not available.

Specific diagnostic criteria are not well established. The diagnosis should be suspected when the characteristic clinical triad and a subacute onset (less than 6–12 months) are present, especially if cortical signs such as aphasia are lacking. Incontinence and apractic gait are rare early in the course of other causes of dementia, so their presence at the onset of dementia, especially in the absence of upper extremity neurologic abnormality, should raise the possibility of NPH. Imaging studies (CT, MRI) show enlarged ventricles and minimal cortical atrophy. A lumbar puncture in which withdrawal of 20 cc or more of cerebrospinal fluid (CSF) transiently improves the gait disorder supports the diagnosis. Continuous CSF pressure monitoring sometimes reveals a characteristic pattern of intermittent, elevated pressure waves and predicts the response to shunt surgery.

Treatment is surgical and consists of placing a tube into the ventricle to drain CSF into the abdomen (peritoneum) or a central vein. In older studies the response rate to surgery was between 25% and 50%. With more conservative selection of subjects, response rates may be higher. From 5% to 9% of patients develop serious postsurgical morbidity or die within the next year. The response can be dramatic, with complete reversal of symptoms in some cases.

Epidemiology

Based on data from referral centers, the prevalence is approximately 0.6 per 100,000 per year. However, the lack of a valid set of diagnostic criteria and the rarity of the syndrome have limited epidemiologic study.

Risk factors for NPH include subarachnoid hemorrhage and meningitis. In most cases, a risk factor or precipitant is not found. By definition, the risk of cognitive impairment and dementia in NPH is 100%, but cases in which gait disorder and incontinence are prominent and cognitive impairment is minimal are reported. Specific criteria for the diagnosis of NPH-associated dementia are not available, so we favor the use of the dementia criteria presented in Table 1.1.

Pathology and etiology

The pathophysiology of NPH is poorly understood. Continuous monitoring of CSF pressure demonstrates an exaggeration of normal intrathecal (within the spinal fluid space) pressure waves even though CSF pressure measured on lumbar puncture is normal. These pressure waves presumably result in mechanical pressure on the subcortex surrounding the lateral and third ventricles and likely cause brain tissue destruction when the elastic properties of the brain tissue are exhausted. This may be why not all patients recover after sustained reductions in pressure.

Multiple sclerosis

Clinical syndrome

Multiple sclerosis (MS) is a chronic neurologic disorder caused by demyelination (loss of cells surrounding nerve tracts) in the central nervous system. Its etiology is unknown. The clinical course is described as "multiple lesions in time and space." That is, the diagnosis can be made with confidence when there is evidence that demyelination exists in at least two separate points in the nervous system and the patient's history suggests that these events occurred at two distinct times. Magnetic resonance imaging scanning has dramatically changed the diagnostic process, since the demyelinating lesions have a distinctive character on MRI scans and can be found even without a corresponding clinical history or evidence on exam of a neurologic abnormality. The mean age of onset is the late 20s. Women are affected three times more often than men.

The course of MS is variable. The disease is classified into three subtypes based on its clinical course. The most common subtype is the relapsing/ remitting type, in which neurologic impairments develop intermittently and in which there are also periods of months or years in which the neurologic defects remain stable. This type affects as many as half of MS patients. Approximately one-third of patients are affected by the secondarily progressive form of MS, which begins as the relapsing/remitting type but develops into a steady neurologic decline. The third subtype is progressive from its very onset. Patients with this form have the worst prognosis and the highest likelihood of developing dementia.

Given that MS is a demyelinating disease and that myelinated tracts are subcortical in locations, it is not surprising that the MS-associated dementia follows a subcortical pattern, with impairments in information processing, memory retrieval, executive function, and dysregulation of mood.

Clinical series suggest that 16%–20% of MS patients have mood disorders, the majority suffering from major depression. A smaller percentage (4%–5%) suffer from panic disorder. Sustained euphoria, irritability, and hypomanic syndromes occur but are infrequent. Delusions and hallucinations are rare.

An emotional state characterized by lack of concern is associated with the dementia of MS. Called *eutonia* by the British neurologist Kinnier-Wilson and often incorrectly referred to as *euphoria,* this mood state is uncommon but is associated with poor adaptation, probably because it is associated with a lack of awareness of the extent of impairment.

Epidemiology

The population prevalence of MS is 170 per 100,000. In community settings, 4% of MS patients suffer from dementia. This percentage rises to 8%–10% in clinical settings. As many as an additional 20% of patients with MS have measurable but mild cognitive impairments, but their impact on functioning is relatively small.

The main risk factor for dementia in MS is involvement of specific white matter areas in the brain: the corona radiata, the insula, and the hippocampus. No other clear risk factors for dementia in MS have been identified. Criteria for dementia in MS have not been published.

Pathology and etiology

The pathophysiology of MS is thought to be autoimmune damage of the myelin sheath of nerve tracts, perhaps triggered by a viral illness that occurred earlier in life. Not surprisingly, the location of white matter lesions is crucial to the development of dementia symptoms. The scattered nature of the subcortical lesions explains the variable clinical picture. For example, patients present with executive dysfunction or unconcern if frontal/anterior white matter areas are affected but with memory disorders if lateral temporal areas are involved.

Human immunodeficiency virus infection and acquired immune deficiency syndrome

Clinical syndrome

Cognitive impairments have been associated with human immunodeficiency virus (HIV) infection since acquired immune deficiency syndrome (AIDS) was first identified in 1981. The AIDS-associated dementia can be divided into two types. Opportunistic brain infection or lymphoma causes a mixture of cortical and subcortical symptoms, depending on the site of injury. For example, brain toxoplasmosis usually causes a subcortical pattern of dementia, while brain cryptococcosis is usually associated with a mixed pattern of language disturbance, affective change, and executive dysfunction.

The second type of AIDS-associated dementia is caused by the HIV virus itself. It is a subcortical dementia with memory loss, slowed mental processing, and executive dysfunction. It usually develops in an insidious and progressive fashion. Reduced motor speed and impaired nonverbal memory are prominent. In the early stages, the most serious impairments are found on tests of planning, which are detected on the Grooved Pegboard or the Trail-Making Test.

The most common noncognitive symptoms of HIV dementia are personality change, apathy, social withdrawal, and uninterest. The HIV dementia is associated with the development of manic syndromes in patients with no genetic or personal risk for mood disorders. From 10% to 15% of patients develop a new episode of depression in the 12–18 months before developing AIDS.

The HIV dementia is associated with a motor disorder characterized by poor coordination, slowness of movement, extrapyramidal symptoms, postural instability, and falling. Prior to the development of multiple-drug therapy, AIDS dementia had a poor prognosis. With retroviral therapy, the cognitive decline can be reversed or slowed. Without treatment, AIDS dementia portends a poor prognosis and rapid decline, with typical survival being 6 months or less.

The main risk factors for HIV-associated dementia are low hemoglobin, low body mass index, high prevalence of constitutional symptoms, and older age at onset. Reduction in pre-AIDS hemoglobin is the most significant predictor. Cognitive impairment becomes much more prevalent after the CD4 cell counts drop below 100.

Epidemiology

The prevalence of HIV infection varies throughout the world, with Western industrialized countries and South American countries being least affected. The most rapid increases in prevalence are in Africa and Asia, especially Southeast Asia. The World Health Organization estimates that as many as 30 million persons worldwide will be infected by the virus by the time the pandemic has reached its peak. In the United States, it is estimated that about 750,000 people are infected with the HIV virus. Well over 400,000 cases of AIDS have been reported, more than half in the last few years. There has been a decline in new AIDS cases in the United States since 1995, when new powerful antiviral therapies were introduced.

Up to 60% of AIDS patients experience cognitive difficulty prior to death, but a prominent dementia syndrome is present in approximately 15%. The incidence of dementia in HIV-infected patients is 7% per year. The most widely used current criteria for HIV dementia are the DSM-IV dementia criteria in Table 3–1 (modified for HIV).

Cognitive impairment has been reported in the early stages of HIV infection when the CD4 cell count is greater than 500. However, longitudinal studies have found that these cognitive impairments are not progressive. This suggests that these impairments existed prior to the HIV disease.

Pathology and etiology

The HIV virus initiates and sustains the dementia through direct infection of brain macrophages or microglia cells that normally fight infection in the brain. Neurons and other brain cells, such as glial astrocytes, are not directly infected. Thus, brain injury and dementia are not the direct result of virus-induced neuronal death. Rather, two indirect neurotoxic processes are involved. In one, the virus induces the expression of viral proteins on the surface of macrophages that are toxic to neurons. A second and more destructive mechanism is immune dysregulation in the brain. The infected microglia produce several cytokines or proteins that are directly neurotoxic. How and why this process becomes localized in the subcortex is not known.

The HIV virus enters the central nervous system early in the course of infection. Opportunistic infections are commonly associated with the later stages of HIV disease and include toxoplasmosis, cryptococcosis, tuberculosis, and syphilis. Additionally, there is an increase in brain lymphomas that can cause cognitive impairment. At autopsy, as many as 80% of patients have pathologic markers indicating HIV infection in the brain.

Dementia associated with mood disorders

Clinical syndrome

The mood disorders are characterized by abnormalities in mood, self-attitude, and vital sense or physical well-being. Depressed individuals of all ages complain of cognitive difficulty, but measurable cognitive impairment is seen primarily in the elderly. We refer to this form of mood-associated thinking impairment as *depression-induced cognitive impairment* (DICI) since not all patients fulfill the criteria for dementia.

The clinical picture of DICI approximates the phenomenology of a subcortical dementia. Patients with depressive dementia have impairments in free recall, delayed recall, and verbal delayed memory but typically have intact delayed visual memory and intact recognition memory. Some depressed patients have decreased verbal fluency, slowed responses, and difficulty with naming.

A reversible motor disorder consisting of bradykinesia and stooped posture has been described in some patients with depression. This, too, occurs predominantly in the elderly. Since these features simulate the syndrome of PD, this motor disorder may be due to impairments in basal ganglia function. Mania is accompanied by impaired cognitive performance, but there has been so little study of this condition we will not discuss it further.

Depression is also prevalent in many irreversible dementias, including AD, vascular dementia, PD and HD, and is probably induced by the neuropathology of these diseases. It is sometimes the first or presenting symptom of these disorders. The pattern of the dementia is that of the underlying disease.

The concept of *pseudodementia*—that is, depression imitating dementia—has been replaced by the recognition that the co-occurrence of depression and dementia often presages a progressive dementia but can indicate a reversible dementia due to major depression. Criteria to distinguish these conditions must be validated by long-term follow-up studies. The hypothesis that there are two broad syndromes of depression-associated cognitive impairment has been confirmed in one postmortem study in which 42% of a small sample of patients with "affective psychosis" had neuritic plaques and neurofibrillary tangles consistent with AD, while the remainder had normal neuropathology. A growing body of research also demonstrates that brain vascular disease contributes to some cases of late-life-onset depression. Called *vascular depression,* this form of depression is characterized by prominent executive dysfunction and extrensive white matter disease on MRI scans.

Depression is associated with increased mortality, but no studies have determined whether depression increases the mortality rate associated with dementia.

Epidemiology

The incidence and prevalence of dementia associated with mood disorder are matters of considerable debate. Among hospitalized patients whose onset of depression is late in life, 30%–40% evidence symptoms of DICI during the depression. The prevalence is much lower in outpatients.

Pathology and etiology

The etiology of dementia in depression is not well understood. Computed tomography and MRI studies find more cortical atrophy in patients with major depression than in elderly controls, and some studies find a greater number of white matter hyperintensities in depressed individuals. These changes are most marked in patients whose depression has begun in late life. Thus, the development of cognitive impairment in a patient with depression can be explained in three ways. First, major depression with onset in later life can be the first symptom of a degenerative or vascular dementia. Second, depression and dementia may have the same cause, but both manifestations may not always be present. Alexopoulos (1997) has suggested that the term *vascular depression* be applied to late-onset cases with evidence of brain vascular disease. Presumably, this pathology also contributes to the development of cognitive impairment. Finally, aging may diminish the brain's reserve, and this could be further "unmasked" by depression. That is, depression might place a physiologic burden on the brain systems that underlie cognition and induce impaired performance only when the depression is present. We believe that each of these mechanisms is at work and that more than one of them may contribute in a single patient.

Cerebrovascular disease

Clinical syndromes

Strokes due to cerebrovascular disease are the second leading cause of death in the United States, and cerebrovascular disease is the second most common cause of dementia. In the past, this type of dementia was referred to as *multi-infarct dementia* or *stroke-related dementia*. At present, the term *vascular dementia* is preferred because aspects of brain vascular disease besides frank stroke (e.g., hypoxia) may be responsible for the cognitive impairment. Table 4.1 contains the National Institute of Neurological Disorders and Stroke/ Association Internationale pour la Rechorde et l'Enseignement en Neurosciences (NINDS/AIRENS) diagnostic criteria for vascular dementia.

Vascular dementia presents in two broad clinical subtypes. The first is related to multiple small and/or large thromboembolic brain infarcts. The characteristics of the clinical syndrome depend on the location of the infarcts; mixed cortical and subcortical features are common. Prevalent symptoms include amnesia, receptive or expressive aphasia, constructional or other types of apraxia, and dysfunctions associated with injury of the frontal lobes, including executive disturbance. These impairments reflect the anatomy of the cerebral vasculature and the frequent occurrence of strokes in the temporal, parietal, and frontal cortical regions.

The second subtype of vascular dementia results from the degeneration of subcortical white matter, referred to as *leukoareosis,* and is presumed to be due to long-standing vascular insufficiency in deep brain areas. Memory disturbance, executive dysfunction, apathy, and amotivation are prominent. Brain imaging and gross pathologic studies show extensive white matter loss (leukoareosis). The extreme form of this condition is known as *Binswanger disease* and is associated with chronic, poorly controlled hypertension.

Multi-infarct dementia has been said to progress in a stepwise pattern. However, many pathologically documented cases of multi-infarct/vascular dementia have followed a slowly progressive course. An insidiously progressive course is more common in the leukoareotic type of vascular dementia. Patients with vascular dementia tend to die sooner and become debilitated more rapidly than patients with AD.

Vascular dementia is associated with several noncognitive impairments.

TABLE 4.1. Criteria for Vascular Disease-Causing Dementia

1. Dementia
   Decline by examination and objective testing
   Deficits in memory *plus* two other areas of cognition
   Functional impairment

2. Cerebrovascular disease by history, examination, or imaging

3. A relationship between AA and AB
   Dementia onset within 3 months of cerebrovascular accident
   Cognitive change in stepwise, abrupt, or fluctuating
   Strokes affect critical areas

4. Supportive features
   Early presence of gait disturbance
   Early presence of urinary frequency or incontinence
   Typical neurologic examination findings

5. Intact consciousness

A depressive syndrome affects 50%–60% of patients. A variety of personality changes can be seen. In the disinhibited type, socially inappropriate behaviors or intermittent but frequent mood swings occur with minimal or no provocation. Stimulus-bound behavior, that is, an inability to stop responding to a stimulus (e.g., grabbing food whenever it is seen or urinating in trash cans), is a common associated problem. Apathy, profound slowness, uninterest, and resistance to care can also be seen in vascular dementia. Delusions and hallucinations are also common, especially in association with strokes of the nondominant hemisphere.

The presence of other neurologic features, such as paresis (weakness), paralysis, cranial nerve changes, visual field loss, sensory defects, or seizures, depends on the location of the stroke.

Epidemiology

The risk of dementia after a clinically evident stroke is not fully known. One study suggests that after 3 months, as many as 13% of those with a new stroke suffer from dementia. Another study provides an estimate closer to 10% after 6 months. Four years after a stroke, as many as 33% develop dementia. Autopsy series of patients with the old definition of multi-infarct dementia indicate that 30%–50% have the pathology of both cerebrovascular accident and AD. Vascular dementia has a median age of onset in the early 70s and may decrease in incidence thereafter. It affects men more often than women.

The primary risk factors for stroke—hypertension, hypercholesterolemia, atherosclerosis, and diabetes—increase the likelihood that dementia will develop after a stroke, probably because a greater number of strokes increases the likelihood that dementia will develop. Controlling these risk factors reduces the incidence and progression of vascular dementia.

Pathology and etiology

Vascular dementia follows the *mass action* principle: the greater the amount of brain tissue affected, the greater the likelihood and severity of dementia. Dementia is likely when 50 cc of brain tissue is infarcted. The pattern of symptoms depends primarily on the location of injury.

There are several mechanisms of stroke, and each causes a different form of dementia. In embolic strokes, an atherosclerotic plaque breaks off from larger arteries (most often the carotid arteries in the neck) or the heart, travels to the brain, and blocks the blood vessels at the point at which the diameter of the plaque exceeds the diameter of the artery. This causes sudden death of tissue "downstream" from the blockage because cells are deprived of blood and oxygen. Thrombotic strokes are due to the formation of a clot in the artery, usually in association with an arteriosclerotic plaque. The clot closes off blood flow downstream, leading to tissue death. Both embolic and thrombotic strokes occur suddenly. In hypertensive vasculopathy, smaller penetrating arteries of the subcortex become narrowed due to long-standing high blood pressure. This leads to oxygen and nutrient starvation and probably demyelination. The clinical picture is usually that of a slowly progressive subcortical dementia without localizing neurologic signs. Another stroke mechanism is rupture of arteries or an aneurysm that leads to a hemorrhagic (bleeding) stroke. This can result in massive deficits because of loss of blood flow and the mechanical effects of bleeding into a closed space. Stroke can also occur if there is a sudden drop in systemic blood pressure, such as during a heart attack or cardiac arrest, or from loss of a nutrient supply induced by hypoglycemia or hypoxia.

Traumatic brain injury

Clinical picture

The clinical features of dementia after traumatic brain injury (TBI) vary with the site of the injury. Cortical, subcortical, and mixed patterns of impairment may occur. In closed head injury, the most common feature is amnesia, with difficulty learning new material. Frontal lobe dysfunctions are frequent as well. Loss of highly learned motor skills, executive dysfunction, language disturbance, inattention, poor concentration, and apraxia can occur. After a penetrating head injury, the impairments are often more focal and relate to the areas where penetration occurred.

Personality change and mood disturbance are the most common behavioral disorders after TBI, occurring in 50%–75% of cases of moderate to severe head injury. Symptoms include disinhibition, apathy, loss of motivation, depression, explosiveness, trouble concentrating, and memory loss.

The *postconcussion syndrome* consists of headache and inattention. It is a common sequela of mild head injury. Depressive syndromes and mania also occur after head injury in the absence of dementia and can worsen cognitive performance. Depression afflicts as many as 25%–30% of patients in the first year following TBI, and mania affects up to 5% of patients. Most studies suggest that the mood and cognitive syndromes are independent. Delusions and hallucinations are uncommon. Neurologic impairment after TBI relates to the region of injury.

Epidemiology

More than 500,000 cases of head trauma occur yearly in the United States. Perhaps one-third to one-half of all TBIs are moderate to severe. While as many as 40% of patients develop transient or permanent amnesia after moderate or severe head injury, a smaller percentage, about 8%–10%, develop a dementia syndrome.

Specific risk factors for dementia after TBI have not been identified, but it is likely that indicators of a poor outcome after TBI increase the risk for dementia. These include a low initial score on the Glasgow Coma Scale (a measure of injury severity that grades the clinical status of the patient at the time of the original injury), older patient age, high-velocity closed head injury, injury to other body areas, brain lesions before the injury, increased intracranial pressure at the time of the injury, longer duration of coma, longer in-hospital stay after the injury, and poor premorbid cognitive state. The criteria for dementia in Table 1.1 are best used.

Pathology and etiology

A variety of mechanisms contribute to trauma of the brain after a blow to the head. Penetrating injuries, in which objects such as bullets or spokes enter through the skull, cause a focal or tract-type mechanical injury. Rapid acceleration and deceleration of the head cause movement of the brain within the skull and lead to two types of injury. Mechanical injury to brain areas next to the skull is caused when the relatively plastic brain strikes the immovable skull. This damage tends to be most severe in the orbito-frontal area, because the brain rubs against the floor of the skull in the front, and in the inferior temporal areas, where the brain can hit against the petrous bones. Acceleration and deceleration can also cause stretching of the axons of the descending and ascending nerve fiber tracts and result in injury to them.

Mechanical trauma and axonal shearing also cause hemorrhage, inflammation, edema, and mass effects that combine to cause damage or death to brain structures. Further injury can result from epidural, subdural, and intracerebral hematomas. The principal determinants of damage are the amount of energy imparted to the brain, the amount of brain tissue directly injured either through coup (the site of the blow) or countercoup (the brain hitting the opposite side of the skull) injury, and the location of the injury. Global cognitive syndromes such as inattention, headache, and difficulty concentrating may be the result of *mass action,* that is, a diffuse disruption of brain cell function, but it is more likely that the specific features of dementia in any individual are closely related to the location of the most severely affected areas of the brain. For example, after coup/countercoup acceleration and deceleration injuries, memory disturbance results from injury to the temporal lobe, executive dysfunction from frontal trauma, and inattention/poor concentration from damage to the reticular activating and related systems.

Toxic dementias

Several substances have been associated with central nervous system toxicity. Alcohol is the most widely used such substance. Other substances with a propensity for inducing abuse and dependence that may cause cognitive impairments with chronic use include cocaine, opiates, marijuana, sedative-hypnotics, and solvent inhalants (benzene, toluene, turpentine). Heavy metals such as lead, arsenic, mercury, manganese, and thallium are also injurious to the brain.

Clinical picture

The clinical syndrome of alcohol-related dementia is varied. A mixture of cortical and subcortical features is common, with the most prominent impairments occuring in memory, with recall and recognition being equally disturbed, and executive dysfunction. The inhalant substances, such as glue and toluene, may cause executive dysfunctions predominantly. Early recognition is important since some or all of the deficits can reverse with abstinence and good nutrition.

Epidemiology

The epidemiology of alcohol use and of other substances of abuse is beyond the scope of this chapter. Alcoholism afflicts 15%–20% of the U.S. population, and the combined prevalence of other substances of abuse, excluding nicotine and caffeine, is approximately 5%. The epidemiology of heavy metal intoxication in adults is much less well known, but occupational exposure is a clear risk factor. In children, exposure to lead remains a major public health problem. As many as 10% of those who develop alcohol use disorders develop dementia. Dementia related to alcoholism accounts for fewer than 2% of all dementias, however.

Risk factors for developing dementia in the context of chronic alcoholism are not well understood. Duration and amount of alcohol abuse are major risk factors, and a family history of alcoholism may be contributory. Alcohol abuse predisposes to repeated head trauma and nutritional deprivation, both of which can cause dementia. The incidence and prevalence of cognitive disorders in persons with polysubstance abuse, inhalant abuse, and heavy metal and solvent exposure are not well established

Pathology and etiology

The pathophysiology of dementia syndromes due to toxins is poorly understood. It is not clear if alcohol itself is the cause of the dementia or if the nutritional disorders and head trauma associated with alcohol abuse are the primary culprits. All probably contribute variably in different individuals. Autopsies of persons with alcoholism and dementia reveal damage to the mammillary bodies, dorsomedial nucleus of the thalamus, nucleus basalis, hippocampus, amygdala, and cerebellum. The associations between these pathologic findings and the dementia syndrome is suggestive but not definitive. The brain atrophy on CT and MRI scans seen in patients with alcohol abuse can be reversed with abstinence. The Wernicke-Korsakoff syndrome, characterized by amnesia, gait disturbance, and impaired eye movements, is due to a thiamine deficiency that damages the dorsomedial nucleus of the thalamus and the mammillary bodies. It is likely caused by malnutrition secondary to alcoholism and occurs in genetically vulnerable individuals.

Little is known about the neuropathologic and neurophysiologic changes that contribute to the development of dementia caused by the use of and exposure to other toxic substances. It is plausible that inhalants enter the brain through the cribriform plate at the base of the frontal lobes and cause executive dysfunction by a direct toxic mechanism, but this has not been proven.

5

OVERVIEW OF DEMENTIA CARE

The care of patients with dementia is based on six general principles (Table 5.1). Each of these rests on the belief that knowledge of the patient's wishes and goals prior to the illness should guide care. This is easy in the abstract but can be difficult when problems are persistent or severe. It is also easy to lose sight of the fact that small changes can be of great value and provide meaningful improvement in patients' quality of life, as well as that of their caregivers.

GOALS OF CARE

The goals of treatment are determined by the needs of the individual patient and his or her caregivers. Table 5.2 lists the most common needs of patients and families and the goals that follow from them. An accurate diagnosis is usually the first goal. This is met by determining that dementia is present, classifying it, and identifying its cause (Chapters 4 and 5). When new problems develop, whether cognitive, medical, psychological, behavioral, or functional, accurate reassessment and diagnosis of the new problems become a priority.

We refer to the next goals as the *four pillars of dementia care*: (1) treat the disease; (2) treat the symptoms; (3) support the patient; and (4) support the caregiver. Each of these can be achieved in a systematic way, as presented in this book. Clinical trial evidence now strongly suggests that proper delivery of this "package" of dementia care has significant positive effects in

TABLE 5.1. Six Principles of Dementia Care

1. People with dementia are individuals.
2. People with dementia have the same needs as others.
3. People with dementia have the same value as other adults.
4. People with dementia can be healthy and happy.
5. Small changes can have great practical value.
6. Something can always be done to help.

terms of symptom reduction, quality of life, and delay of disability, as well as substantial benefits to caregiver mood and quality of life. Dementia care also appears to delay institutionalization when delivered to people living in their homes or other community settings.

The first pillar is to treat and, if possible, cure the disease that has caused the dementia. Unfortunately, cure is rarely possible at present. However, some interventions are available that may slow the progression of AD (see Chapter 10) and possibly other dementias. If patients have vascular disease or vascular risk factors such as hypertension, cerebrovascular disease, and atrial fibrillation, aggressive management and control of these conditions may well delay dementia progression. There is debate about the right level of systolic blood pressure control that may affect dementia progression. There is good evidence to support keeping systolic blood pressure below 160 mmHg and some evidence that keeping it below 140 mmHg is important in delaying dementia progression. More and more studies are suggesting that medical co-morbidity is a major factor in dementia progression. Keeping cholesterol under control, controlling blood sugar in diabetics, and keeping medical co-morbidity well controlled may also delay progression of many dementias.

As presented in Chapter 10, there is increasing hope that more effective disease treatments will become available. These may slow the progression of the underlying disease, but may not necessarily reverse the symptoms since the latter are due to the brain damage caused by the disease and may be irreversible. Thus, new disease treatments are likely to be most effective when dementia is mild, hence the increasing emphasis on early diagnosis by experts in the field.

The second pillar of dementia care is symptom relief. Reaching this goal requires an understanding of the specific symptoms of each patient and creativity in devising treatment approaches. Three types of symptoms are evident in most dementia patients: cognitive, functional, and behavioral. Each should be addressed, sometimes separately but sometimes with a single approach.

TABLE 5.2. Needs of Dementia Patients and Their Families

Patients Need:	Families Need:
Accurate diagnosis	Education about the diagnosis and
Treatment of the disease	Prognosis
Treatment of cognitive symptoms	Guidance in decision making
Treatment of noncognitive symptoms	Emotional support
Provision for needs and wants	Referral to community resources
Meaningful activity	Physical and emotional well-being
Personal safety	Socialization
Adequate physical and dental health	Time for themselves
A supportive, stable environment	

In AD, cognitive symptoms can be improved in the short term by medications (Chapter 10). Functional and behavioral symptoms can be treated in many dementias. These are discussed in Chapters 8, and 9.

The provision of appropriate supportive care to the patient is the third pillar of dementia care (Chapter 6). This includes ensuring meaningful activity and personal safety and addressing physical and dental health needs. Good supportive care requires knowledgeable caregivers and a supportive, stable environment.

The fourth pillar of dementia care is the support of the family and other caregivers (Chapter 7). It is achieved by educating them about the diagnosis and prognosis of the patient's condition, providing guidance in decision making, helping families adjust to the changes brought about in their own lives, and referring them to community resources. Family members also need to attend to their own physical, emotional, and social well-being.

Appendix B contains a scripted *psychosocial intervention* that can be used to deliver the last two pillars in a systematic way in almost any clinical setting. Information is provided about how to deliver this intervention, along with supportive materials in the form of guidelines for caregivers and useful checklists. This material in Appendices A–C can easily be copied and used in day-to-day clinical practice. Chapters 6 and 7 provide supportive detail on how to deliver these supportive interventions.

TREATMENT PLANNING

The treatment plan provides a blueprint for care. Table 5.3 lists the attributes of an optimal dementia treatment plan. It must be rational and realistic. Recommendations should be based on a thorough assessment of each patient and caregiver at every point in time. Although much is known about

TABLE 5.3. Five Attributes of
a Treatment Plan for Dementia

Realistic
Flexible
Anticipatory
Comprehensive
Hopeful

the course of dementia, there is variability among patients. The use of interventions should be based on a realistic sense of their likelihood for success.
False hope can be as destructive as no hope. The optimal treatment plan
should be dynamic and flexible—it must change if the patient's or caregiver's
condition changes. If a crisis occurs, ready access to the appropriate professional is crucial. Since much day-to-day care rests on trial and error, the plan
must be flexible enough to address the unexpected.

An effective treatment plan should be anticipatory. Preventing a problem
before it develops is ideal, although not always possible. For example, providing a medical alert bracelet and keeping recent photographs available in
case a patient wanders away can save the patient's life. The plan should prepare for most eventualities that are common to dementia. Informing family
members that swallowing problems are beginning to develop will allow
them to consider the benefits and burdens of tube feeding well before they
are faced with the need to decide about this issue. Teaching family members
that behavioral symptoms can be due to the dementing disease may encourage them to seek help for distressing mental symptoms and prevent them
from taking personally something said by the patient as the result of a delusion or memory impairment.

The optimal treatment plan should also be comprehensive and focus on
as many aspects of the patient's care and the caregivers' needs as possible.
Since caregivers carry out the treatment plan, communication between them
and the clinician is a necessity. It is sometimes best if there is a spokesperson
for the family, but the key to success is continued communication among the
interested parties.

A comprehensive dementia plan should include day-to-day activities for
the patient, indicate which signs and symptoms should be brought to the attention of a professional, provide a list of which professionals are involved
in the patient's care and what aspects of care they are addressing, and spec-
ify the plan for future transitions, such as nursing home placement.

A critical element of the treatment plan is the conveyance of hopefulness.
The plan should assume that short-term improvement is possible but should
recognize that, in most cases, long-term decline is inevitable. As is true in the

care of a person with any chronic illness, the focus is on maximizing functions and minimizing disability by identifying those impairments that can be treated.

IMPLEMENTING THE TREATMENT PLAN

The implementation of the treatment plan begins with the communication of the diagnosis and treatment options to the patient and family. The most effective way to communicate the diagnosis is in a family conference. This involves inviting into the office or clinic all members of the family who will potentially be involved in caring for the patient.

The discussion of the diagnosis and treatment options should be as clear and concise as possible. There should be time to answer questions and an opportunity for all involved to raise concerns. By meeting together, all family members hear about the specific difficulties the patient is experiencing and how they are a product of the disease. Sometimes family members who are not providing direct care do not appreciate how arduous caregiving is. The clinician should listen for this and clarify misunderstandings on this issue. We usually meet without the patient first, since many family members do not ask questions if the patient is there and because the patient usually becomes "talked about" rather than being included. We then have the patient join the meeting and review the treatment options, allowing the patient to set the pace of discussion.

Many family members benefit from written instructions and information. In Appendix A, the Johns Hopkins Dementia Care Guidelines for Families are provided. Similar guidelines and information pamphlets about dementia are available through the Alzheimer's Association in the United States, and similar information is available in other countries from comparable societies. Many websites also provide such information that can be shared with caregivers (e.g., www.alz.org).

Several questions are frequently asked. One is "How was the diagnosis established?" Clinicians need to explain the process of diagnosis, as presented in Chapters 3 and 4, emphasizing its systematic and time-tested nature. A review of the results of cognitive testing, such as specific items or scores on the cognitive mental status examination and neuropsychological testing, is sometimes useful since they objectively identify deficits. Patients and families sometimes explain deficits on single items, such as difficulty knowing the date or doing the serial sevens, by saying that the patient was anxious or "never could do this" or using statements such as "No old person can do this." We find it helpful to remind families that it is important to look at the big picture ("Yes, one or two problems on the examination might be due to anxiety, but not ten items"), that these tests are generally well normed by age ("Most older people score above 25 on the MMSE"), that declines are more relevant than absolute scores ("Your husband was a college graduate who likely would have scored 28 to 30 on MMSE years ago, so a score of 22 today is a decline"), and that all patients tested in the clinic are anxious but that anxiety rarely accounts for consistently poor performance.

Other frequently asked questions at the time of diagnosis include "How sure are you of this?," "What can be done?," and "What does this mean for the future?" Patients and families should be reminded that the diagnosis of dementia is based on the presence of a clinical syndrome and can be made with very high confidence, while the accuracy of a diagnosis of the *specific cause* of dementia varies, ranging from around 100% for posttraumatic dementias, to 90% for some cases of AD, to less than 50% for vascular dementia without AD. When discussing what can be done, the clinician should review the treatment recommendations, options, and expected outcomes of each.

Providing information about the future course of the disease (prognosis) is more difficult. We believe that clinicians should provide an estimate of progression if they have an opinion but should be very clear about the limited ability of any clinician to predict the future. The prognostic assessment becomes more accurate as patients are followed over time and their course becomes evident. The rate of worsening in dementia is intimately tied to its cause. Alzheimer's disease patients who are untreated decline on average 3–4 points on the MMSE every year. Patients with vascular dementia may not decline at all in a given year, even though the decline is more rapid than with AD on average over longer time periods. The rate of decline in AIDS dementia has slowed since the development of antiviral therapies.

Involving the patient with dementia in the treatment planning process is important. This begins with establishing a relationship with the patient (see Chapter 6). However, many patients with dementia, particularly those with AD, lack insight into their cognitive deficits. This lack of insight is called *nosoagnosia*. Persistent attempts to convince patients without insight that they suffer from dementia are rarely useful and often may lead to distress. Confrontation almost never helps. Some patients are aware that something is wrong and complain that "I'm not right and need to be put back together" or that "There is something different about me" but deny having a memory problem. We recommend telling them once that they have a memory problem but, if they deny it, then going on to tell them that you will do your best to solve their problem. If patients have a different complaint, it should be responded to as much as possible. On the other hand, if patients accept that something is wrong because their spouse says so, it is usually not necessary to persuade them that they have dementia.

Communication among caregivers is obviously important. Caregivers vary in their time availability, devotion, energy, and resources. The clinician's primary responsibility is for the well-being of the patient, although the well-being of the caregiver and patient are inextricably intertwined. We try to be direct with caregivers and to communicate freely. We are not always successful, but we believe that the themes of this book—being informed about dementia, focusing on problem solving, acknowledging and addressing the emotional impact of dementia, and reexamining the patient's condition when problems arise—are keys to good communication.

Caring for dementia patients often requires a multidisciplinary team. The team may include primary care physicians, medical specialists (psychiatrists, neuropsychiatrists, neurologists, geriatricians), psychologists, nurses, social workers, counselors, activity therapists, occupational therapists, and physical therapists. It is important that all professionals involved in treatment participate in the development of a plan. Regular communication between team members is necessary. At times of crisis—for example, when a patient is hospitalized—it is useful to have a face-to-face meeting of the treatment team.

Every member of the treatment team has unique skills (nurses, psychologists, physicians, social workers, activity therapists, nursing assistants, respite care workers, day-care workers, and many others). This need for several care providers has led to the suggestion that a care coordinator be appointed for each patient to coordinate the professionals. In practice, the family or a family spokesperson, in collaboration with a physician or nurse, becomes the care coordinator for most patients.

Clinicians should strive to include rather than exclude practitioners from different backgrounds and to see all different practitioners as colleagues. It is often a relief for professionals to be reassured that they are not expected to know, understand, or do everything. Sometimes the family must be reminded or encouraged to use practitioners who have specific backgrounds. They may need legal, financial, medical, social, or transportation resources. Social workers are an important source of knowledge about the community since they may know who can provide information about specific problems. If there is a local Alzheimer's Association chapter or a similar organization, it, too, might provide information about specific agencies who are able to help. In most cases, the medical care of patients with dementia can be managed in the community by a primary care physician in collaboration with other professionals. Occasionally, specialists need to be consulted.

The treatment plan's implementation should address the setting in which the patient is treated. Care is provided in settings as diverse as outpatient medical clinics, supported housing (assisted living, residential care, life care, group homes), adult day care, hospital wards, psychiatric inpatient units, or nursing homes. It is important to consider how the patient's needs are being met by each site and to understand how the strengths and weaknesses of the setting interact with the patient's needs (see the discussion later in this chapter).

Care providers should try to anticipate the issues that may arise when moving to a different care setting. Transitions in housing are particularly challenging, and are often associated with increased confusion and behavioral disturbance. These usually remit as patients become familiar with the new setting. A frequent question about moving is whether it is better to move a person earlier or later in the course of the illness. This question is best addressed on an individual basis, but often there is no single right answer.

GOOD CLINICAL PRACTICES

Table 5.4 presents a list of good clinical practices professionals should keep in mind when they care for dementia patients. This book provides some basic facts about the most common diseases causing dementia, but further reading may be necessary in complicated cases. An appreciation of the natural history of the disease assists the clinician in determining whether a problem is related to disease progression or if an alternative cause should be sought. For example, if a patient with AD declines more rapidly than expected, the clinician should look for a cause—such as depression, a urinary tract infection, or an emerging medical problem—to explain the decline.

Knowledge of the current status of each patient requires an adequate diagnostic evaluation and formulation, as well as regular updates about how the patient is doing, who the involved caregivers are, and which other professionals have been consulted. Careful record keeping in the patient's chart helps keep the care providers abreast of changes in the patient's condition. We recommend a routine visit approximately every 6 months. This is an optimal interval for following the progression of the disease and keeping the clinician aware of the patient's current status.

Good practice also includes knowing the available local resources. This is easier for those who specialize in dementia care, but most practitioners come into contact with relatively few patients with dementia. Knowing who to refer to can substitute for knowing specific resources. A local chapter of the Alzheimer's Association or the local county Office on Aging are reliable in identifying local resources for patients with dementia. Other useful resources to know include social workers or rehabilitation experts (occupational/physical therapists) who specialize in dementia; local specialty or university clinics specializing in dementia; and specific service programs such as adult day-care programs, senior centers, supported living environments, and nursing homes that cater to patients with dementia.

TABLE 5.4. Good Clinical Practices in Dementia Care

Know the natural history of the disease.
Know the specific case.
Know the available local resources.
Use a team approach.
Use persistent trial-and-error problem solving.
Think of how to deal with a crisis before it happens.
Be as specific as possible.
Look for and react to sudden, even subtle, changes.

Trial-and-error problem solving is a crucial element of dementia care. Even the most experienced clinician is confronted with situations that seem daunting. No obvious solution may be at hand or the problem may require time to solve. Almost always, something can be done to improve a situation. Therefore, the clinician should be ready to try several things, to be persistent, to recognize failure when it occurs, and to try new alternatives when failure does occur.

An important aspect of good clinical practice is to identify changes in the patient's state and to teach caregivers how to do this. Many changes are an inevitable part of dementia progression; others are not. A sudden change should alert the family and caregiver to the likelihood that a new problem has occurred. In the patient with AD, the development of a new problem should raise questions about a new medical condition (e.g., constipation, urinary infection, upper respiratory infection, pain, a dental problem), medication toxicity, or a new brain lesion such as a stroke. Any sudden change should be considered medically treatable until proven otherwise. When a significant change occurs, it is good practice to review in detail all changes that occurred in the patient's environment over the past month or 6 weeks. The addition of a new medicine, changes in the routine of a day-care program, a new caregiver, illness in a caregiver, or hidden injury from an unwitnessed fall can all cause the patient to change.

Clinicians should be prepared to deal with crises. Crises in dementia care seem to happen at the most inopportune moments and often inconvenience everyone. When they occur, the first step is to get as much information as possible as quickly as possible. How much of the crisis relates to the patient, how much relates to the care provider, and how much relates to the environment should be determined. The next step is to engage the caregiver in a conversation (often on the phone) to help him or her calm down and to problem-solve. This conversation should review what the caregiver has tried and note what has and has not helped. Determining the availability of other caregivers may be important. Even though caregivers don't always do what is advised, talking to a professional on the phone can help deescalate the situation, introduce logic, and offer possible solutions.

Medical emergencies must be attended. It may be necessary to have the patient evaluated at an emergency room or hospitalized, particularly if there is evidence that something dangerous is about to happen. Emergency department visits should be viewed as a *last resort* because these facilities are not well equipped to handle patients with dementia and will often restrain or overmedicate them due to lack of staffing or inexperience.

DEMENTIA IN SPECIAL POPULATIONS

The symptoms of dementia depend on the disease causing it but are modified by the characteristics of each individual. A knowledge of features common to many individuals forms the basis for effective care, but some groups of patients are different enough to require special discussion.

Dementia in the young

Dementia is uncommon before age 65. It is extremely rare in early adulthood because most of the diseases that cause dementia in the young are rare genetic conditions. One major difference between dementia in the young and in the elderly is the effect on the family. If the patient has young children, the disease often has a devastating effect on their lives. Marital relationships are more likely to be disrupted, perhaps because the couple may not have developed sufficient bonding to survive the devastation of the illness. Since younger patients are more likely to be working, a change in work performance is sometimes the first symptom. Loss of a job may occur before the dementia is recognized as the cause of declining ability, depriving them of disability income. Even with disability insurance, they will have had less time to accumulate savings, so financial problems are much more common in young patients. There is some debate as to whether people with dementia who are below age 60–65 are best cared for in specialty clinics for young dementia patients. In our experience, this is neither necessary nor additionally helpful. About 10%–15% of patients in our memory clinics are in this younger age group, and we have no reason to think that their care is less thorough, as long as the primary clinicians are mindful of the special issues younger dementia patients and their families face, as articulated earlier.

Cultural and ethnic backgrounds

Few studies have looked at how cultural and ethnic backgrounds affect the clinical presentation of dementia, but anecdotal writings and clinical experience suggest wide variation. In some cultural groups, dementia is not seen as an illness but rather as an aspect of growing old. In others, it is seen as the result of lifestyle. It is important for the clinician to recognize how memory loss and cognitive decline are viewed in persons of different cultural and ethnic backgrounds and to use this knowledge in devising a care plan.

Cultural and economic status also influences the availability of and willingness to use resources. If there is mistrust of traditional medicine, individuals may be reluctant to use desired or necessary services. The appropriateness of support groups also varies significantly by culture. While it is sometimes said that support groups are a uniquely American phenomenon, there are many cultural groups in the United States for whom speaking in public about ill family members is not acceptable, especially if strangers are present. Other supports will probably benefit such families more.

The adult with mental retardation

Individuals with lifelong cognitive incapacities such as mental retardation are at greater risk for dementia. In Down syndrome, for example, the onset of AD is common in midlife. Variations in the initial presentation and course of dementia are among the challenges of identifying and treating dementia in the mentally retarded. Early changes in behavior are sometimes wrongly attributed to changing life circumstances when they are the result of the onset of AD. Conversely, changes in behavior due to depression or a reaction to a change in life circumstances may be misinterpreted as due to dementia.

DEMENTIA IN SPECIFIC ENVIRONMENTS

Day programs

Many day programs, sometimes referred to as *adult day care,* have been developed to provide activities, supportive care, and supervision for impaired older persons. A substantial proportion of persons in adult day care suffer from dementia. One controversy is whether it is better to keep healthy elders and persons with dementia in separate programs. Our experience suggests that combined programming is not appropriate and often is beneficial to neither the cognitively normal older person nor the person with dementia. The hope that the mingling of persons with dementia and those with normal cognition will provide a better understanding of dementia and provide stimulation for the person with dementia is far outweighed by the need of individuals with dementia for more direction and cognitive support. However, we know of no studies that support this or the opposing position.

Another controversial issue is whether there should be a single program for all dementia patients or whether different programs should be provided for persons with milder and more severe dementia. The answer to this question depends on the particular center and the individual participants. As dementia progresses, many patients become less able to participate in activity programs. Inability of the facility to adapt to this changing need is one reason leading to discharge from day programs. We believe that facilities that have the resources and an adequate number of participants function better with programs that vary activities based on the severity of the person's illness, but financial and size limitations often prevent the provision of more than one group at a time.

Group and assisted living homes

In the past 10 years, there has been a rapid increase in the number of group home and assisted living facilities marketing themselves as appropriate for dementia patients. These settings are often attractive because they look less institutional and almost always cost less than a traditional nursing home. Like day centers, these environments are very diverse and are licensed differently in different states. Since licensure determines the amount of oversight that is provided by local health departments, this is an important issue. The Maryland Assisted Living Study, the most comprehensive study of its kind, has found that dementia occurs in 70%–75% of residents of any assisted living facility, not just in "special care" dementia units in these settings. And dementia has major effects on the quality of life, disability, and ability to age in place of assisted living residents. This requires group homes and assisted living facilities to have mechanisms in place to monitor patients' mental health needs and to provide necessary care. Smaller group homes may lack structured activity programs, and day care should be considered if this is the case.

Nursing homes

From 60% to 80% of individuals in nursing homes suffer from dementia. As with assisted living settings, the principles and practices discussed in this book are universal and apply to the long-term care setting as well as to dementia patients in the community. The residents of long-term care facilities have a wide range of physical, social, behavioral, emotional, and cognitive impairments, and this presents a major challenge to the staff who provide care and design treatment programs. There is no convincing evidence that "special care" units are necessary to provide the appropriate level of stimulation and support for persons with dementia, but specific programs that address the activity, emotional, and physical needs of such persons are needed.

Special care units may be better able to care for the more seriously behaviorally impaired dementia patient, but this has not been adequately demonstrated. Programs that address the needs of the cognitively normal residents are also necessary. Staff training in caring for dementia patients and managing behavior is a critical aspect of care for any nursing home.

Emergency departments

Acute changes in behavior or cognition are the most common reasons a patient with dementia is seen in an emergency department (ED). Searching for an underlying physical cause of the behavior disturbance is crucial. History from knowledgeable informants can help the emergency team more quickly discover the cause or causes of the patient's change in status. Atypical presentation of physical and psychiatric illnesses is common in the elderly, so lack of elevated temperature and other signs of illness should not dissuade the team from performing a thorough evaluation. Treatment with sedatives or neuroleptics should be avoided if possible until a cause has been identified or ruled out. Having someone who knows the patient stay with him or her at all times, and repeated frequent explanations of what is happening, can lessen the need for sedation. Thus, EDs that treat many patients with dementia can prevent a lot of problems associated with restraint and overmedication of these patients by training their staff in behavioral interventions (perhaps by reading the relevant chapters of this book), by allowing families to stay with dementia patients in their ED rooms, and by having available "sitters" to provide one-on-one supervision and support to dementia patients.

Acute hospitals

The majority of individuals in acute general hospitals are elderly. Individuals with dementia are prone to certain medical conditions that may lead to hospitalization. These conditions include delirium, hip fractures, arthritis, stroke, cancer, diabetes, hypertension, heart disease, and others. Therefore, it is no surprise that 15%–20% of persons over 65 in acute care hospitals suffer from dementia. Dementia prolongs the length of stay on the typical medical or surgical unit by an average of 4 days. Patients with dementia in the acute care hospital should be monitored carefully for delirium due to medication intoxication, metabolic instability, or the complexities of their medical condition. Many will require constant reorientation and reminders about why they are in the hospital, what they should be doing, and what is planned for the future. If 24-hour support can be provided by family members or a nursing aide, this should be done before problems arise. If this is not possible, frequent brief interactions with staff, or the use of one-on-one sitters, should be used to remind and reorient patients. This will diminish patient distress and lessen problematic behaviors including wandering, climbing out of bed, and calling out. The prevalence of dementia is high enough that acute care general hospitals should develop methods for identifying patients with dementia at the time of admission. This will improve the assessment and management of their special needs, and improve the patients' and families' experiences in the hospital. It may also reduce the length of stay and the likelihood of restraint use.

Acute psychiatric units

The treatment of behavioral and mental disturbances in patients with dementia sometimes requires acute psychiatric hospitalization. Given the stigma associated with psychiatric treatment, it is best to mention the possibility of hospitalization to family members early in the treatment course if this is being considered. Because elderly patients with dementia have unique needs, they should be admitted to psychiatric units that have specifically trained, knowledgeable staff.

Hospice and end-of-life palliative care

Patients with late-stage dementia who have been cared for at home are being referred for hospice care with increasing frequency. The care of patients with dementia at the end of life is addressed in a later chapter. This approach can be applied in the hospice setting. Hospice services are provided to persons having less than a 6-month life expectancy. This includes patients who are dependent, who are not eating and drinking, and whose families have agreed to forego medical treatment of acute illnesses unless it would improve the patient's comfort. Hospice care is sometimes provided at a designated hospice unit, but sometimes the hospice team comes into the home and provides comfort measures for the patient and support for the family.

6

Supportive Care for the Patient with Dementia

The goals of supportive care are to maintain the patient's quality of life and prevent morbidity. This chapter focuses on the general approach to the patient, issues in day-to-day living, safety and supervision, and health maintenance.

Approaching the Patient

Establishing a relationship

The first step in dementia care is forming a relationship with the patient. This begins with the initial contact, which should include time alone with the ill person to appreciate his or her experience of the illness. Taking a personal history as outlined in this book from the patient at the initial evaluation typically accomplishes this goal. The situation of patients is best understood by taking into account their lives before the illness and the changes the illness has forced upon them.

One of the great challenges in caring for patients with dementia is maintaining their dignity as individuals in the face of cognitive impairment that may be progressive. This includes being sensitive to their feelings, adapting one's approach to their needs, and providing an environment as similar as possible to that previously experienced. Respecting the dignity of patients involves not laughing at them, but laughing with them when the situation warrants. It involves understanding that privacy is desirable but recognizing that there are times when danger requires it be overridden. It also includes the responsibility to report to authorities any inappropriate conduct on the part of caregivers.

The time spent appreciating the life that occurred before the illness helps the clinician appreciate the patient's current emotional state and sets the stage for an empathic relationship throughout the course of the illness. In the early stages of dementia, many patients express fears about losing their abilities. Most moderately to severely impaired patients have no appreciation of their impairment. This lack of insight is the result of the dementing illness and should not be viewed as psychological denial. Therefore, we do not recommend arguing with individuals who have dementia when they make incorrect statements (e.g., saying "My mother is coming to pick me up" when she has been dead for years) or resist a medically necessary action such as stopping driving or bathing. It is almost always better to empathize ("I'd be upset too") or respond supportively ("While we're waiting, could you help me?") rather than confrontationally.

Communication

Impairments in communication are major impediments to establishing and maintaining a relationship. Patients with cortical dementias develop difficulties in making themselves understood (expressive aphasia) and in understanding others (receptive aphasia). They may substitute a word that sounds similar to the one they cannot remember. They may describe the function of an object they cannot name, for example, "I need the thing for drinking" instead of "I want my coffee cup." Patients typically retain the rhythm, intonation, prosody, and gestures of speech long after they lose the ability to communicate with words. These aspects of speech are called the *pragmatics*.

Paying attention to the pragmatics of speech can enhance one's ability to understand what the patient is trying to say. Such was the case with a patient who spoke only in numbers. When greeted in the waiting room of the clinic with the words "Good morning, Mrs. E. How are you?," she would make eye contact, smile, reach out to shake hands, and respond, "Twenty four, three seventy one!" The pragmatics of her talk communicated that she was responding and telling the greeter that she was fine. Prosody and pragmatics also help patients understand what is being said to them. Unfortunately, some caregivers use an approach that minimizes prosody. Raising one's voice and using a monotone to say "How are you?" eliminates prosody and makes communication even more difficult.

Taking time to listen for key words can also help the clinician understand what patients are attempting to say. Some patients are embarrassed by their difficulties in communication and become withdrawn from their families and from social groups. Careful listening and observation can help restore morale and help patients become more functional.

An issue that experts disagree on is whether patients should be addressed by first names or more formally ("Mr. X"). Some patients respond only to their first name. Many women with dementia forget their married name but respond to their maiden name. Therefore, the choice of using first or last names is a question that depends on the particular caregiver and patient. We suggest that clinicians introduce themselves as Dr. _____, Mr. _____, or Ms. __ and address the patient by his or her last name. If the patient doesn't respond, then the first name should be used. Some caregivers, particularly those who spend many hours with patients, are most comfortable and find patients most responsive when first names are used. This seems quite appropriate to us, particularly when the care providers use their own first names. For example, "Hi, Bill, it's Esther. Let's go down the hall and join the sing-along."

It is important to be cautious about using terms of endearment when speaking with patients. It is quite natural for husbands and wives to call each other "honey" or "sweetheart," but it is *rarely* appropriate for a professional care provider to use that form of address with a patient. The use of such informal terms of endearment can be especially confusing to patients with dementia, who may respond in kind, assuming a more familiar relationship (inappropriately), or who may feel frightened, overwhelmed, and unable to communicate their mistrust.

It is helpful to make eye contact before beginning to speak. Clinicians should ensure that patients can see and hear them by putting on the patients' eyeglasses and keeping their hearing aids in working order. Dentures can help people speak more clearly. Clinicians should bend down or kneel to speak to and maintain the attention of seated or lying patients. A gentle touch can gain and maintain the attention of a patient who is easily distracted. Other noise and distractions should be kept to a minimum, and radios and televisions turned off.

Clinicians should ask only one question at a time and give the patient time to respond. Patients with PD, HD, and other subcortical dementias often need more time. If English is their second language, patients often revert to their first language as they become more impaired. Clinicians should speak slowly and use short, uncomplicated sentences. If patients are struggling to find a word, the clinician should offer a guess.

Directions that are given one step at a time will improve the ability of the patient to understand and cooperate. If the person doesn't seem to understand directions, a gesture might be given. Clinicians should use nouns and names frequently. When speaking about a third person, use the name rather than *he* or *she*. Similarly, use nouns when possible. For example, ask "Do you want cake?" rather than "Do you want it?" A positive approach to communication is usually more helpful than a negative one. For example, when patients attempt to leave a safe area, they will respond more readily to an invitation to engage in a pleasant activity than to being told "You can't go out there."

Nonverbal communication becomes increasingly important as the dementia progresses. Caregivers will pay even more attention to facial expressions and gestures, and patients will respond to a smile and a gentle touch even if they cannot understand any words. When patients do not seem to understand something, the care provider should try to regain their attention and speak slowly and quietly rather than more loudly. These general steps in successful communication are summarized in Table 6.1. Appendix A also contains, as part of the Johns Hopkins Dementia Care Guidelines for Families, a specific guideline that clinicians can use to teach family caregivers how to communicate with patients.

SUPPORT IN DAY-TO-DAY LIVING

Maximizing function and identifying abilities

The day-to-day living of patients should be structured to maximize their remaining abilities and function. This preserves their dignity, makes life easier for caregivers, and possibly encourages abilities to persist for longer periods of time. Clinicians should work with caregivers to find settings and environments in which limitations are minimized and remaining abilities maximized.

When structuring the day-to-day living of patients, the clinician should consider their prior interests, wishes, and usual activity level. Among the questions to be asked are: Were they always active with other people, or did they typically do things in small groups or alone? What specific things did they like to do? How did they pace and structure their life? In what ways did they derive pleasure and enjoyment? How important were routines and predictability?

One difficult aspect of maximizing function is the fluctuating nature of some patients' abilities. They may be able to do some of their activities one day but may resist and be overwhelmed by them on another day. Sometimes these fluctuations can be explained by environmental, medical, or psychological events, but usually a specific cause is not identified. Thus, the maximization of function is an important goal, but this is not always possible.

Periodic reassessment is important. As impairments accumulate, it can be helpful to focus on activities and functions that remain of interest to the patient. For example, patients who are able to perform basic ADLs but show

TABLE 6.1. Tips for Communicating with Language-Impaired Patients

Addressing the Patient	Responding to the Patient
1. Address the patient by name and identify yourself.	1. Listen for key words.
2. Make eye contact; sit or kneel for seated patients.	2. Observe and respond to the emotional tone of the communication.
3. Reduce distractions: turn off the radio and television.	3. Observe and interpret body language, rhythm, and rate of speech.
4. Make sure that the patient is using eyeglasses and functioning hearing aids.	4. Offer a guess.
5. Speak slowly in a low tone of voice. Give commands one step at a time. Use visual cues and gentle physical guidance when needed.	

limited interests in participating in other activities will be more active if their day is structured around ADLs.

A place to live

A variety of living arrangements and environments are available for patients with dementia. Early in the disease, most continue to live in their homes. Others move into the homes of their children, either fully integrated or in special living spaces developed for them, such as additions, renovated basements, or attics. Some patients live in assisted living environments. Assisted living is becoming increasingly available in the United States. It provides meals and some direction but sometimes requires that persons be able to take medication on their own. Facilities range from small "mom and pop" operations, usually housing a small number (fewer than 6–10) of individuals who may have dementia, to larger, more corporate operations sometimes referred to as *new model* facilities. Finally, there are nursing homes and skilled nursing facilities where dementia patients may reside, either integrated with residents who require general nursing care or in special areas designed for the care of dementia (special care units). The best place for individuals is determined by their level of functioning and their available resources.

A common question that usually arises early in the course of dementia is whether the patient is able to live alone. This is possible for individuals who can perform their ADLs well, can safely provide their own nutrition, hydration, and basic activities, and know what to do if an emergency arises. If there is any doubt about a patient's ability to live independently, an assessment by an occupational therapist can provide useful information. Two types of information are typically needed, one regarding the *level of care needs* of the patient and the other regarding the *safety of the home environment.* Occupational therapists use standardized methods of determining the level of care and types of support needed by dementia patients at home. One such method used at Johns Hopkins is the Assessment of Motor and Process Skills (AMPS). Occupational therapists and other professionals also conduct rigorous safety assessments in the home environment and assist dementia patients and their families in safety-proofing their homes. In addition, several books are available on the topic of safety-proofing the homes of persons with dementia. Safety-proofing, which is discussed at length later in this chapter, may involve removing unsafe objects (e.g., throw rugs), reducing fire hazards (disconnecting the stove and arranging for microwave-only cooking), making arrangements for dealing with emergencies (portable call buttons that access remote operators on the phone), or introducing assistive devices in the bathroom (grab bars and toilet commodes).

Some patients are able to live alone safely for a period of time if their home is safety-proofed, if they are provided help with meal preparation and medication supervision, and if they are checked regularly by telephone or in person. Participation in an activity program outside of the home, such as at a senior citizen center or adult day program, can prolong their ability to live independently. Patients who are not able to live alone might do well if they have a companion living with them part- or full-time. This could be a family member or a hired aide. Many individuals move in with children or other family members.

Patients with dementia require environments that are safe, stable, and able to accommodate their cognitive, functional, behavioral, and medical impairments. The environment should be neat and clutter-free, because this enhances the ability of the patient to focus on the task at hand. For example, a dining room table that has only a place setting on a contrasting table mat is preferable to a table that has newspapers, daily mail, and toys. Likewise, a bathroom sink that has only a toothbrush and toothpaste visible enables the ill person to pay attention to these specific cues rather than to bottles, lotions, laundry, and other objects. Photographs and familiar objects throughout the house or in a room provide many cues and orient the patient to his or her past life.

Nutrition and hydration

Maintenance of adequate nutrition and hydration can be a challenge for several reasons. Dementia impairs the ability to plan and prepare meals, to differentiate fresh from spoiled foods, to eat a balanced diet, or to remember to eat at all. Because these impairments are common, meals often must be organized and monitored by the caregiver. Inedible garnishes should not be used and decorative wax or plastic fruits should be eliminated from the home. It is better for the caregiver to offer condiments to the patient rather than leave them on the table.

The dignity of the patient can be preserved by preparing plates of food in the kitchen and cutting that food out of the view of others. Many foods can be prepared to be eaten as finger food for patients who can no longer use utensils. Tough meat should be avoided. Since some patients eat rapidly and choke, the caregiver should learn how to perform the Heimlich maneuver. Small amounts of food can be offered gradually to avoid gorging. Weekly or monthly weigh-ins can be used to monitor intake and identify weight problems.

Fluid intake should be monitored carefully. Patients may misidentify a dangerous liquid, such as a cleaner or paint, and drink it when thirsty. To ensure adequate intake, fluids should be offered every 2 hours. Caffeinated beverages should be avoided and fluid limited in the evening to minimize nighttime awakenings caused by the need to void. Appendix A also contains, as part of the Johns Hopkins Dementia Care Guidelines for Families, a specific guideline that clinicians can use to teach family caregivers how to provide nutrition for patients.

Sleep hygiene

Adequate rest is an important factor in assuring optimal functioning. Day-night sleep cycles can be easily disturbed and even reversed in dementia. If sleep cycles become abnormal, then the behavior of dementia patients may be affected the next day, with agitation or apathy related to fatigue. Also, abnormal sleep cycles lead to insomnia at night that can be exhausting for patients and especially caregivers. Thus, meticulous attention to sleep hygiene is critical. Appendix A contains, as part of the Johns Hopkins Dementia Care Guidelines for Families, a specific guideline that clinicians can use to teach family caregivers how to ensure the sleep hygiene of patients.

Establishing a routine of activities leading up to bedtime facilitates adequate rest. Daily mild exercise, such as mall walking, and exposure to bright light (at times by using bright light devices) can assist in maintaining normal sleep cycles. Keeping the patient awake in the evening is a challenge for many families. Scheduling evening activities that patients enjoy can prevent them from wanting to go to bed too early. When complaints about sleep are raised, caregivers should be asked to monitor the patient's total sleep in a 24-hour diary. The patient who naps during the day often needs less sleep at night and resists going to bed at night. Keeping patients dressed during the day and in bedclothes at the same time each night can further cue the patient to prepare for sleep.

The temperature of the bedroom should be comfortable, and night clothing should be loose-fitting. Night lights are helpful to some patients, but the shadows that result can be frightening. Some medications, including beta blockers and antidepressants, can cause frightening dreams that disturb sleep. Other medications, such as diuretics, may awaken patients at night or lead to nocturnal incontinence, and thus should be avoided in the evening if possible. For patients who tend to get up to go to the bathroom at night, consideration might be given to limiting fluids within 3 hours of bedtime and making sure that patients empty their bladder before going to bed. Sleep medications should be avoided, if possible, as they can impair the sleep/wake cycle and cause increased confusion. Further discussion of management of sleep disturbance is presented in Chapter 9.

Establishing a daily routine

Because the dementias reduce flexibility and adaptability, the vast majority of patients do better in a stable, predictable environment, even very early in the illness. Ideally, these routines should be patterned after those that the patient and family has followed for years. There are plausible reasons why a stable, unchanging routine is helpful and supportive to many people with dementia. First, a predictable pattern of activity is likely to maximize the ability to learn. The more routines are repeated and the more they are reinforced by the environment, the greater the likelihood that the patient will learn. This is called *implicit learning* or *learning by doing*. Patients with dementia even at very advanced stages may be capable of learning in this way. For example, many patients learn where the bathroom is several weeks or months after moving into a nursing home, presumably because of repetition. A second reason that daily routines help patients is that they provide predictability. If patients associate taking medication with mealtime, for example, they are more likely to learn that they will eat right after they take their medicine and to be more cooperative with both.

Establishing a predictable and repetitive routine is not always easy. Nevertheless, it must be a *very high priority*, and the clinician must spend adequate time making sure that caregivers develop routines for the patient and themselves. The psychosocial interventions presented in Chapter 5 guide clinicians in how to do this with caregivers.

Activities and situations can change and necessitate an alteration in schedules. Conversely, the goal of establishing regularity should not prevent the development of new activities or routines. This is important since the maintenance of an interesting and stimulating life sometimes requires the introduction of new activities. Ideally, new activities will draw upon previously learned and enjoyed activities. For example, holiday parties in nursing homes generate the same kind of excitement that they do at home or among schoolchildren in the classroom. Some of this excitement comes from staff and families, but patients also get caught up in the fun because holidays involve rituals and behaviors that have been lifelong. Even very impaired individuals can participate and actively enjoy the excitement and pleasures of celebrations.

Successful activities

Activities should stimulate as many of the patient's remaining capacities as possible. They provide pleasure, keep people occupied, strengthen muscles, and help people feel useful. Getting dressed and making the bed are activities and opportunities for success as much as a ball toss or arm stretching. With activities viewed in this way, time can be organized to make life pleasurable and meaningful for both the patient and caregiver. Appendix A contains, as part of the Johns Hopkins Dementia Care Guidelines for Families, a specific guideline that clinicians can use to teach family caregivers how to develop activities.

Family members often ask how to determine if an activity is a success or not. The outcome to look for is interest and involvement on the part of the patient. At Copper Ridge, we have found that success in an activity can be reliably assessed in three simple areas: participation, need for cueing, and apparent enjoyment. If patients participate, require little cueing, and seem to enjoy themselves, then in all likelihood the activity is a success. The Copper Ridge Activity Index can be used in long-term care settings if professionals are interested in gauging success for their residents.

For patients who are very impaired and who have limited attention spans, simply being in a room with others and observing an activity such as dinner preparation may be enjoyable and convey that they are still part of the family. Even though patients may not recall an activity or event later, they can enjoy it while it is occurring.

Providing activities for a person with dementia can be very time-consuming. We suggest that a schedule of activities be written down on a calendar (e.g., the calendar in Appendix C) and put in a prominent place such as on the refrigerator. A written plan will also assist in providing continuity when more than one caregiver is involved. Having a scheduled routine can also help caregivers by allowing them to set aside times to attend their own needs.

Emotional support

Patients with dementia have the same need for emotional support as any other person. This need increases when difficulties with day-to-day living are encountered or when bad news such as the illness or death of a friend or spouse is learned. Emotional support may take the form of spending more time with ill persons, encouraging them, and listening to their distress. Occasionally, professional support in the form of individual counseling or group psychotherapy is necessary. Patients with milder dementia are better able to benefit from these sorts of professional intervention. In institutional settings such as assisted living and nursing homes, the need for emotional support can get lost in the rigid structure of the institutional routine because the caregivers and professionals do not have much time to sit and listen.

However, many patients with dementia are aware that they are losing their memory and their ability to think and become distressed. These feelings should be directly addressed by acknowledging their upset, validating the source of the distress, and encouraging them to refocus their thinking on things that they can accomplish. Establishing tasks and goals that can be accomplished, implementing them, and having successes over a period of time are important steps in remoralizing patients with dementia who feel that they are losing the ability to control themselves and their environment.

Some patients with dementia are upset by anticipating the future. Again, support can be provided by allowing them to express their thoughts and feelings, providing emotional support, helping them identify and maintain positive aspects of their life, and providing information about the ability to preserve and maintain their dignity even with advanced dementia. Clinicians in any environment and of any professional background can provide this support to dementia patients.

Travel

Travel can be desired or necessary for many reasons: visiting family, moving closer to family, or continuing regular travel that has been part of a couple's retirement plans. Significant events that occur in a patient's life such as weddings, graduations, and funerals may require traveling long distances.

Unfortunately, travel with a person who has dementia can be quite difficult. Nevertheless, it is possible, even in advanced stages, if the appropriate steps are taken. First, start by deciding if the travel is necessary or beneficial for the patient. For example, a visit to a recently born grandchild can directly benefit a patient who has the capacity to appreciate the event. On the other hand, a spouse may wish to take a patient on a cruise but may not realize that the patient has lost the ability to enjoy the cruise.

Once it is clear that travel can be beneficial to the patient and that the patient wants to go, consider the means of travel. It is best to travel the fastest way (usually by airplane), to travel to as familiar an environment as possible, and to provide distraction and personal time for the patient during the trip. If a patient is to travel by air, inform the airline that a dementia patient will be traveling. Most airlines will provide preferential seating to dementia patients—for example, close to the bathroom or on the aisle with more leg room. They can be escorted onto the airplane earlier than other passengers and given wheelchair assistance if needed.

During travel, minimize what is expected of the patient. Luggage should be taken care of by the person accompanying the patient. Driving to and from airports and train stations should be limited as much as possible by using the closest and quickest destination. Scheduling travel for times that are least busy such as midday, midweek can lessen overstimulation.

During the trip, make sure that the patient remains adequately hydrated and fed. Planned activities—for example, being read to, listening to a portable tape player, or playing a card game—can distract and engage the ill person. After arrival, it is better to rest and relax rather than immediately become involved in another exciting or stressful activity. One-on-one attention from a familiar person is ideal. If travel across time zones is involved, the family should talk to their physician about the use of a sedative-hypnotic pill that will help the patient sleep upon arrival.

Placement

Patients who are unable to live alone or whose spouse or children cannot provide care are candidates for moving into an organized, supported living situation. This is referred to as placement and can be particularly difficult for family caregivers, since placement is often lifelong. Some caregivers see placement as a failure on their part, but we see it as a necessary step for many individuals because of the impairments caused by the disease.

The need for placement usually results from one of four reasons. First, cognitive impairment may be such that the patient is no longer able to recognize or interact with his or her environment. The second is functional decline that causes the patient to be dependent on others. Impairments in dressing, bathing, feeding, toileting, and ambulating are major reasons for placement. The development of chronic behavioral disturbances that are hard to treat or manage and that require constant supervision is a third common reason. Finally, there are co-morbid medical disorders that require specialized nursing care. Table 6.2 lists some of the factors that necessitate long-term care placement.

The transition between living situations is an important aspect of sup-

TABLE 6.2. Common Reasons for Out-of-Home Placement in Dementia

Patient Factors	Family and Resource Factors
Need for 24-hour supervision due to wandering	Lack of an available caregiver
Aggression during care on a regular basis	Caregiver is impaired: frail, depressed, demented,
Dependence on others for basic living activities such as eating	Death of the primary caregiver
Complex co-morbid medical illnesses	Respite unavailable for the caregiver:
Unpredictable behavior	cannot afford day care or assistance,
Constant pacing	other family member not available
Confinement to bed	Unsuitable home or caregiving location

portive care. Patients who need to move out of their house, who can no longer live alone, or who are about to be placed in assisted living or a nursing home will face a period of adjustment. They will usually have little say in such a transition, although they will most likely go along with it because others tell them that it is appropriate. When possible, transitions should be planned well ahead of time so that they can happen in an organized fashion. If the patient's level of insight and ability to appreciate the need for the transition is impaired, it is usually necessary to limit his or her involvement in planning and executing the transition. (See the discussion in Chapter 13 regarding the ethical issues that this situation raises.)

Unanimity among family members and clinicians can make a move smoother. Patients who cannot appreciate the need to move may do better if the time period that they have to brood or worry over the move is limited. On occasion, it is best if the patient is not told about the move until the last minute.

Preparation of the new environment is important. Whether the patient is moving into the home of a relative or into an institution, having familiar objects in sight and regular routines established can smooth the transition. Many individuals benefit from a tour of the facility before the move, but in some instances this is more upsetting than beneficial.

For some patients, having frequent visitors is calming and positive. For others, however, it is better to limit visits until the patient becomes adjusted to the new environment and new staff. Some patients who move into a new setting have difficulty sleeping at night and benefit from a sedative-hypnotic medicine for a short period of time (typically less than a week). This can prevent disruption of the sleep/wake cycle during the transition. Most patients who move are able to adjust within a month. If adjustment problems last longer, an alternative explanation should be sought since new behavioral disturbances or medical disorders can cause similar problems.

Safety and Supervision

Several safety issues must be addressed in caring for a dementia patient. Driving and falls are discussed in Chapter 9 and will not be considered here.

Household accidents are common. Some are minor and unrelated to having dementia, but most are caused by the dementia. Some result from loss of memory—for example, leaving the stove on, allowing food to spoil outside of the refrigerator and eating it anyway, or forgetting to lock doors.

Wandering and getting lost are serious problems that need to be considered with every patient at every point in the illness. At the very least, all patients should wear an identification bracelet with their name, their address, and an emergency phone number. The Alzheimer Association's Safe Return program (www.alz.org) is an option available to all dementia patients at a low cost and has saved thousands of lives.

Smoking is less prevalent than in the past but is still an issue. Whenever possible, efforts should be made to help the patient quit, perhaps with the use of a nicotine patch to ease the transition. If total abstinence from smoking is not possible, then observation during smoking is necessary. Hunting and access to weapons are prevalent in some areas. Like driving, hunting is an activity that has often been lifelong and symbolic of achieving independence. After the onset of dementia, access to guns has at times led to tragedies. Finally, financial and personal victimization, particularly in patients who maintain their own finances or who are left at home unsupervised, can also be problems. Limiting patients' control over their assets is often the best protection.

Prevention and safety-proofing

In the home

One of the challenges in caring for demented patients is making the environment safe *before* an accident happens. Families should be told that patients can be unpredictable and do things they would not have done before becoming ill. Even though they can still read labels on containers, patients lose the ability to sense what is appropriate to eat or drink and what is unsafe. Because of visual agnosia, patients lose the ability to see hazards around them. They are at risk of climbing out of an upper-story window or over the safety rails on a bed, or of wandering out into traffic. Many patients will not recognize the significance of a car horn, a smoke detector alarm, or the smell of smoke. They are at risk of scalding themselves if they lose the ability to regulate the water temperature appropriately prior to taking a bath. Adequate lighting can increase the ability of patients to perceive what is around them. Stairwells should be brightly lit, day and night, as should the doorway to the bathroom. Hand rails on stairs must be secured into the studs to prevent a patient from pulling them out, thus possibly falling and becoming injured. Exposed radiators and hot water pipes should be insulated to prevent their burning the patient who touches them or sits on them. Baby gates across stairwells and doorways are useful only if they prevent the patient from crawling under or climbing over them. Many families use two baby gates to prevent a patient from entering an area that would be unsafe. Inexpensive motion sensors can be placed to alert a caregiver when patients attempt to enter a room where they should not be, or when they get up at night and need to be escorted to the bathroom and back to bed.

Clinicians must assume that a dementia patient might eat or fiddle with anything. Potentially toxic plants should be removed from the environment, cleaning solutions kept under lock and key, and power tools locked up and kept inaccessible to the patient. Even salt and pepper shakers may need to be removed and put out of sight. We have known patients to eat hearing aids, flowers, or a bowl of shells (perhaps perceiving it as a bowl of snack food) or to drink a bottle of paint (perhaps thinking it was fruit punch).

It is essential that patients wear identification such as a bracelet or pendant on a necklace. These are available through Medic Alert and the Alzheimer's Association. They can be made attractive for persons who are bothered by the appearance of such items. Keeping a recent photograph readily available at all times will aid in finding an individual who gets lost. People who are agnosic and anxious may need only a moment of turning away from their care provider to become frightened and rapidly walk away. Putting labels in clothing can help identify a person who does not have a wallet or purse. One creative family whose grandfather wore a baseball cap put his last name in bold letters on the cap so that he could be easily identified if he wandered away at a county fair.

Patients may not perceive hazards in front of them and trip on them. In the home, clutter should be eliminated, rugs tacked down securely, and low pieces of furniture that the patient may not notice removed. For patients who have a diminished perception of depth, a contrasting strip of tape on the edge of steps may increase contrast or depth perception and help the patient see the edge. Obviously, swimming pools should be securely fenced and the patient's ability to get to ponds or streams should be prevented.

Cigarettes, cigars, pipes, and matches must be secured in a locked cabinet away from patients, and their use should be supervised at all times. Gas or electric stoves should be turned off to prevent a patient from attempting to light a cigarette on the burner.

A "No Solicitations" sign on the door may be somewhat helpful in keeping salesmen away from the home. However, the best protection from financial victimization is to limit the patient's access to money, bank accounts, and other resources.

Bathrooms can be hazardous in many ways. Medications, razors, bars of soap, and scissors should be secured away from the patient's view and access. A bath mat is essential to prevent falling on a slippery, wet floor. Urine and water must be wiped up immediately to prevent falls. It is important to turn the thermostat down on the hot water heater so that patients cannot scald themselves. Caregivers should either reverse or remove bathroom locks or tape open the bathroom door so that patients don't lock themselves in. Windows should be securely locked or capable of being opened only 6 inches to prevent patients from crawling out. Pull cords on shades, blinds, and draperies should be pulled up and secured out of the view of the patient, and electric cords must be securely tacked down.

In the kitchen, families can have a master switch installed on the stove so that they can turn it off when unsupervised. Similarly, coffee pots and irons that have an automatic shutoff can be invaluable. Sharp instruments such as carving knives should be stored out of sight or locked away. Families must be vigilant in observing what is in the refrigerator of patients who live on their own since they may lose the ability to determine which food is fresh and which is spoiled. Finally, guns and related weapons (e.g., hunting bows) must be removed from the home. Clinicians should ask about such weapons to prevent tragedies, such as a dementia patient accidentally discharging a weapon or killing others in response to a delusion.

In the nursing home and other institutional settings

The same cautions apply in long-term care settings. The potential to ingest harmful substances is a particular hazard. All staff, including housekeeping employees, must be educated to ensure that hazardous substances, whether cleaning supplies or condiments, are not available to patients. Thus, items such as bottles of Betadine and craft paint must be kept away from the patients. Supplies in arts and crafts classes, including magic markers, must be nontoxic. Electric socket covers, such as those used in child-proofing, are useful in preventing electric shock; those that are clear plastic will be much more difficult for patients to remove.

Items such as shaving cream and razors, whether blade or electric, should not be left in patients' rooms. Additionally, rooms in a nursing home should be routinely examined to see if the residents are hoarding food, which can become spoiled and then eaten. Windows should be set to open no more than 6 inches to avoid a patient's crawling through them. In outdoor areas, protective fences should be high enough to prevent patients from climbing over or being boosted over by other patients. Garden furniture should be heavy so that it cannot be moved to a wall to be used as a climbing aid.

Motion sensors and key padlocked doors are very useful in nursing homes, as are wander guards. Low flat-heeled shoes of the right size will aid greatly in promoting gait stability. Conversely, sashes that hang down or pants that are too long will place a patient at increased risk for falls. Remove items from the pockets of patients' clothing before laundering since patients have been known to eat shredded paper and other substances after they have gone through the washing machine.

Patients who have full or partial dentures are particularly at risk for choking because bread or other soft foods can become entangled in the denture, leading patients to attempt to swallow them. Patients who eat very rapidly should have their food cut into small pieces before serving and be kept away from other persons' dinner plates. Pacing the rate at which food is presented can avoid choking. Staff should be trained in the Heimlich maneuver in the event that a patient chokes. Ornaments placed on holiday decorations such as a Christmas tree should be made of edible substances such as cookie dough or a string of licorice with Fruit Loops on it. Christmas lights should be eliminated. At other holidays, such as Easter, decorations that might be perceived as edible should be edible. Real or candy eggs are safer than plastic or papier-mâché decorations, for example.

If patients persistently try to leave a facility, it is preferable to place them in a secure setting such as a locked area rather than to sedate or restrain them. Patients need sufficient area to wander about safely, and restraints are not an acceptable alternative to a safe environment. The design of modern facilities has generally accounted for this need, providing adequate wandering space. Bed rails are generally hazardous to patients with dementia since patients often try to climb over them.

Leaving patients alone

Given the wide-ranging safety concerns discussed above and the fact that safety-proofing does not always prevent problems, it is reasonable to ask whether any individual with dementia can be left alone. Clearly, in more advanced dementia, patients cannot be left alone because they are at high risk of harm. However, for many patients, some degree of independence is desirable, as this maintains their dignity, privacy, and quality of life. These benefits must be balanced against the risks of being left alone. Rather than all or nothing, this is often best viewed as a graded issue: some patients can be left alone for part of the time or with limited supervision. Table 6.3 provides a list of questions to ask when determining whether an individual should be

TABLE 6.3. Should the Patient Be Left Alone?

A NO answer to any of the following questions may suggest that it is unsafe to leave a patient with dementia alone at home:

1. Can she make phone calls?
2. Can she recite her full name, address, directions to her house, and telephone number?
3. Can she recite what she would do if a fire started?
4. Can she recite what she would do if she fell down or became suddenly ill?
5. Can she identify persons who should be allowed to enter the house and those who should not?

A YES answer to any of the following questions may suggest that it is unsafe to leave a patient with dementia alone at home:

1. Does he say that he "wants to go home" when he is at home?
2. Has he often wandered out of the house unexpectedly?
3. Has he been lost in the neighborhood?
4. Does he often misidentify the caregiver or members of the family?
5. Does he smoke cigarettes, a pipe, or cigars in a careless manner?

left alone. The final decision depends on clinical judgment and requires extensive family input.

MAINTAINING HEALTH

Purpose and coordination

Patients with dementia are susceptible to developing delirium in response to minor changes in their physical homeostasis and are vulnerable to becoming upset, distressed, or explosive in reaction to what appears to be a small or minor discomfort. It is common that changes in medical status first manifest as a behavioral disturbance before presenting with more typical symptoms of the medical illness (e.g., incontinence or pain). There is also evolving evidence that medical co-morbidity is a major contributor to functional and cognitive impairment in dementia as well as to dementia progression.

Unfortunately, most patients with dementia are not able to coordinate their own health care and must rely on a caregiver for help. It is important that each patient have a primary care physician who has an understanding of dementia and can respond to acute changes in the patient's physical and behavioral status. The caregiver should know the medical diagnosis of the patient and the medicines he or she takes, including the dose frequency, administration route, purpose, and potential side effects.

Basic hygiene and preventive care

The maintenance of good dental health presents a major challenge. Early in the course of dementia, many patients lose the ability to perform adequate oral hygiene and need help brushing and flossing daily. Patients should have their teeth cleaned every 3 to 6 months at a dental office. These cleanings offer the opportunity for close inspection of teeth and gum conditions. As the dementia progresses, the need for vigilant inspection increases since resistance to routine care often results in broken teeth, abcesses, and dental caries.

Denture care is also important. Patients with dentures may forget to insert them properly or to clean them. Having a routine place to soak them at night and supervision for insertion in the morning will minimize the chance for loss of dentures. Proper insertion with appropriate adhesives will also ensure that eating is comfortable and lessen the likelihood that dentures will be thrown away. Properly fitting dentures also allow appropriate appearance and speech.

Preventive care also includes attention to the skin and feet, which is most easily done during bathing. Caregivers should inspect patients' skin for any erosions, rashes, or bruises. These may indicate malfitting clothing or previous falls. Any redness in a skin fold can cause discomfort and can be treated with cornstarch. During winter, lotions should be applied to the skin to prevent dryness and itching. Periodic podiatric care will ensure that feet are free from infection and nails are appropriately cut. Gentle application of lotion to the skin and feet also provide a source of pleasure and relaxation for patients.

Attention to hearing and vision will ensure that patients can function maximally. Glasses should be kept clean and worn with a cord to secure them. Hearing aids should be kept in working order and put away at night.

Careful attention to elimination patterns is important. Patients may not complain of trouble urinating or moving their bowels due to forgetfulness or poor judgment. The caregiver should be taught to monitor bowel movements and ensure their occurrence at least two to three times per week. Over-the-counter stool softeners, such as senna and fiber supplements, or other medications may be necessary if dietary regulation does not ensure regular bowel movements. Caregivers should be reassured that preventive use of even moderate doses of over-the-counter supplements to maintain regularity far outweighs the potential risks. Caregivers should also monitor for bladder infections whose only sign may be increased confusion, unexpected incontinence, or frequent bathroom use.

Other aspects of preventive care include the monitoring of co-morbid chronic illnesses and annual visits to the primary physician for flu shots, mammograms, Pap tests, and prostate exams. Caregivers should be encouraged to participate in the visits to provide information and to record any instructions.

Medication administration

The primary caregiver should take responsibility for medication administration since the risk of patients' forgetting to take prescribed medications and the risk of taking too much because they have forgotten is high. As is the case for any older person, the medication regimen should be organized so that *only essential medicines* are given on a schedule that is acceptable to the patient. A dosing schedule that minimizes the number of times the medication needs to be given is ideal. Given the many demands of caregiving, many family members use a calendar to check off when medications are given. This can be incorporated in the daily structure as "medication time." Because of the potential for accidental misuse, medications, including over-the-counter drugs, should be kept safely out of the reach of patients. Child-guard caps may not be sufficient to ensure that patients do not open the bottles. Appendix A contains, as part of the Johns Hopkins Dementia Care Guidelines for Families, a specific guideline that clinicians can use to teach family caregivers how to deal with the medications of a person with dementia.

Some patients may resist taking medications or have difficulty swallowing pills. Caregivers may need to be taught how to crush medications and disguise them in pudding, applesauce, ice cream, or other sweet foods the patient will accept, but they should check with the physician to make sure that this is appropriate. Medications that are available in liquid form are often easier to administer. Optimally, such medications should be given with food as part of a meal, thus minimizing the need to convince patients to take them. This is especially helpful with patients who are suspicious that their medications have been tampered with.

Procedures/surgery

In general, dementia is not a contraindication for any operation. However, it is important for any dementia patient and/or caregiver to consider the risk–benefit equation prior to agreeing to an operation. It is important to determine the purpose of any procedure, as well as its potential risks and benefits. The impact the dementia may have on choosing to have the procedure or on managing the patient after the procedure should be explicitly discussed.

For example, patients with very advanced dementia who are preterminal and have symptoms of cancer may not be candidates for a CT scan of the chest if nothing will be done to treat their cancer. The potential benefit to patients need to be weighed carefully. One of our patients with very advanced dementia had a prolapse of the uterus into the vagina and developed the belief that she was pregnant, which was very distressing to her. The problem was resolved after a successful vaginal hysterectomy.

Once the decision has been made to proceed with a procedure or operation, it is important to focus on reducing the adverse effects of the procedure by using anesthetic agents with as short a half-life as possible and by minimizing medication and restraint during recovery. There is also some evidence that regional or spinal anesthesia is less likely to lead to delirium or cognitive decline in people with dementia.

If major surgery is being contemplated, it may be wise to ask the dementia care specialist to discuss the matter with the surgeon and the anesthesiologist. Additionally, it is important to appreciate that postoperatively, after even minor procedures, many dementia patients develop a delirium that can last for several days. The best way to address this issue is to provide one-on-one supervision by a familiar person throughout the hospital stay. It is important to attempt to avoid restraints, to be reassuring, and to use medications judiciously, as these may prolong delirium. The section on delirium in Chapter 8 provides information about the management of a delirium.

7

SUPPORTING THE FAMILY AND THE CARE PROVIDER

THE FAMILY CAREGIVER

More than two-thirds of individuals with dementia live at home, and the majority are cared for by family members. Compared to people who live at home, individuals living in long-term care facilities are more physically ill, more frail, older, less likely to have the ability to feed and dress themselves, and less likely to have living relatives. These differences demonstrate that many individuals are admitted to nursing homes because their families can no longer provide the level of care they need or because there is no one else available to provide care. The average age of caregivers is 57 years. This highlights the fact that spouse caregivers are also elderly and that daughters and daughters-in-law may also be employed and have responsibilities for their own nuclear families.

Who are the care providers for the elderly still living at home? In the United States, most are women. About one-half are wives, and another one-third are daughters or daughters-in-law. Husbands provide 10% of the care, with the remainder provided by other relatives, such as sons, nieces, and nephews, or by hired aides.

Much of what we know about family care providers comes from people who have taken a relative to a dementia evaluation clinic or who have joined a family support group. Many individuals who care for someone with dementia at home have not sought help from a medical or social service professional or from informal support groups. Since caregivers who have been studied are probably quite different from those who have not sought professional attention for their relative or themselves, we know little about the concerns and needs of many caregivers.

Providing care for a person with dementia is both rewarding and stressful. We tend to hear little about the rewards and a great deal about the stresses. In this chapter, we will emphasize the problems that caregivers have, because this is a book about helping distressed or ill individuals. It is important to remember, though, that many (probably the majority) care providers are doing well emotionally. In one study done by our group, more than 60% of families did not report significant emotional distress. Therefore, a majority of caregivers may not require any type of assistance beyond that which they have been able to obtain themselves through family, friends, social service agencies, hired individuals, community resources (such as day-care centers), or a health professional.

How Common is Distress in Caregivers?

More than one-third of families who join a family support group or have their relatives cared for in a dementia center are experiencing significant levels of emotional distress. This has been demonstrated in many studies using many different methods. Studies that measure depression or distress in caregivers report that rates of these symptoms are two to three times higher in dementia caregivers than in the general population. Other studies have shown that tranquilizer and sedative use is higher among caregivers than in the general population. Still others reveal that social isolation and family disagreements are more prevalent than in similar families who are not caring for someone with dementia.

What kinds of emotional problems do caregivers have? The majority of those who are distressed experience a mixture of feelings; frustration, anger, sadness and irritability are all common. Often these feelings fluctuate and depend on how well things are going that day or week. Twenty percent of caregivers in some studies report that distress is present much of every day. Many caregivers also report feeling physically exhausted, having difficulty sleeping, or lacking their normal level of energy. It is not easy to decide whether these feelings result from overwork or demoralization, but it is likely that both contribute. Research has not demonstrated that care providers have poorer physical health than the population at large, though many believe that this is the case. Clearly, ill health is a common reason for caregivers to stop providing direct care for an ill person.

Surprisingly, the few studies that have followed caregivers over time have found that they tend to do *better* emotionally over time even though the dementia becomes more severe. This finding suggests that many people can use their innate psychological strengths and external social and financial supports in times of difficulty to adapt to and overcome many problems. Caregivers likely have more needs than others, but most do not need constant emotional, physical, and social assistance. The following sections will discuss in more detail some of the negative feelings that caregiving engenders. As already stated, these feelings frequently coexist and often fluctuate, depending upon the circumstances of the moment.

Grief

Many professionals who help caregivers have invoked the concept of grief as a way of understanding the emotional experiences of family carers. The word *grief* refers to the universal human emotional state that follows the loss of a person or object that is important to the individual. Grief is characterized by a variety of feelings that come and go. Sadness is the emotion that most people associate with grieving, and it usually comes on suddenly ("a welling of grief") when the person is reminded of the person or thing that has been lost. In the grief associated with the death of a loved one, physical symptoms such as difficulty falling asleep, low energy, and diminished appetite are common.

Studies show that the majority of grieving individuals report significant diminution in these symptoms by 3 months after the death of a loved one. However, even after a year, intermittent wellings of sadness are common, usually brought on by reminders of the deceased person. It is common for a photograph, special object, or anniversary to trigger a memory of the deceased and rekindle the feeling of loss.

Another aspect of grief that is well known through the writings of Elizabeth Kubler-Ross, Murray Parkes, and others is that grief follows a typical course. Numbness and anger are common in the early phases of grief, while acceptance usually emerges later, often after several months. It is important to note, however, that these feeling states intermingle and do not occur in specific, time-limited, sequential steps.

Emotional experiences similar to those seen in grief are reported by *some* caregivers. This has led some to speculate that caregivers experience *chronic grief*. Research to date has shown that caregivers, as a group, remain distressed for many years, but no study has found that there is a consistent pattern to this emotional distress. Anger and guilt appear to diminish over time in many caregivers, but some individuals report that they adapt emotionally to one set of symptoms, only to become demoralized again when a new set of disabilities or symptoms develops in their loved ones. This fluctuating "roller coaster" of feelings is similar to the emotional state of acute grief. Thus, some caregivers do experience a state similar to chronic grief even though the ill person is not deceased. Supportive counseling is likely to benefit individuals who experience this chronic form of grief.

Anger

Anger is a common experience of caregivers. Many report that they have been frustrated, angry, and irritated with the ill person, the disease, friends, and family members. Anger can also be directed at professionals, institutions, or society. Some caregivers are embarrassed or distressed by this anger. Knowing that it is not only common but almost universal emphasizes that it is an understandable response to a sad, frustrating, uncomfortable, and unfair situation. Anger commonly arises around loyalty conflicts—for example, if there have been several marriages or if the caregiver has been married to the ill person only a short time. Contributing elements include children from separate unions who may not feel it is their responsibility to step in and help and relatively recently married spouses who do not consider care for chronic medical problems a part of their marital agreement.

Anger can have an undesirable or dangerous side. If expressed physically, it can lead to physical, psychological, or financial abuse of the ill person. Anger can also be expressed by neglect, thus placing the ill person at risk of harm. If unexpressed, it may increase the emotional turmoil experienced by the caregiver. Therefore, it is important to help caregivers appreciate that *frequent frustration and anger are warning signs of being overwhelmed.* Caregivers who are experiencing more than occasional anger outbursts should seek help. Acceptable settings in which these feelings can be expressed include discussions with friends or families, support groups, and counseling sessions with clergy or health professionals. Relief from some direct caregiving responsibilities (sometimes called *respite*) by paid professionals, family members, or friends is also helpful in reducing anger. A combination of these may be most beneficial.

Demoralization

The words *sadness, depression, discouragement,* and *demoralization* are used interchangeably to describe an unhappy mood state. Unfortunately, the word *depression* has several meanings that are sometimes confused. *Depression,* as in *clinical depression,* is used by professionals to refer to a condition such as major depression or manic-depressive illness in which the mood "takes on a life of its own." In this type of depression, individuals are sad almost every minute of the day for weeks or months. This low mood is often accompanied by a feeling of low energy, decreased appetite, poor sleep, and self-deprecatory beliefs. This type of depression is uncommon in dementia caregivers. It will be referred to here as *clinical* depression to distinguish it from other depressed states.

Demoralization, in contrast, is a feeling of sinking low mood, upset, and distress that occurs when facing a problem without an easy solution. Almost all individuals have been demoralized at some point in their lives. Demoralization can be brief or long-lasting, and is often accompanied by a feeling of loss of control over circumstances. Many caregivers report feeling demoralized by the caregiving situation. A common comment is "The future only holds more decline. There is nothing to look forward to."

Demoralized feelings usually fluctuate and are worse when caregiving becomes more frustrating. These feelings of discouragement often intermingle with the belief that things are going well or as well as they could be. Indeed, we suspect that caregivers who claim that they have never been discouraged by caregiving are either unaware of these feelings or fooling themselves. Research suggests that being able to talk about frustration and distress with a close friend or relative (sometimes called a *confidante*) is one important way many people get through periods of demoralization. It is probably for this reason that many caregivers do not require any specific professional, ministerial, or outside help even though demoralization and discouragement are universal feelings and are probably unavoidable when providing care for a person with dementia. Individuals who experience persistent demoralization should seek help. Support groups, pastoral counseling, professional counseling, respite, vacations, and hobbies are resources that can relieve or diminish the hopelessness that accompanies demoralization.

Some individuals realize on their own that they are becoming discouraged, demoralized, and frustrated and that they probably need to use available resources better or find additional ones. However, others do not see that their current emotional state is a problem. When this is the case, a frank supportive discussion will often move them to seek the help they need.

Guilt

Guilt refers to a feeling of responsibility for something combined with the belief that it could or should have been handled differently. Defined in this way, guilt is common in dementia caregivers. In our research, guilt is more common in family members who care for someone with dementia than in family members who care for a person with another chronic illness. This research has also found that guilt declines over time in the caregivers of persons with dementia. Why should guilt be more common in caregivers of the demented? We can only speculate, but several explanations seem plausible. Dementia, unlike most other chronic illnesses, ultimately impairs the ill person's capacity to understand current circumstances and plan for the future.

This is not true in every person with dementia, but the majority, particularly those with AD, are unaware that their memory is deteriorating and that they are less able to care for themselves. This combination of lack of awareness and impaired decision-making capacity puts family members in a very difficult position; it forces them to make difficult decisions for another adult. Frequently, these decisions involve choices that neither the ill person nor the family would have made before the dementing illness. Even worse, they are often actions that the ill individuals dislike, such as being told that they cannot drive or go out for a walk on their own; having their checkbook taken away; being taken to a day-care center; being admitted to a nursing home; or being brought to a doctor to have their memory evaluated. Each of these actions may be necessary and is being done for the benefit of the ill person. Nonetheless, many families feel guilty that they have to decide such important matters for another adult, even when they know that they are doing the right thing. The fact that the ill person may disagree or is often unable to say "thank you" makes these actions even more difficult and more guilt-provoking.

Some writers and thinkers have referred to this act of making decisions for a parent or spouse as *role reversal*. We agree with Elaine Brody that this term is inaccurate because it misses the dilemma experienced by the caregiver. It is more accurate to say that many family members are *conflicted* about the changes forced upon their relationship with the ill person. The child who has to tell a parent what to do, the husband who can no longer rely on his wife's advice about children or grandchildren, and the wife who must tell her husband that he can no longer drive all face the awareness that they must act differently toward the ill person than they did prior to the dementia. It seems incorrect to say that the relationship (parent, child, spouse, lover) has been reversed since the long- term emotional bond is still present. What *has* changed is that the healthy person must act differently toward the ill person. This can require a change in some aspects of role (decision maker, planner, food preparer), but there is almost never a complete reversal of the prior relationship. Whatever one calls it, though, this *change* in role is a common source of guilt.

Guilt can also arise because caregivers feel they have failed to uphold a long-standing belief or desire. Most cultures share the belief that it is the family's duty to care for a disabled family member. This value is sometimes transformed into a belief that it is *wrong* to seek help from others. As a result, some caregivers perceive that asking for help from family, friends, or professionals, placing a loved one in a long-term care facility, or using others to bathe, dress, and feed a loved one means that they have failed. This feeling is made worse if the ill person believes that help is unnecessary and resists it. Since AD causes an inability to appreciate the need, unwarranted guilt in the caregiver commonly follows.

Fatigue

Some patients need to be dressed, fed, and bathed. Others develop balance problems and need help walking. Some become unable to walk. Since most caregivers have multiple responsibilities that go beyond physical care, and because many are older and frail themselves, these requirements can become overwhelming. The fatigue that results worsens demoralization and robs the caregiver of the ability to derive enjoyment from other activities. Fatigue may even become a health problem for the caregiver. Therefore, tiredness, low energy, and poor sleep are indications that caregivers need more help than they are currently receiving.

THE NONFAMILY CAREGIVER

In the United States, 30%–50% of dementia patients receive care from nonfamily caregivers. Some are aides or nursing assistants hired directly by the family to care for someone in a home setting. Others work for home-health agencies, assisted living facilities, retirement communities, hospitals, or nursing homes. Most are aides, practical nurses, licensed nurses, or geriatric assistants. Many have little or no training in the care of persons with dementia.

The small amount of research that has examined these nonfamily caregivers suggests that they have the same emotional responses to caregiving as do family caregivers, even though they tend to work in shifts and usually do not have long-term personal involvement with the patient. Being attentive to one's emotional needs and knowing how to approach the problems that arise in care are as important for the professional caregiver as they are for the family caregiver.

HELPING THE FAMILY AND PROFESSIONAL CARE PROVIDER

Even though almost all of the dementias are currently irreversible, a great deal of help is available. This is an important message for caregivers and the public at large because the emphasis placed on cure and prevention by the U.S. health system implies that chronic, progressive diseases like the dementias are unimportant and untreatable.

It is important to realize, nevertheless, that there are limits on what can be done to treat dementia. Some symptoms don't respond to the treatments we try and others improve only partially. Furthermore, the emotional, physical, social, and financial resources of patients, families, and society are limited. In spite of these challenges, the principles outlined in Chapter 5 are powerful and compelling reasons to provide treatment and to include the caregivers/families as a focus of care.

Since not all caregivers need professional help, should we wait until people become distressed and overwhelmed before we offer them help? The answer is clearly "no." Research is beginning to help us identify which caregivers are at high risk of having a difficult time with caregiving and for whom preventive interventions may be especially helpful. One study has shown that a series of meetings with caregivers in the weeks following diagnosis results in long-term mood improvement in the care provider and a delay in nursing home placement.

Research also shows that caregivers who feel supported by their spiritual or religious beliefs are less likely to be distressed and less likely to become demoralized over time. These studies also find that being able to find spiritual meaning in difficult situations is more important than actual attendance at religious services. This may be true because many caregivers who are unable to attend formal services because of the dementia are still able to find meaning in this difficult, adverse situation.

One unexpected finding from research is that greater severity of dementia does not increase the caregiver's need for emotional support or help. Perhaps this is why an intervention early in the course of dementia can have benefits years later. Most studies have also shown that it is the caregiver's *perception* of whether a particular issue is a problem, rather than the objectively measured severity of a specific symptom, that determines whether the caregiver needs help. As stated previously, there is no direct relationship between disease severity and burden. Professionals must therefore directly ask about caregivers' perception of stress.

The importance of caregivers' perceptions of the situation and of their ability to give meaning to the situation demonstrates that each caregiver must be treated as an individual. Caregivers' innate psychological resources, in combination with their interpersonal, intellectual, and financial resources, are major determinants of how distressed they are likely to become. It is the professional's job to elicit information about each of these factors, to integrate this information with the assessment of the patient's needs, and to recommend a treatment plan that is most likely to help that family.

Regular reassessment, ideally every 4–6 months, is helpful. This can help the clinician develop a long-term relationship with the caregiver and can make it easier for the caregiver to ask for help when needed. Reassessment should also be triggered by major changes in the patient's clinical status, the caregiver's status, or caregiving circumstances (e.g., a housing move).

GENERAL APPROACHES

Although we emphasize the unique aspects of each caregiver's situation, there are some approaches that we use frequently.

1. *Repeat information.* Families and patients receive a great deal of new information from clinicians, friends, and the media, much of it in the form of bad news. It is not surprising, therefore, that they do not absorb everything they are being told. For this reason, clinicians should try to identify situations in which they haven't "gotten through." Specific, direct information is most likely to be understood, but repetition is often necessary. Providing written information in the form of brochures and books can complement a discussion and reinforce what is being said. Clinicians should ask if there are questions but keep in mind that many people are intimidated by professionals and do not ask questions or acknowledge that they don't understand. Therefore, anticipating common questions ("a lot of people ask about . . . ") and offering to repeat things are strategies that make it easier to provide the repetition some people need.

2. *Give caregivers a feeling of hope.* The demonstration that things can be done to improve a situation is important. Clinicians who identify the symptoms that may improve and acknowledge that some cannot generate realistic optimism and help caregivers begin to accept the parts of the illness that cannot be changed.

3. *Listen for myths and misunderstandings.* Society, individuals, and professionals share many incorrect ideas about the dementias. The clinician should listen for these and attempt to correct them if they arise. For example, some caregivers worry that the ill person will "go crazy." This is such a broad statement that it has very little meaning, but it usually reflects the concern that the ill person will become violent or aggressive, that his or her behavior will be unpredictable, and that nothing can be done to help. It is important to point out that agitated behavior does occur but only in a minority of individuals. More importantly, most patients who develop such symptoms can be helped with available treatments. Some people believe that inactivity, life style, diet, or particular behaviors can cause AD. There is no evidence that these are significant risk factors. Another common concern of care providers is that they waited too long to bring the patient to medical attention. Exploration of this issue usually reveals that earlier diagnosis would not have made a significant difference to the patient or family.

4. *Help the caregiver recognize that frequent distress in the patient is a sign that changes are necessary.* Patients with dementia usually signal when something is beyond their ability even if they cannot say so. Indicators that patients are overwhelmed include frequent frustration, catastrophic reactions, and repeated resistance to certain tasks. These behaviors suggest that changes are needed in the environment, the caregiver's approach, or both.

5. *Encourage caregivers to use available resources.* No single clinician can provide all the necessary legal, financial, medical, and resource information. The evaluating clinician should refer patients and families to a social worker, agency on aging, family support organization such as the Alzheimer's Association, or family community resources when issues arise about which they do not have expertise. Some families have a lawyer who can be consulted, but they may need advice from an expert in family law or geriatric law. Referral to a social worker, family services agency, financial planner, or geriatric care specialist can provide needed information. Families often resist such referrals, particularly when the symptoms of dementia are mild. It may be helpful to point out that an early awareness of available resources can delay or prevent problems from arising later.

6. *Organize a family meeting.* A meeting of family members, both those who are directly involved in caregiving and those who aren't, can accomplish several goals. It is common for those not directly involved in care to underestimate the stress of caregivers. The meeting allows for all involved to hear of the diagnosis, and current and future needs of the patient and primary caregivers. Often primary caregivers are reluctant to ask directly for help. The leader of the meeting can facilitate enlisting the help of others.

7. *Listen for misdirected anger.* Anger can be generated by many issues: the disease, the ill person who does something "wrong," family members who do not help more, professionals who do not make the proper diagnosis or are not being supportive enough, or society for not providing needed resources.

   However, anger can be misdirected. A caregiver may be frustrated by one thing but end up expressing it toward something or someone else. This happens in many situations in life. A person may be frustrated at work or disappointed in a relationship with another person and yet explode later at someone who has nothing to do with the disappointment. Among caregivers, anger at the disease, their situation, or other problems may manifest as anger toward the ill person or other care providers.

   Sometimes it is neither possible nor appropriate to express anger directly at its source. If the anger arises from an action of the patient, it is usually not appropriate to express the upset directly to the ill person since he or she cannot respond appropriately. In this instance, it is helpful to have other outlets. It is often a relief just to express the anger in words to another person. Many people find that talking to a close friend or relative (a listening ear), participating in a support group, or keeping a journal are healthier ways of letting out anger. Persistent angry feelings are usually an indicator that a person needs time away from caregiving or at least time away from a specific individual or situation. If anger persists after several attempts to correct misperceptions and redirect it, referral to a counselor or support group should be considered.

8. *Provide caregivers with a nonjudgmental setting in which they can express feelings.* Some caregivers are frightened or overwhelmed by their feelings of guilt, demoralization, or anger. It is usually helpful to be able to express these feelings openly. A supportive listening ear can help caregivers understand that their feelings are common among caregivers and do not make them a bad or uncaring person. Talking openly about feelings can provide relief in itself and may help caregivers think about *why* they are distressed. For example, some caregivers have not considered the fact that they are losing or have lost a loved one. Being able to discover a cause for feelings is helpful to many individuals.

9. *Be available in a crisis.* It should be anticipated that the disease will progress and crises will occur over time. Assuring caregivers of the availability of the clinical team can inspire great confidence. Such contact in the event of an acute change such as sudden changes in behavior also allows for appropriate triage, evaluation, and treatment.

UNDERLYING PRINCIPLES OF INTERVENING WITH CAREGIVERS

Three pillars underlie good care: education, symptom reduction, and addressing the emotional needs of caregivers. Each of these is combined in a prescription that may constantly change but that works best when all elements are present. For simplicity, they must be discussed separately. Professionals who provide care are like symphony conductors, knowing when to bring in and emphasize one or two elements but also knowing that the balance among these approaches is what makes the overall care work best.

Table 7.1 contains a list of interventions that must be considered for all caregivers, family, and professionals.

TABLE 7.1. Caregiving Interventions

Education
  Dementia
    Cognitive impairments
    Functional impairments
    Noncognitive symptoms
  Diagnosis
  Prognosis
  Treatments (Chapters 8–11)
    Cognitive enhancing (Chapter 11)
    Noncognitive symptoms
    Support of the patient (Chapter 6)
  Medications (Chapter 11)
  Dispelling myths
  Genetics
  Keeping up-to-date
  Research
Long-range planning
  Caregivers and responsibilities
  Resources and how to get them
  Residence plans and placement
  Late-stage care
Decision making and advance directives
Resolving family conflict
Coaching on how to approach the patient
Problem solving
Legal-financial issues
Respite
  Individual assessment and treatment
  Attending to personal needs
Emotional support
  Regular meetings and professional teams
  Availability
  Support groups
  Advocacy groups

Note: Italics indicate interventions that may not be necessary with all caregivers.

Education

Well-informed caregivers are best equipped to address the problems that dementia presents. How much education caregivers need depends on their role in the caregiving situation, their ability to learn about a very complex situation, and their interest. Educational needs also vary over time because most dementias are progressive. Furthermore, caregivers' ability to comprehend, learn, and accept information may change over time. Most can absorb only so much information in one hearing, and their ability to learn may be affected by their emotional state.

People learn by different methods. Some learn best by listening, others by reading, and most by repetition. Written material is helpful for many people, and several organizations, including the Alzheimer's Association, provide excellent pamphlets on specific topics.

We believe that being informed about medical facts provides a sense of mastery because the problems of the individual ill person are placed in a framework that explains many aspects of the patient's presentation. However, we do not believe that a general understanding of the illness will explain all or even most of the patient's problems. Helping caregivers identify which of the patient's symptoms arise from the brain injury and which likely have other causes is an important goal of the education process.

Teaching problem-solving skills

Patients with dementia develop many problems that neither they nor their caregivers have faced previously. We find that commonsense problem solving is frequently effective. Even when solutions are only partially successful in resolving a problem, they can provide tremendous support to the ill person and the care provider. One of the benefits of focusing on commonsense problem-solving is that most individuals are able to learn the principles and use them to address new problems when they arise. The problem-solving approaches that we advocate are emphasized in Chapters 8 and 9.

SPECIFIC PROBLEMS

Coaching how to approach the patient

Dementia usually changes the way people relate to each other. Some caregivers, family members, friends, and acquaintances have difficulty recognizing this and benefit from direct instruction about how to approach a person with dementia. There are emotional aspects of this issue that are dealt with in the next section. For many caregivers, knowing that the disease is changing a person's behavior rather than that the person is doing something on purpose provides insight through which they can change their approach. Some caregivers benefit by observing a clinician interact with the ill person and then meeting separately with the clinician to discuss how to approach the person. Occasionally, the clinician will need to demonstrate how particular actions of the caregiver distress or agitate the patient and how a change in approach can alter the undesirable interactions.

Long-range planning

Caregiving for a person with dementia is a long-term affair. When the diagnosis is first made, some caregivers are surprised that there is a problem. As the disease progresses, dementia forces changing roles upon both the caregiver and the patient. Even if the dementia remains stable, there are changes in environment, family makeup, and medical status that require adaptation.

Long-range planning issues include financial resources, legal needs (will, power of attorney), possible change in residence, and end-of-life decisions. While these issues may not arise for months or years, preliminary discussions are almost always beneficial. If they occur early in the course of the illness, the patient may be able to participate. However, it is impossible to anticipate all needs and attitude changes, so patients and families should be counseled to expect some planned choices to change in the future. Caregivers can be helped greatly by knowing that the clinical team will assist with issues as they arise.

Respite: helping the caregiver accept outside help

In our opinion, time away from caregiving is a universal need of caregivers. It is often useful for the professional to point out early in the course of treatment that respite is necessary for all caregivers. It is also important for the professional to point out to other family members that providing help to the primary caregiver and allowing him or her time away from the caregiving situation will benefit all involved, including the ill person.

Respite can include having another family member or good friend spend several hours with the ill person, hiring a person to clean the house, or having someone stay with the ill person while the family member goes out shopping or visiting friends. It is best done on a routine and predictable basis.

Professional respite resources are available in some communities. Therefore, clinicians who do not know what is available should refer the caregiver to a social service agency or a clinician (such as a social worker) who is knowledgeable about available social services in that area. Some facilities provide overnight respite.

Some patients resist having a "stranger" come into the house or resist going to a day-care or overnight respite center. This is less likely if these activities become routine practice early in caregiving, particularly when the patient is able to understand why they are being done. Often, a patient's resistance reflects the ambivalence or reluctance of the caregiver. When this is the case, the clinician should discuss this directly with the care provider. If the patient continues to resist, we suggest that the caregiver say that the respite worker is there to help the caregiver. For example, the caregiver might say, "This person is here to help me" rather than saying that help is necessary because of the illness.

Scheduled respite usually works best. It is sometimes necessary for the professional caregiver to contact other family members directly and emphasize the importance to the primary caregiver of respite care. Making this an issue for the whole family to decide rather than for one individual lessens the burden on the primary caregiver and spreads the care among several family members.

Substitute decision making

Because dementia impairs the capacities that underlie thinking, most dementias eventually rob the patient of the ability to make decisions. At the beginning of the illness, however, many patients have an intact decision-making capacity. In the slowly progressive dementias, decision-making capacity is lost gradually so there is no single time when a person goes from having the capacity to losing it. The ability to make complex decisions becomes impaired first, while the ability to make less crucial decisions is retained until later in the disease.

This gradual loss of decision-making capacity places several demands on the caregiver. Although it is desirable that patients make decisions when they can, it is difficult to know when the capacity to make a specific decision has been lost. This is especially problematic in AD, since most patients with this disease are unable to appreciate that their capacity to decide has become diminished or lost. As a result, family members or legally appointed representatives need to be on guard, especially when complex issues arise, and sometimes overriding a patient's wishes. Professional caregivers can help families decide which decisions the ill person can still make, which decisions the ill person is unable to make, and which decisions should be made mutually.

The caregivers' or guardians' emotional reactions may keep them from making decisions for an ill person. When this is the case, the professional should point out to family members or the guardian the emotional challenges they are facing. Clinicians can help the family member make the necessary decisions but should not impose their judgments on the family. It often takes time for family members or a guardian to consider the issues, and there is often no reason to rush to a decision. The clinician can sometimes help the process by identifying the benefits and drawbacks of various options.

Helping caregivers address personal needs

Caregiving is a time-consuming activity, and some caregivers do not attend to their own needs. Medical and dental appointments, hobbies, meeting with friends and family, and going on vacation are examples of activities that some caregivers need to be reminded to do. Caregivers ignore their own needs so frequently that we routinely raise the issue when we first evaluate patients with dementia. A common reason that caregivers don't attend to their own needs is the prevalent belief that they provide the best care for their loved ones and, therefore, cannot leave the person with friends, family, or paid caregivers. We believe it is important to address this issue directly, and point out to caregivers that it will benefit both them and the ill person if they pay attention to everyone's needs. Guilt and demoralization frequently interfere with caregivers' ability to get away and should be addressed if they are preventing caregivers from attending to personal needs. This is another example of the frequent need to offer both practical solutions and emotional support.

Providing emotional support

While many caregivers report feeling emotionally overwhelmed by the caregiving experience, not all caregivers do. Elsewhere we address the importance of supplying appropriate information about the individual patient, the disease, and available community resources. Many discouraged caregivers also benefit by having direct attention paid to their mood. Research studies demonstrate that the most effective caregivers' support groups are those that provide both emotional support and education, but that providing emotional support alone will reduce caregiver distress more than providing education alone. Therefore, we recommend that caregivers who are emotionally distressed or overwhelmed be provided with both. This can be done in individual meetings with clinicians or in support groups. Many individuals benefit from both. We believe it is important for caregivers to have a setting available in which they can express their frustrations and negative emotions. We also believe it best if the individuals providing counseling and running groups are knowledgeable about dementia so that they can provide support but not incorrect information.

We do not believe there is evidence that any one kind of counseling is more beneficial than any other, but this is a controversial topic. What is important is that the emotional concerns of caregivers are addressed and that practical problem solving is offered when needed. Providing emotional support requires an understanding of caregivers' prior pattern of response to difficulties and having a thorough knowledge of their strengths and limitations.

Support groups

Many caregivers benefit emotionally from support groups. However, we do not believe that support group attendance is necessary or desirable for all caregivers. As noted earlier, some caregivers are doing well and do not seem to need the support and information provided by a group. Others are uncomfortable in a group situation and are better helped if they can meet individually with a clinician, counselor, or social service worker. The ability to benefit from support groups is likely to depend upon the cultural background since support groups have been very successful in the United States but less so in other countries.

Extensive research and clinical experience have identified what makes support groups successful. One important aspect is the establishment of an atmosphere in which participants share experiences with other individuals who have faced the same problems. Another is the provision of a setting in which negative feelings are understood and accepted. Support groups are particularly powerful in helping caregivers recognize that they are not alone in facing a difficult situation, that the emotional challenges dementia has brought to bear on them are understandable, and that help is available to solve the practical problems and social challenges they face. Many caregivers find it easier to accept support and advice about symptom management and the need for respite from other caregivers who are or have been in the same situation.

Several issues about the composition and leadership of support groups have not been fully resolved. Many researchers believe that there needs to be an identified group leader, but some groups appear to run well without a leader. Also controversial is whether the group can be run by an untrained individual or is best led by someone who has been trained to run groups. We do not believe there is adequate scientific evidence to make a definitive recommendation about either issue, but our experience is that having one person in the group who is responsible for including as many participants as possible, calling on new or quiet members, stopping a discussion if most attendees feel it is not beneficial, and keeping time results in groups that are rated as more effective. It sometimes takes the skills of a trained group leader to provide this important guidance.

One question that arises frequently is whether it is useful to provide different groups for "old" and "new" caregivers. People who are attending their first group, or who have a relative or friend who has recently been diagnosed, often have many specific questions about AD or dementia that are not of interest to more experienced group members. Therefore, when practical, having a separate group for carers of persons who have been recently diagnosed is useful. Another reason for having separate groups is that the problems of patients with severe dementia may frighten or overwhelm the caregiver of someone whose loved one has recently been diagnosed. However, experienced caregivers provide information and emotional support that is very valuable, so we generally recommend not having too many specialized groups.

One common problem in groups is the tendency for one or two individuals to monopolize a group. These individuals often feel that they have a great deal to teach the others. A sensitive group leader can be helpful if this happens by directing the conversation to other issues and by involving other caregivers. The leader can also address this problem by gently reminding the person who is monopolizing the group that it is important to hear from others.

Some support groups work well because most important topics are brought up by group members. Often, however, it is helpful for the group leader to have specific discussion topics in mind before the group starts. The leader may not need to raise them if the group is running well or if they come up spontaneously. However, there are important topics, such as feelings of frustration, depression, or demoralization, that may not be addressed unless raised by the group leader. This issue can be brought up by noting that caregivers experience a variety of emotions. Group leaders who feel comfortable discussing their own feelings can provide a model that other attendees may follow. A common and important type of problem the group leader may need to address is an unreasonable belief, idea, assumption, or demand on the part of one group member. For example, some caregivers place unreasonable expectations on themselves or other family members (e.g., "I'll never place my husband in a nursing home"). Others put off difficult decisions or have unrealistic expectations of treatments, therapies, or institutions. Support groups can point these out and do so in a manner that is supportive ("I did that too, and now I realize it was a mistake" or "I felt the same way").

The skilled group leader listens for common themes and makes sure that the group addresses them when they do arise. The power of support groups comes from the realization that many of the experiences of caregivers are shared by most group members. This can be a remoralizing and renewing insight.

Resolving family conflicts

In one study, 56% of caregivers reported significant disagreement among family members. This is not surprising since many of the problems discussed in this book are difficult ones and affect various family members differently. The issues contributing to family discord include relationships prior to the development of dementia, the emotional resources of individual family members, the geographic proximity of caregivers (it is a common experience that children who live outside of town underestimate the severity of the dementia and the challenges faced by the caregiver), involvement of multiple families (when there have been prior marriages), and the current economic, cultural, social, and religious values of individual family members.

The primary goal of resolving family conflicts in the context of dementia is to help the family provide the environment that will be best for the ill person and for family members. Therefore, it is useful to distinguish between conflicts that predate the dementia and those that have emerged because of the dementia. Even though this distinction is complex and often difficult to make, they are important. It is often helpful to make this distinction explicit to family members. Focusing on current problems keeps the emphasis on trying to solve problems directly relevant to the dementia. Ideally, all involved family members should meet together, but this is not always possible. It is important to begin by making sure that all family members have an adequate understanding of the disease and of the ill person's condition at that time. The clinician should help the family identify the nature of the disagreements and focus the discussion on solving these problems. It is important to be knowledgeable about prior and current relationships among family members, since this often makes the current problems more understandable and provides guidance in resolving whatever conflicts exist.

It is important to identify the opinions of all attendees. Sometimes the clinician needs to be directive and make specific suggestions. It is usually better for family members to come up with solutions themselves. The long-term goal is to help the family develop problem-solving skills so that they can better address future difficulties. When long-standing problems are identified that predate the dementia, the clinician should suggest to the family that they seek other counseling.

One common source of conflict is that what is in the patient's best interest may conflict with what is in the family members' best interest. Making this explicit can help family members weigh potential drawbacks and benefits and enable them to resolve challenging dilemmas.

Placement

When a diagnosis of dementia is made, the course cannot be predicted with any certainty. We urge all family caregivers not to make any promises to the ill person about long-term living arrangements; many patients with dementia require more care than family members can provide. Therefore, we tell families that a wide variety of caregiving options are available and that they cannot know ahead of time which will be best for the ill person.

Long-term care outside of the home is frequently necessary in later-stage dementia. The decision-making process is less challenging when financial, emotional, and practical issues are addressed directly, when information is provided about the range of realistic options, and when there is recognition that this is a major life decision that may take weeks or months. Long-term care options include day care, in-home respite by family and friends, in-home respite by paid professionals, brief out-of-home overnight respite in facilities that provide this service, assisted living, and nursing home placement. It is important for the professional to recognize that the use of long-term care is not a failure and to convey this to the family.

Placement outside of the home is appropriate when the patient's needs are greater than can be provided by the caregiver in the home setting. There is rarely a single reason for or precipitant of placement. Most commonly, a combination of functional decline and cognitive impairment makes it necessary. Unmodifiable behavioral disturbance is a frequent contributor as well. We believe the decision to place the ill person in long-term care depends upon the needs of the patient and the family. Among the effects of dementia on the family that need to be considered are adverse effects on children, the need of family members to work, and the constant emotional and physical burdens on the caregiver.

It is sometimes appropriate for clinicians to give direct recommendations about placement. Some caregivers need "permission" to place the patient in long-term care, especially if they are not aware of how severe the illness has become or do not recognize that placement would be best for the family.

We generally recommend that family members visit a variety of facilities and suggest that they do so before a crisis arises. Since it is rare that any single facility is right for every patient and family, many elements need to be considered. In addition to the elements discussed already, financial resources, travel time to the facility, the physical environment, and the background interests of other residents are factors to consider.

In choosing a facility, families should ask staff about their training in and knowledge of the care of patients with dementia and inquire about the availability of expert consultants. It is especially important that an activity stimulation program be present on site and that any resident who is able to participate be encouraged to do so.

Once long-term placement has occurred, families should monitor care and raise concerns about problems when they arise. They should also be encouraged to express positive feelings when these are appropriate.

Many dementias ultimately lead to death. Chapter 12 discusses the challenges raised by the physical care of late-stage disease. Common ethical dilemmas that arise in late-stage care include placement of feeding tubes and treatment of new-onset medical illnesses. (These are discussed in Chapter 13.) Families' and patients' wishes regarding these issues can be discussed in advance, but we find that opinions and decisions often change over time and that families sometimes make different decisions when a problem actually rises.

Addressing questions about genetics

The role of genetics in AD and other dementias is an area of active research. Many questions are unanswered, and the knowledge base is changing so rapidly that we try to avoid making generalizations. In our opinion, a discussion of the genetics of AD and other dementias is appropriate in some circumstances, but it is helpful for the clinician to know current information about genetic risks and influences. At present, we do not recommend genetic testing for unaffected individuals, but this is an area of ongoing debate. Genetic testing is discussed in depth in Chapter 14.

ADVOCACY GROUPS

Advocacy groups have been important sources of information about heart disease, cancer and many other illnesses for over 60 years. In the United States, advocacy groups focused on dementia have been in operation since the 1970s. The many services these groups provide include information about the disease, up-to-date reviews of research findings, and suggestions about management of day-to-day problems. Many local Alzheimer's Association chapters offer support groups and provide information about respite resources within their community.

Many advocacy groups are active politically and seek funding for research, medical services, and social services. An important role of these groups is advocating before legislative bodies for improved funding of research and care. We believe positive advocacy is an important task of these associations, but we do not think it is appropriate to advocate against other groups ("disease A gets too much money—more of that should go to disease B").

8

Noncognitive Behavioral and Neuropsychiatric Disorders

Impairments in cognition are the defining characteristics of dementia. However, much of the debility that patients experience derives from the functional impairments and disturbed behaviors that often accompany dementia. One major theme of this book is that dementia can be treated and managed by systematically addressing these impairments. Chapters 8 and 9 present a systematic approach to the assessment and management of both functional impairment and noncognitive neuropsychiatric disturbances in dementia patients. The primary assumption of this approach is that distinguishing among different problems guides the development of appropriate interventions and improves outcomes. We call this the *4D approach*. It is presented in Table 8.1.

This approach is grounded in several principles. First, the impairments seen in dementia have multiple causes that can be distinguished from one another. Second, identifying the sources or causes of an impairment can lead to treatment strategies that are effective and beneficial to both the ill person and the care provider. Third, there is usually no one best treatment for any functional impairment or behavioral disturbance. As a result, discovering the most effective intervention for a particular individual is often a trial-and-error process.

As outlined in Table 8.1, the first step of the 4D approach is *define and describe*. The main purpose of this step is to define the clinical problem as specifically as possible. This requires a careful assessment of the patient and the environment based on information derived from the history, discussion with caregivers, physical examination, and laboratory studies.

TABLE 8.1. Overview of the 4D Approach to Mental, Behavioral, and Functional Disturbances

---

Define and Describe

Describe the phenomenology of the problem.
When, where, how, with whom, and after what does the problem arise?

Decode (What are the contributing causes?)

Cognitive disorder (aphasia, apraxia, agnosia, amnesia, executive disturbance)
Recognizable psychiatric syndrome
Medical or neurologic illness or medication
Environment
Caregiver approach

Devise a Treatment Plan and Implement It

Does the problem need to be treated? Why?
Which of the contributing causes can be removed or modified?
Are there empirical or anecdotal treatments that can be tried?
Are there commonsense treatments or interventions that can be tried?
Who will do what and by when?
How will emergencies be addressed?
What are the target symptoms?
What is the anticipated time course of the treatment response?
What is the fallback plan?
What untoward effects of treatment are expected and how will they be monitored

Determine If the Treatment Works

In the second step, *decode,* the potential contributing causes to and precipitants of the problem at hand are identified by systematically examining five areas. First, because all patients with dementia suffer from a cognitive disorder, the effects of the specific *cognitive impairments* associated with each patient's dementia must be assessed. The second area looks for the presence of recognizable *psychiatric disorders* such as depression or delusions that might be causing or contributing to the current clinical problem. The third area is *medical illness* and its symptoms. Medical side effects, urinary tract infections, upper respiratory infections, pain, visual impairment, hearing impairment, constipation, arthritis, dizziness, headaches, and the exacerbation of existing chronic conditions such as diabetes, heart disease, and stroke are common contributors to disability. The fourth area to consider in the decoding process is the *environment.* Is it too cold? Too noisy and stimulating? Is there enough structure? Finally, the approach of the caregivers is reviewed. Do they have a good understanding of dementia? Do they approach the patient carefully? Do they rush the patient?

In the third step, clinicians and caregivers first *devise* a management plan that flows out of the decoding process by trying environmental, behavioral, and pharmacologic approaches. It should be clear why an intervention is being tried, what the goals are, and who will do what, in what sequence, where, when, and for how long.

The second part of the third step has to do with making sure that the plan is implemented as outlined. This is crucial to the process of problem resolution. In our experience, many well-thought-out plans fail because they are not implemented consistently. The likelihood of success is maximized when plans are communicated clearly to those who will implement them, most often family caregivers and nursing assistants. In long-term care facilities, one major challenge is to ensure that all caregivers on all shifts implement the plan, whether they are agency staff or visiting family members.

The fourth step, *determine,* is as critical as the preceding steps. It involves setting a goal that is realistic and achievable, followed by ongoing monitoring of progress toward the goal. Since it is common for the first intervention to fail or be only partly successful, it is important to know when it is time to stop an intervention and try something else. Some interventions fail because they have not been implemented consistently rather than because they were ineffective. Having a goal sometimes enables the practitioner to see that partial progress has been made and that persistence is in order

Chapters 8 and 9 are structured around the 4D's. They discuss the more common clinical problems but certainly not all. The discussion in these chapters illustrates the approach to clinical problems and can be applied to many other problems in dementia care.

Catastrophic Reactions

Define and describe

The term *catastrophic reaction* refers to a sudden expression of negative emotion (such as crying or yelling) that is precipitated by an environmental event or a task failure. The term is useful because it expresses the idea that a person is behaving as if a catastrophe has happened even though the precipitant or stressor is a seemingly minor event. However, the term is awkward because its meaning is not obvious and because it exaggerates what is occurring. Catastrophic reactions are associated with brain injury from any cause. These are common in individuals who have experienced head trauma or stroke and in persons with developmental disabilities.

Catastrophic reactions almost always begin suddenly. There is often a warning, however, so astute clinicians and caregivers can anticipate them or know that one is coming. The premonitory signs vary from person to person. Common warning signs are motor restlessness, a facial expression of distress, increasing resistance to care, or a change in the tone of the person's voice. Sometimes a warning is observable but difficult to put into words. Catastrophic reactions often stop as abruptly as they begin.

The emotions expressed in a catastrophic reaction range from unhappiness and crying to anger and rage. Catastrophic reactions are often accompanied by heightened physical activity and sometimes by aggression. Several of the behavioral problems discussed in this chapter, including physical aggression, running away, intermittent yelling out, and crying, can be manifestations of catastrophic reactions.

The occurrence of frequent catastrophic reactions is a sign that the environment is overwhelming for the patient. It is important, though, not to conclude that the environment is at fault. For example, catastrophic reactions can be precipitated by necessary activities such as bathing, feeding, or dressing. Sometimes a careful assessment and the patience to try several approaches during these activities may decrease the frequency of catastrophic reactions or totally prevent them. There are many instances, though, when the best that can be done is to decrease the severity and frequency of the catastrophic reaction by reducing exposure to precipitants.

Frequent catastrophic reactions may indicate that expectations are too high or that an activity that a patient was previously able to perform and enjoy is now overwhelming. The repeated occurrence of catastrophic reactions later in the day suggests that the person is fatigued and that a change in schedule is indicated.

Decode

Cognitive disorder

Catastrophic reactions can be precipitated by an inability to remember. An example is the patient who becomes frantic when a caregiver leaves the room. The inability to express needs or wants or to comprehend what is being said (aphasia) is also a frequent cause. An inability to perform an action that was previously easy to do (apraxia) is one of the most common causes of catastrophic reactions. Many of the problems that involve dressing, bathing, or grooming are catastrophic reactions, and many of them are precipitated by apraxias. Since catastrophic reactions reflect a loss of usual control of emotional expression, it is likely that damage to the frontal lobes, which play a major role in emotional and behavioral inhibition, attention, and appreciation of social cues, contributes significantly to their occurrence and persistence. Catastrophic reactions also occur with injuries to limbic (also called *emotional*) circuits deep within the temporal lobes.

Psychiatric disorders

Catastrophic reactions are common manifestations of depression, illusions, hallucinations, delusions, and mania in patients with dementia. Delirium can cause disinhibition of emotional control, so catastrophic reactions may signal the onset of a new medical illness.

Medical disorder

Any medical disorder, ranging from an exacerbation of a chronic disorder to the development of a new illness or medication toxicity, can be a cause. Pain is a common precipitant. Sources of pain that should be considered include gum erosion, broken teeth, cavities, hip fracture, osteoarthritis, spine fractures, constipation, burning on urination, a beginning decubitus ulcer, a skin rash, and a cold. Therefore, a thorough physical examination is indicated whenever catastrophic reactions develop or increase in frequency.

Environment

Environmental precipitants range from a minor change in routine to a change in residence. Loud noises, such as from fire alarms, construction, television, and overhead paging systems, can trigger catastrophic reactions. Common causes in long-term care facilities include loud staff meetings, the calling out or yelling of other residents, a busy, noisy dining room, and overcrowding.

Caregiver

Caregivers who rush patients, insist that they do activities they can no longer perform, make critical statements, or speak too rapidly or too loudly can provoke catastrophic reactions. Touching or moving close to patients without having gained their attention is another common precipitant. It is important to avoid making caregivers feel guilty when catastrophic reactions occur; it is better to help them recognize their role in causing such reactions and to use this recognition to diminish the frequency of precipitating their occurance if possible.

Devise

The identification of situations that are likely to precipitate catastrophic reactions leads to a care plan that seeks to lessen the frequency of the precipitants and subsequently of the catastrophic reactions themselves. If *cer-*

tain individuals are present when catastrophic reactions occur, it is important for them to assess what they are doing and how they are doing it when the reaction occurs. If catastrophic reactions occur at *certain times* of the day, an attempt should be made to perform potential precipitating activities at other times. For example, if most catastrophic reactions occur later in the day, it is best to schedule doctors' appointments, trips, or visits in the morning.

Catastrophic reactions often occur in *certain places* such as the bathroom. This is probably because most adults are used to performing bathroom functions in private, but the small size of bathrooms may also contribute. Apraxias that cause an inability to toilet, brush teeth, or bathe are frequent precipitants and are examples of causes that cannot be avoided. We recommend decreasing the frequency of bathing if this is a precipitant.

Understanding that task failure is a common precipitant of the catastrophic reaction can lead to innovative ways of preventing task failures. For example, if a person is no longer able to use a knife to cut food, others can cut the food in the kitchen. If trouble using buttons is a precipitant, the provision of clothing that does not require buttons or zippers, for example pullover shirts or Velcro fasteners, may decrease frustration and lessen the frequency of catastrophic reactions.

When catastrophic reactions are just beginning, several steps can be taken to stop them or lessen their severity. First, individuals around the person should remain calm. Second, care providers should make it clear, in a supportive, firm way, that they are in control. A statement that explains what is happening and at the same time provides reassurance is an effective way of doing this. For example, saying, "Don't worry, Bill, I can help with that. It's not so bad. We can finish this together," demonstrates the recognition that the patient is upset, shows that you will provide help, and makes it clear that control of the situation is not lost.

Distraction is an important tool in defusing a catastrophic reaction. If the precipitating stressor can be removed, the catastrophic reaction may be avoided, stopped, or diminished. Often the care provider is able to stop the dressing, bathing, feeding, or other precipitating activity. However, there are times when it is best to quickly finish what is being done, all the while talking the patient through the activity. For example, "Ellen, we almost have your blouse on. Now straighten your arm. Let me pull it over your head. We're almost finished. I know this is hard for you, but I'm helping you and we will be done in a minute."

It is rarely necessary to physically restrain a person, and this should be avoided unless there is clear, imminent danger. For example, when a person is about to run into the street or is holding a sharp object, then physical restraint might be needed. However, distraction, talking the patient through, emotional support, and removal of the stressor are almost always more effective and less dangerous.

Catastrophic reactions are often frightening to caregivers and to others around the ill person. It is sometimes helpful, after the fact, to explain to the other individuals what happened and why. It is important for caregivers to appreciate that their own emotional state and those of others can precipitate or worsen catastrophic reactions.

The avoidance or diminution of catastrophic reactions embodies many of the principles discussed in Chapters 5 and 6. Early recognition may help prevent them. A careful assessment of who, what, when, and where they occur may lead to commonsense solutions. Several interventions are often necessary before a successive one is found, and catastrophic reactions cannot always be prevented or stopped. Since some precipitants cannot be avoided, understanding that catastrophic reactions arise from the brain injury and are precipitated by the environment is a crucial insight. However, failure to prevent them does not necessarily mean that the environment is unsupportive, inappropriate, or at fault.

Medications are prescribed when catastrophic reactions are frequent and dangerous and have not responded to environmental approaches. We know of no medication treatment study that specifically addresses catastrophic reactions. In our experience, antipsychotic drugs are modestly effective in diminishing aggressive behaviors, some of which are probably catastrophic reactions. Alternative treatments are mood stabilizers or selective serotonin reuptake inhibitor (SSRI) antidepressants (see Chapter 10). In our practice, medication treatment is used only as a last resort. When catastrophic reactions are related to depression, mania, or delirium, appropriate treatment should lessen their occurrence.

Determine

Counting and charting the number of catastrophic reactions and rating their severity serves as the basis for determining if they are decreasing as a result of treatment. Successful strategies may fail in time. When catastrophic reactions increase in frequency, the process of assessment should begin anew, since this usually signals a change in cognitive, psychiatric, medical, or environmental status. If medications are prescribed, no more than 4 weeks should be allowed for a given agent or dose to show benefit. The documentation of catastrophic reactions can be seen as an additional burden by staff. The use of readily available behavior monitoring sheets or a simple piece of graph paper can minimize the burden and maximize available information.

UNCOOPERATIVENESS AND RESISTANCE TO CARE

Define and describe

The definition of *uncooperativeness* varies in relation to where it is occurring, who the caregiver is, and the specific situation. The words *uncooperative* and *resistant* are unsatisfactory because they imply that the behavior is deliberate. In fact, resistance to care is often the result of multiple factors. Problem behaviors can be willful—patients may not want to do something they fear—but most commonly they result from or are influenced by the impairments caused by the dementia. For example, patients who resist bathing may be unable to wash, recognize the caregiver, or recognize their own disabilities. Uncooperativeness may result from an apraxia or agnosia or from the distress of a person being undressed by someone perceived to be a stranger. In spite of the awkwardness of the term *uncooperativeness,* we will use it because it is a common complaint, identifies problem behaviors that can be further broken down and specified, and serves as a model for how rational interventions can be devised. We cannot define *uncooperativeness* or *resistance to care,* however, because each reflects the caregiver's perspective rather than a specific set of behaviors.

The threshold for defining a particular behavior as uncooperative often depends on the setting in which it occurs. In caregiving situations where there are no time pressures and caregivers can approach and reapproach a task, the problem of *restlessness* can be avoided. In a nursing home where a nursing assistant is caring for 8–10 residents, a behavior may be labeled as *uncooperative* if it delays the care process.

Uncooperativeness in a person still able to do the tasks in question should be distinguished from the inability to comply with requests because of an inability to hear or to comprehend. It is important to note whether the problem is intermittent or constant and whether it is associated with certain activities, events, or times of the day.

Caregivers frequently conclude that resistance to care—for example, repeated undressing, grabbing the sink and refusing to enter the shower, calling out ("help, call the police"), or slapping at the caregiver or the air—is being done deliberately to frustrate them. While this is certainly possible, it is uncommon in our experience. Careful assessment almost always reveals that these difficult behaviors are a result of the person's deficits, the environment, and the emotional reactions of the ill person and the caregiver.

One aspect of dementia that contributes to the use of the terms *uncooperative* and *purposeful* is that behavior problems vary in frequency from day to day, from one caregiver to another, and even from minute to minute. Often this inconsistency seems to make no sense. For example, a person may urinate in waste baskets or on the floor but use the toilet when taken to the bathroom. Understanding that many behaviors result from the disease leads to strategies that can avoid them and defuses the frustration and anger that many caregivers experience.

Cultural expectations and family values shape how a behavior is interpreted. Patients who pick up food with their hands can be viewed as difficult or rebellious ("Why can't he eat like an adult?") or embarrassing ("She always had such good manners"). While such a behavior may be embarrassing to care providers or may increase their workload, it is rarely done to deliberately cause these feelings.

Other elements that influence how a behavior is interpreted include time pressures and the demands of competing responsibilities. For example, patients who take 45 minutes to dress may be late for breakfast or miss a doctor's appointment, so that the slowness is identified as problematic. In this instance, the slowness is interfering with eating or going to doctors, but the problem is the need to rush the patient.

Decode

Cognitive disorder

Amnesia can cause patients to forget that they have already done something or that they are supposed to do something. They may not even remember that they have dentures and will resist attempts to remove them and clean them ("I'm 35; how could I have false teeth?"). Aphasia interferes with the ability to understand verbal or written instructions and is a common reason that requested actions, especially when complex, are not carried out. Apraxias are among the most common causes of uncooperative behavior. They can be difficult to recognize because a patient may be able to do part of an action or may be able to do the activity intermittently. Apraxia should be suspected whenever patients do part of an activity and then become upset or uncooperative, do an activity out of sequence (e.g., try to pull on pants before their feet are in both pants legs or put a slip on top of a dress), or do an activity incorrectly (put toothpaste on a finger rather than on the toothbrush.) Apraxias can impair simple activities (getting into and out of a chair or car) as well complex ones (using a microwave oven, cooking a meal). Apraxias can be difficult to recognize in dementia because they begin subtly and progress slowly. As a result, they may be noticed only when the whole activity becomes impossible. Another reason for not recognizing an apraxia is that the caregiver has compensated for it without realizing it. This sometimes occurs to such an extent that the loss of ability is not recognized as a problem until the impairment is so severe that the patient can no longer do any elements of the task. Agnosias impair the ability to recognize caregivers, places, and objects (pills, clothing, food). They also impair the ability to recognize that one is ill and needs help. Each of these conditions can contribute to the appearance of uncooperativeness.

Apathy causes a lack of motivation to engage in activities a person is capable of doing. It is a frequent source of frustration for the caregiver and is often interpreted as intentional resistance. A grasp reflex may be misinterpreted as resistance if the patient grabs and holds on to bed rails, the care provider's clothing, or a hand and does not respond to a request or command to let go. The grasp reflex is activated by stimulating the inner surface of the hand (palm or fingers). It becomes stronger as someone or something pulls against it.

Psychiatric disorder

Depression is a common cause of apathy and withdrawal, and may lead to resistance and negativism. In addition, depression can result in delusions that lead to resistant behavior. Examples of depressive delusions that interfere with function include the beliefs that a person cannot do things she is capable of doing, that she should not do something because she is bad, that someone is out to harm her, that activities are hopeless or that something bad will happen if she does a particular activity. Suspiciousness and delusions such as the belief that the food is poisoned or that a stranger is in the home can lead to a refusal to eat, take medications, participate in activities, or follow instructions. Hallucinations may lead to behaviors such as fleeing the house, calling the police, or refusing to go to bed because a stranger is in the room or bed. Mania causes overactivity, pacing for hours, refusal to eat, overconfidence, and irritability, all of which may lead to uncooperativeness.

Medical disorder

Behaviors that result from pain, hearing deficits, visual impairments, incontinence, and weakness may be misinterpreted as uncooperativeness. Pain is particularly difficult to recognize in severely ill nonverbal patients. Withdrawal, guarding, or pushing others away may be the only sign that a person is in pain. Akathisia may cause patients to pace or move when they are asked or told not to do so. We are aware of no specific medications that cause uncooperativeness, but medications that impair cognition are likely to contribute to behavioral resistance.

Environment

Environments that are overstimulating and noisy (e.g., television, overhead paging systems) exacerbate the effects of cognitive impairments and precipitate catastrophic reactions that are labeled as uncooperativeness. Common examples include busy dining rooms or activity areas with unfamiliar or confusion stimuli (e.g., medication carts), poor contrast, and dim lighting. Soft, low chairs can contribute to resistance because they are difficult to arise from.

Caregivers

Resistance to care is more likely when the caregiver is rushing, being demanding and critical, has unrealistic expectations, gives complicated multistage commands, or does not get the patient's attention before starting an activity or making a request Resistance can be reduced or eliminated when the approach is tailored to each individual's strengths and limitations.

Devise

The principles that underlie the management of resistance to care and uncooperativeness are those that run throughout this book: Identify the problem as specifically as possible, determine potential causes and contributors, devise strategies that address the causes, and regularly reassess success and failure. Specifically, for each problem labeled by a caregiver as uncooperativeness, it is helpful to ask: (1) What is the specific problem?; (2) Where is it occurring and what other activities are going on?; (3) When is it occurring? For example, is there one time of day when the problem is usually occurring; (4) With whom is the patient uncooperative? Is it everyone or just some individuals?

When uncooperativeness is intermittent, it is important to review situations in which the patient was cooperative. If one caregiver is more successful than another, his or her approaches should be studied and replicated. It may be useful to have another person watch an activity when resistance is a routine occurrence. The observer may be able to identify subtle problems and recognize strategies that facilitate cooperation.

If resistance to care arises from amnesia, aphasia, apraxia, or agnosia, it is sometimes helpful to tell patients what is about to happen and then to talk them through each step, giving one instruction at a time. If simple language and repetition do not help, then nonverbal communication, such as touching the patient and helping to guide the activity, may be attempted. Sometimes a patient can imitate an activity if the caregiver demonstrates it.

When apraxia is present, the task should be broken down into its most basic steps. Physical assistance should be provided. Instructions should be given one step at a time ("Let's open the toothpaste tube . . . put it on the brush . . . put it in your mouth . . . move it back and forth, up and down"). Encouragement and praise should be provided frequently in a supportive tone ("Good job . . . you're doing fine . . . we're almost done"). Imitating the task sometimes helps the patient get started, and the activity then proceeds normally.

When it is clear that patients are unable to perform part of a task, caregivers should do it for them. This works best if patients are told that the caregiver will help them and then informs of each step as it is being done. Agnosias are best managed by caregivers saying who they are, using a supportive tone of voice, keeping the task in the patients' line of sight, reminding them several times what is being done, and using both verbal (words and inflection) and nonverbal (touch, visual) cuing.

Making requests in the form of a statement rather than a question or order, saying, for example, "It's time for your shower" rather than ordering a person to "Take a shower" or asking "Do you want to take a shower?" may lessen resistance. Distraction sometimes helps. For example, a pleasant conversation, a favorite food, or another person may momentarily take a resistant person's attention off a task; when it is started again several seconds or minutes later, the task might proceed without difficulty.

The identification of contributing psychiatric and medical conditions is an essential step in addressing uncooperativeness. Even if the condition cannot be immediately treated, caregivers may more easily empathize with the patient if they understand that the resistance is coming from a recognizable condition such as apathy, paralysis, depression, or pain.

Resistance to taking medication is common. Potential solutions include using liquid forms of medication, crushing pills, and putting them in applesauce or a drink (if it is appropriate for the medicine to be dissolved), encouraging patients, "bribing" patients ("I'll take you to the sing-along as soon as you take this"), deceiving them ("Just try it this one time"—see Chapter 13 on ethics), or giving medication only once a day at the patient's best time of day.

When patients become uncooperative or resistant during an activity, the activity should be stopped if possible and the patient distracted. If the task needs to be done, it can be attempted later. The process of care should be reviewed in the hope of finding a way to avoid or minimize the recurrence of the behavior

Uncooperativeness due to a strong grasp reflex is best managed by very slowly removing the clothing, bed rail, or hand from the patient's grasp. Distraction may lead to a spontaneous release of the grasp. Giving the person something else to hold on to may enable the caregiver to complete whatever needs to be done. Offering an alternative to occupy the person's hands, such as another article of clothing, can avoid a struggle. On occasion, the grasp is so strong or persistent that the finger needs to be pried off the object. This should be done gently and *very* slowly to avoid injury.

Medication should be considered when all other approaches have failed, when the patient, caregiver, or others are at risk of harm, or when a specific psychiatric symptom or syndrome that is known to respond to the medication is present. Even when medication is indicated, it is usually more effective to combine it with a behavioral/environmental approach.

Determine

Goals need to be realistic. While some problems can be easily solved, others can only be partly improved or take months to solve. Failure of one strategy does not preclude success with another. It is important to set a specific time frame for the determination of success or failure of a particular strategy. If a strategy is partly effective, it may need to be modified. It is difficult to generalize about how many different strategies should be tried, but sometimes partial success is all that can be realistically achieved. Occasionally, a problem is reduced only with the passage of time, presumably because the disease process has progressed.

AGGRESSION/AGITATION

Define and describe

Agitation and *aggression* are nonspecific terms used to describe a variety of disturbances. When a patient presents with agitation or aggression, it should first be clarified what is meant by the term. For some, *agitation* refers to an activated state in which patients are overactive and distressed. *Aggression* is defined as any act that leads, or threatens to lead, to harm to any person or object. Most cases of aggression in dementia involve verbal aggression such as yelling, screaming, or threatening through body posture. Occasionally, patients with dementia engage in physical aggression such as hitting, pushing, or shoving. Some people limit the use of the word *aggression* to instances in which harm is the intended outcome, but this is not universally accepted as necessary. However, the words *agitation* and *aggression* are used so differently by people that we prefer to focus on the specific behavior—for example, "hits when being bathed." A purely behavioral description is not always possible, however, and seemingly unprovoked aggression and agitation do occur. Most often, however, a precipitant or provocation can be identified and a specific behavior focused upon. Aggression and agitation are serious problems in dementia because they can lead to injury, distress in patients, and distress in others.

When confronted with aggression, the clinician should describe the form the aggression takes, against whom it is directed, the context in which it occurs, and its consequences, such as injury. The time of day, the frequency of aggression, and what the patient says also needs to be determined.

Decode

Cognitive disorder

Patients with aphasia may become verbally or physically aggressive as part of a catastrophic reaction (see earlier in Chapter 8) when frustrated by being unable to express themselves or to understand something being said to them. Patients who have agnosia and do not recognize a person who is approaching them may become aggressive and strike out in self-defense. Executive disorder contributes to aggression by removing the usual inhibitions of aggressive urges.

Psychiatric disorder

Aggression in dementia is a common consequence of delusions and hallucinations. Depression, mania, and sleep deprivation can also lead to agitation and aggression.

Medical disorder

New aggression in an otherwise stable patient is often due to delirium secondary to a new medical problem. Pain, constipation, and visual or hearing impairments predispose to the development of aggression, especially in patients with impaired communication. Steroids and dopamine agonist (e.g., L-dopa) medications may predispose to aggression. Even a seemingly minor discomfort such as a rash can result in significant changes in behavior and the emergence of aggression. Thus, a thorough physical examination should be conducted when aggression occurs.

Environment

Overstimulating environments, understimulating environments, and environments that lack adequate structure and activity are associated with aggression and agitation.

Caregiver

Being rushed, approached from behind, or inadequately communicated with may provoke aggression. Conversely, caregivers who are supportive and attentive are less likely to provoke aggression even in stressful situations.

Devise

The identification of cognitive, psychiatric, medical, environmental, and caregiver precipitants dictates the general strategy for prevention. If aphasia, apraxia, agnosia, or executive dysfunction are contributing factors, caregivers should modify their approach to lessen the misperceptions caused by the symptom and the distress that they cause in the patient. The discussions under "Catastrophic Reactions" and "Agitation/Aggression" provide specific suggestions.

Since aggression and agitation are frequent manifestations of catastrophic reactions, the removal of a precipitant, distraction of the patient, and calmness on the part of the care provider can help defuse acute aggression and agitation. Avoidance of harm and protection of the frail are of primary importance. If there is a meaningful risk of harm, then the care provider must act to stop the behavior even if this means grabbing the patient. Many individuals with dementia are frail, so caution must be used in the rare event that force is used. Most often, though, the development of a catastrophic reaction can be stopped before physical aggression occurs.

If a particular psychiatric symptom or syndrome such as delusions, depression, or mania is present, it should be treated. The same is true for an acute medical problem. Appropriate environmental modifications should be made. Caregivers should be educated about identifying precipitants of aggression in the patients they are caring for so that if the patients become irritable or otherwise upset, they can attempt to distract them or calm them to prevent an aggressive episode. Increasing staff or caregiver time with the patient, providing activities, and structuring the day also can reduce aggression and agitation. If aggression or agitation is occurring exclusively in the context of providing care, the professional and caregiver should review the process of care provision and modify it on accordingly. Caregivers may need to learn how to protect themselves against violent patients by blocking arm swings, getting out of holds, or controlling patients' hands.

If these approaches fail, management of aggression necessitates a consultation with a psychiatrist or another behavioral management expert. Occasionally, inpatient psychiatric care is appropriate because of the danger to others or the need for close supervision of medication trials.

If aggression is unprovoked or unexplained after careful evaluation, or if the danger to either the patient or another person is significant, pharmacologic treatment is appropriate (Chapter 10). First-line agents have traditionally been the antipsychotics, such as quetiapine, olanzapine, risperidone, aripirpazole, or haloperidol. Second-line agents include anticonvulsants (divalproex sodium and carbamazepine), followed by SSRI antidepressants. At times, a combination of more than one of these might be used. Since clinical trials have now demonstrated that neuroleptic antipsychotics and anticonvulsants are effective in lessening the occurrence of aggression, a trial comparing these two classes of drugs is needed before a recommendation can be made regarding comparative efficacy. If the aggression seems driven by disinhibition, amantadine, stimulants, or levo-dopa might be used. If sexual aggression is present, progesterone or leuprolide might be used. Some clinicians believe that failure of the above, alone or in combination, can lead to consideration of electroconvulsive therapy (ECT), but its efficacy has not been adequately studied and we do not believe aggression by itself is an indication for ECT.

Determine

The primary goal of aggression management is complete resolution of aggression. If this is not possible, the secondary goal is minimization of the aggression's consequences. The latter is especially appropriate when aggression occurs only during the provision of care.

Interventions to manage aggression require as much as 1 month to succeed. Pharmacologic treatment may require several medication trials in sequence and can take longer. At all times, it should be clear who is responsible for each intervention, how the response to treatment is being assessed, and how long a trial will be allowed before calling a given intervention a failure. On rare occasions, the process of controlling aggression can take months and require repeated hospitalizations.

WANDERING AND PACING

Define and describe

Wandering is defined as moving about physically without a goal that is obvious to an observer. Individual patients often exhibit a pattern characteristic for them, for example, wandering aimlessly about while looking calm and content, wandering back and forth between two places, or wandering in a repetitive circular pattern around the perimeter of the nursing unit or a particular room.

Pacing, in contrast, is driven, rapid walking. Pacing individuals often appear unable to stop or relax. The description of wandering and pacing behavior should include where, when, and how often the patient moves about.

On occasion, wandering or pacing presents risks to the patient or others. Elopement is the most common reason an intervention is needed. If patients attempt to leave safe surroundings such as their own home or a nursing home, they must be redirected if they may have lost some or all of the ability to recognize hazards such as stairwells, windows, or traffic, or are at risk for falls and other injuries. Intervention is also appropriate for patients who repeatedly wander into other people's rooms in long-term care or assisted living facilities. This is problematic because it is an intrusion into the privacy of another and can lead to physical or verbal retaliation against the wanderer.

On the other hand, individuals who simply wander around the perimeter of a room or up and down a hallway do not need to be stopped as long as they do not disrupt others. An occasional patient may pace to exhaustion or may be at risk for a fall or serious injury from wandering. Experts cannot agree on whether it is appropriate to restrain such patients in order to enforce periods of rest and nourishment or to prevent falls.

Decode

Cognitive disorder

Amnesia can prevent patients from learning where they are and why they are there. This can lead to their repeatedly looking for deceased relatives, home or family, and wandering about to find them. Aphasia impairs the ability to ask for something or to understand what one has been told; it may result in patients wandering about looking for what they want (food, clothes, or people). Apraxia of gait can increase the risk of falls and self-injury and necessitates an intervention. Agnosic patients are unable to recognize familiar places and people. They may wander about as they look for something or someone familiar.

Psychiatric disorder

Mood disorder may result in variable activity over time. Depressed individuals are usually less mobile early in the day and more active in the afternoon and evening. Depression can cause early morning awakening or frequent awakenings, and these can lead to nighttime wandering. Causes include hallucinations, illusions, and delusions. One patient of ours repeatedly heard a voice (an auditory hallucination) saying "Your children are burning, your children are burning" and paced around the nursing home until she fell to the floor in exhaustion looking for them.

Medical disorders

Hunger, thirst, and the need to urinate are universal human states that may lead to wandering. The need to use the bathroom is suggested by patients' tugging at their clothing and looking anxious. Pain, even due to minor conditions such as a rash, can cause discomfort and lead to wandering. Common causes of pain include headaches, dental pain, sinus congestion, arthritis, constipation, and gynecologic disorders. Wandering may be the first symptom of medical conditions, such as urinary tract infection, urinary retention, hyperthyroidism, or delirium.

Akathisia due to antipsychotic medications causes restlessness and pacing. Patients with PD and other basal ganglia disorders may develop akathisia due to their disease. The chorea of HD sometimes leads to a characteristic lurching walk that resembles pacing. Medications that cause stimulation may increase motor activity and stimulate pacing. These include thyroid replacement therapy, stimulant drugs, pseudoephedrine, and theophylline. Diuretics causing frequent urination may induce wandering. Excessive consumption of caffeine can lead to restlessness, pacing, and wandering.

Environment

Wandering may be a response to an overstimulating, noisy environment or to the yelling or calling out of others. Wandering at shift change in a nursing home may be cued by seeing the nursing staff leave, either because it suggests that it is time to go home from work or as the result of less observation by staff. Other visual clues that can suggest to patients that they try to leave are coats and hats, passing cars, or visitors leaving. Ironically, lack of stimulation can also induce wandering. For example, the person who is left alone may wander outside to look for someone or something to do.

Caregiver

Patients may wander in an effort to get away from caregiving that upsets them. A more common problem, however, is the caregiver who attempts to interrupt pacing or wandering and precipitates a catastrophic reaction or an aggressive act.

Devise

Specific causes of wandering or pacing, such as akathisia or other medical or psychiatric disorders, should be treated appropriately. There should be a review of the patient's daily routines and his or her response to activity and distractions. Caregivers should be educated about wandering and reminded of the hazards associated with trying to stop it. When possible, caregivers can walk along with the patient or provide adequate space for the behavior to occur.

If the wandering is an effort to communicate a feeling or need, caregivers should observe and recognize cues promptly; for example, caregivers should ensure that appropriate food and drink are available throughout the day and should not assume that patients can find food and water when they need them. Increasing scheduled activities is one of the best methods for decreasing wandering.

Unwanted cues should be kept out of sight. If overstimulation is contributing to wandering, noise and lighting should be decreased or the patient taken to a less busy environment. Patients might be sheltered in an area where they cannot observe the coming and going of staff. Small changes in the environment, such as moving to another corridor of a nursing home or to a new setting, can result in wandering about for days or weeks, but the behavior often lessens over time.

The risks and benefits of wandering should be reviewed with caregivers. Windows should have stops so that they can be opened only 6 inches, and doors should have locks that are out of the patient's sight—for example, a hook-and-eye lock at the very top or bottom of the door. Many nursing centers and adult day-care centers have outside wandering gardens for patients to have freedom of movement. Even with the best design, however, a patient can occasionally climb a fence and escape. Thus, patients must be supervised even when they are in seemingly secure areas.

Medications to reduce wandering are rarely beneficial and are best avoided. Restraints are indicated for wandering only when the risk of harm is significant.

Determine

Most interventions to treat wandering, other than those where a cause may be identified and treated, aim at permitting the wandering to occur in a safe and contained manner. Necessary environmental modifications and caregiver education can usually be provided over a period of weeks. Safety modifications should be made as soon as possible, however. In cases where safety is compromised and physical restraint considered, a careful review of the potential risks and benefits should be carried out with the family or guardian and, if implemented, reassessed regularly. Medications have not been shown to be of benefit in treating wandering specifically, and in our experience their use for wandering tends to lead to more harm than good.

Delirium

Define and describe

The hallmark of delirium is an impairment in the level of consciousness or sensorium. This includes distractibility, inattentiveness, disorientation, and an inability to sustain a conversation or activity. Delirium is usually accompanied by a range of mental symptoms such as irritability, visual or auditory hallucinations, misperceptions, delusions, affective lability, depression, euphoria, and social withdrawal. Some patients are hypervigilant, active, and easily startled. Others are lethargic, withdrawn, or hard to arouse. Most cases of delirium begin suddenly, and the symptoms usually resolve with treatment of the underlying cause. An acute general medical condition is the most common cause. The assessment and recognition of delirium can be complicated in patients with dementia because the impairment in cognition sometimes makes it difficult to determine whether or not sensorium is impaired. In cerebrovascular dementia and dementia of the Lewy body type, the cognitive impairment may wax and wane, giving the impression of fluctuations in sensorium.

Decode

Cognitive disorder

Memory impairment is common in delirium, but aphasia, apraxia, agnosia, amnesia, and executive disorder are not. However, delirium will worsen these symptoms when they are already present. A waxing and waning level of alertness, the hallmark of delirium, is paralleled by fluctuations in cognitive performance.

Psychiatric disorder

Delirium can resemble any psychiatric disorder since almost any mental symptom can occur in delirium. Patients with major depression may be inattentive, functionally impaired, and confused, and thus give the impression that they have delirium. The same may be true of patients with delusions or sleep disorders. Thus, while these conditions are unlikely to be causing or contributing to delirium, they need to be distinguished from it.

Medical disorder

Delirium is invariably caused by a condition or substance that is toxic to the brain as a whole. Thus, when delirium is diagnosed, there must be an underlying physiologic cause, and a detailed physical examination and laboratory tests must be performed. The most common causes of delirium are medication toxicity and urinary tract infection. Dehydration, constipation, malnutrition, and other infections are other common causes. Many cases of delirium are due to multiple concurrent physiologic disturbances, each contributing to its development. Delirium typically resolves when the cause is corrected, but this may take days or weeks. Delirium should be distinguished from sleep apnea, in which daytime drowsiness is common because of frequent nighttime awakenings. Snoring is a common symptom of sleep apnea.

Environment

Environmental influences rarely cause delirium, but they commonly influence its presentation. For example, dark or noisy environments increase the likelihood of hallucinations. In the past, it was thought that environments lacking stimulation, activity or windows cause delirium but this does not appear to be the case.

Caregiver

Caregivers cannot cause delirium directly, but inattentive caregivers may allow exposure to toxins or medications, or risk dehydration by not encouraging adequate fluid intake. Caregivers who are not attuned to fluctuations in a patient's mental state or behavior may not recognize a delirium until it is more severe.

If the decoding process identifies the medical problem(s) or medication(s) that is (are) likely causing the delirium, the treatment is their modification or elimination. However, in up to one-half of cases of delirium, a definite cause is not found. In this situation, it is usually best to stop or lower the dosage of as many medications as possible. Appropriate supportive care, good lighting, one-on-one attention, frequent reorientation, explanation of circumstances, and meticulous attention to the patient's personal care needs are essential aspects of the management of delirium. If delirium is persistent and accompanied by marked sleep disorder, the treatment of the sleep disorder with the use of light therapy or medication can provide symptomatic relief (see Chapter 10).

Pharmacologic interventions are warranted if patients are persistently aggressive, engaging in dangerous behaviors, or suffering from delusions and hallucinations. Antipsychotic neuroleptic drugs are preferred, haloperidol being the most commonly used agent. Alternative agents include risperidone, olanzapine, and other high-potency antipsychotics such as fluphenazine (see Chapter 10). Benzodiazepines should generally be avoided in patients with delirium, as they may worsen the delirious state and further disinhibit the patient, but they may be used on occasion when sedation is the primary goal.

Determine

The primary goal in treating delirium is its resolution, which is usually accomplished by treating and correcting the underlying cause. Improvement should occur within days or weeks, but patients with dementia may require an even longer period of time to recover fully. This is an important issue in patients with dementia who undergo surgery since postoperative delirium is common and prolongs the recovery time after surgery.

When an underlying cause cannot be identified and the delirium becomes chronic (often in more advanced dementia), management is complicated. Patients can live for many months in a delirious state. They require intensive supportive medical care but rarely need physical restraints for protection. Medication is sometimes necessary to alleviate distressing symptoms. Chronic delirium signals a poor prognosis.

YELLING, CALLING OUT, AND SCREAMING

Define and describe

Vocalizations such as yelling and constantly calling out are common in patients with moderate to severe dementia. These vocalizations include screaming, repeatedly calling a person's name, asking for help, or asking for something specific such as food. They also include repetitive sounds or syllables, moaning, or unintelligible noises.

Vocalizations may occur intermittently but often follow a diurnal pattern, usually worsening in the afternoon or evening. Vocalizations are particularly disruptive in institutional settings, such as nursing homes, because they affect a large number of people. However, even when only one caregiver is involved, they may produce significant distress in the care provider. They may also be distressing to the person calling out, although many patients who call out repetitively say that they are not distressed when asked. In long-term care facilities, vocalizations often trigger calling out by other residents, thus escalating the adverse effect on the environment.

Vocalizations are of concern to care providers because they indicate suffering in the patient. They also place the patient at risk of being hit or retaliated against by other residents in a nursing home. In addition, they induce stress in caregivers and visitors to the home or nursing home. Distressing vocalizations can lead to the ill person's being removed from a nurisng home area in which the majority of residents spend their time, such as a lounge or living room. This removal can lead to progressive social isolation. Vocalizations may also prevent patients from participating in stimulating or distracting activites. The vocalizations discussed here do not include verbal threats, which are dealt with in the section on aggression.

Decode

Identifying an underlying cause for yelling, calling out, or screaming is especially challenging. Information from direct care providers, such as nuring assistants, is invaluable in identifying any potential cause(s).

Cognitive disorder

Repetitive use of syllables (called *pallilalia*) is almost always seen in patients with severe aphasia. Patients with executive disturbances and frontal lobe damage will also often call out or scream repetitively. Patients who are agnosic or aphasic may call out for help as they try to sort out what is going on in their environment.

Psychiatric disorder

Depressed mood is a common cause of calling out, as are fearfulness, suspiciousness, paranoia, hallucinations, and delusions. In depression, calling out may follow a diurnal pattern (usually worse in the afternoon or evening) and is accompanied by other evidence of depression. If a patient appears fearful, delusions or hallucinations should be suspected.

Medical disorder

Physical discomfort, delirium, and pain are common causes of repetitive calling. Dental pain, unsuspected hip pain, shoulder or vertebral fractures, skin rashes, gastrointestinal distress, arthritis, constipation, and urinary tract infections are all common causes of discomfort, yelling, or calling out. Immobility itself may lead to discomfort and calling out. Thirst and hunger result in calling out, especially in patients who are unable to ask for food or drink for whatever reason, including aphasia. Visual or hearing impairment can lead to calling out, either because of fear and isolation or because of the inability to communicate.

Environment

Noisy environments in which a radio or television is constantly turned on may stimulate calling out. Environments with significant activity may be confusing or threatening to patients and a source of overstimulation. While the source of the distress may seem minor to caregivers, yelling may be the only means by which some patients can express their distress.

Caregiver

Caregiver contributions to calling out include understimulation, overstimulation, underappreciation of the patient's deficits leading to unrealistic expectations, or caregiver distress that adversely affects the patient.

Devise

If aphasia or miscommunication is contributing to calling out, it is important that all caregivers be instructed about the best approach to the langauge disorder of the particular patient. Patients with severe aphasia or disinhibition may respond to calm, quiet, supportive environments and to nonverbal interventions such as touch or guidance with touch and gestures.

Repetitive statements such as asking for food or believing that something is about to occur (e.g., "My mother is taking me home this afternoon") may respond to redirection or distraction using a confident, calm, tone and manner. Sometimes it is necessary to lie to the patient to reduce his or her distress. (This ethical issue is discussed further in Chapter 13.)

Depression, delusions, and hallucinations respond best to treatments for those conditions. Fearfulness and suspiciousness often respond to a supportive, nonthreatening environment with one-on-one attention. Most often these psychiatric symptoms require a combination of a supportive setting and pharmacotherapy.

Individuals who call out only in the late afternoon may be tired and may improve with a scheduled nap.

Whenever pain is suspected, a complete physical examination should be performed by a physician or nurse practitioner. It is crucial that the skin be carefully assessed, that the teeth and gums be examined, and that the patient be palpated for potential bruises or fractures in the spine, hips, shoulders, and long bones. If delirium is present or possible, medications should be reviewed. On rare occasions, when the patient seems in pain but no source can be found, a trial of an analgesic medication (acetaminophen, a nonsteroidal agent, or possibly a narcotic) is worthwhile. If the calling out diminishes, a renewed search for a source of pain should be undertaken and medication continued as long as it is safe or until a specific cause is found.

If no cause can be identfied, and if the distress to the patient and other individuals is great or the behavior will lead to the patient's being forced to move, medication treatment may be used to help the patient inhibit the calling out or to produce sedation. The SSRI antidepressants (such as sertraline, fluoxetine, or paroxetine), mood-stabilizing anticonvulsants (such as divalproex sodium, carbamazepine, or gabapentin), antipsychotic agents (such quetiapine, risperidone, olanzapine, aripiprazole, or haloperidol), sedative-hypnotics (such as lorazepam), or other agents such as trazodone have been reported to be of benefit but supporting evidence is lacking.

Determine

Yelling, calling out, and screaming are among the most challenging behavioral problems in dementia care. Management failure is common. A combination of treatment approaches is frequently necessary. Treatment goals include the reduction in the frequency or severity of calling out, a reduction in the disruptiveness of calling out to patients and others, and a reduction of

risk that the patient faces as a result of calling out. Typically, a treatment response requires several weeks to months and multiple attempts at different
treatments.

Affective and Mood Problems:
Depression, Anxiety, Irritability, Mania

Define and describe

A variety of mood states are seen in patients with dementia. In *euthymia,* the
mood is generally normal for that person, fluctuating within its usual range
and not persistently or markedly low or high. In *dysthymia,* the mood is sad,
unhappy, blue, or bad. Sometimes, crying, self-deprecation, and hopelessness
are present. *Euphoria,* in contrast, refers to mood elevation. It may be accompanied by *irritability,* a mood state in which patients have a short fuse
and react in a hostile or belligerent way to stimulation. *Labile* mood refers
to frequent, rapid shifts of mood. Low or depressed mood should be distinguished from *apathy,* a state of diminished motivation, initiative, and activity that occurs in the absence of sadness.

Anxiety is a mood state in which individuals are fearful, tense, and physically aroused. It is often accompanied by rapid heartbeat, muscle tension,
and a feeling of panic. *Grief* is a mood state in which patients experience recurrent episodes of sadness (*welling up*) following a loss.

Variations in mood state occur as part of day-to-day living. These fluctuations are usually transient and linked to current circumstances. However,
when a mood becomes extreme, sustained, unresponsive to daily events, or
markedly labile, it is often a source of distress or danger to the patient and
others.

When a mood state is not only abnormal for the individual, but also accompanied by a recognizable set of signs and symptoms, a *mood syndrome*
is diagnosed. Several mood syndromes are associated with dementia. In *major
depressive episodes,* a diminished vital sense (trouble sleeping, trouble eating, trouble with energy, trouble with concentration) and a low self-attitude
(self-deprecation, hopelessness, self-blame, diminished self-esteem, and the
feeling of being a burden to others) are characteristic.

Recent research has suggested that patients with AD develop atypical affective states in which anhedonia (loss of pleasure), anxiety, and irritability
are more prominent than dysphoria and in which about one-third of patients
have delusions. These syndromes have been referred to in the literature as
depression of AD or *Alzheimer-associated affective disorder.* Proposed diagnostic criteria for both have been published and are being validated. Clin-

icians should be aware of the fact that affective and mood disorders in dementia may have different presentations than those seen in elders without dementia. A recent review by Lyketsos and Lee (2004) provides a more in-depth discussion of this issue.

The opposite of depression is the *hypomanic or manic syndrome,* a state of elevated euphoric or irritable mood, increased vital sense (less need for sleep, overtalkativeness, overactivity), and increased self-attitude (over-confidence, poor judgment, or grandiosity and grandiose delusions).

Panic disorder is characterized by recurrent episodes of the feeling that something terrible is about to happen (*panic attacks*) and, often, avoidance of situations in which these panic attacks occur. Panic attacks usually start suddenly and are accompanied by physiologic symptoms such as rapid heartbeat, inability to catch one's breath, numbness, tingling, dizziness, and abdominal discomfort.

These mood syndromes are associated with a variety of adverse outcomes including mental suffering in the patients, deconditioning from the limited activity that accompanies depression, weight loss and dehydration from limited eating, exhaustion and falls from overactivity, victimization due to bad judgment, and suicide.

The abnormal mood states and mood syndrome associated with dementia can be difficult to diagnose. Patients may have trouble communicating their mood or knowing how sustained their mood change has been. Caregivers may not notice or be aware of changes in mood, even if they notice behaviors such as tearfulness, irritability, social withdrawal, or aggression that can signal depression. Depression may not be recognized in persons with dementia because low mood is thought to be the logical result of becoming demented. Statements such as "Well, wouldn't you be unhappy if you had Alzheimer disease?" or "It makes sense that she's crying and not eating; she's unhappy living in a nursing home" indicate ignorance of the fact that abnormal mood states can improve if they are appropriately treated.

Decode

Cognitive disorder

Frustration resulting from specific cognitive impairments (such as amnesia or agnosia) that occur with dementia can cause emotional upset even in patients who lack insight. This frustration is often manifested as a catastrophic reaction but may take the form of *transient* crying, sadness, or self-deprecating comments ("I'm useless"). Frustration should be differentiated from the persistent mood change seen in major or minor depression and from grief. The latter is seen in patients who forget that a loved one has died and become tearful when reminded of this loss. The tearfulness of grief occurs only in the context of being reminded of the death.

Psychiatric disorder

Patients with dementia who have a personal or family history of mood disorder prior to developing dementia are at higher risk of developing depression. This usually represents recurrence of a preexisting disorder or reactions of vulnerable people to the stress of dementia.

The presence of certain delusions referred to as *mood-congruent delusions* should suggest to the clinician that major depression may be present. These delusions include the conviction that a person is a burden to others, not worthy of being helped, that the situation is hopeless ("God should take me"), or that the patient's food is poisoned.

Medical disorder

Medications (steroids, benzodiazepines, beta blockers, reserpine), pancreatic and lung cancer, left frontal stroke or tumor, chronic lung disease (perhaps due to hypoxia), vitamin B_{12} deficiency, and endocrine disorders such as hypothyroidism and Cushing disease are associated with mood disorder. Pain, constipation, and urinary tract and other infections can cause persistent discomfort and present as abnormal mood states.

Environment

Changes in the environment such as moving or changes in the daily routine, misinterpretations of sad television shows, or seeing objects from the past such as pictures of deceased relatives can induce sadness. Most patients adjust to major changes in their life or routine, but this can take weeks or months. Persistent adjustment difficulties may indicate the presence of a major depression.

Caregiver

The approach of the caregiver has a major effect on mood. Being critical, angry, unsupportive, or threatening can cause sadness, crying, or demoralization. Exposing patients to situations in which they are likely to fail increases the likelihood that they will become upset and tearful. There is also evidence that depression in the caregiver is associated with depression in the patient. It is not known which causes the other, but treatment of either the caregiver or the patient can improve the mood of the other. It is important not to blame caregivers and to recognize and treat caregivers who are depressed, demoralized, or overwhelmed.

Devise

When an identifiable cause of the abnormal mood state or mood syndrome, such as a new medical problem, an environmental stressor, or a caregiver difficulty is identified, it should be corrected. Particular attention should be paid to whether the abnormal mood state or mood syndrome appears to be independent of the patient's circumstances and environmental stressors. If the depression is mild, intermittent, or non-life-threatening, environmental and behavioral interventions should be tried first. Increasing structure, activity, and predictability often benefits depressed, anxious, and irritable patients. Research has shown that identifying activities that the patient previously liked and increasing the time that the patient engages in them can improve the mood of both the patient and caregiver. Activities that the ill person can no longer do should be avoided.

When patients become acutely distressed, panic-stricken, irritable, or sad, reassurance should be provided. Distraction can decrease the amount of time spent in the abnormal mood state, but it is time- and labor-intensive because it requires one-on-one attention for long periods of time. When possible, patients with abnormal mood states should be enrolled in day programs since these provide both distraction and structure.

If there is an abnormal mood state or mood syndrome that is not responsive to the above interventions, or if the mood state clearly meets criteria for major depression or one of the Alzheimer-associated mood syndromes, then pharmacologic treatments should be considered. The treatment of depression and other affective disturbances with medications and electroconvulsive treatment is discussed in Chapter 10.

Interventions for mood disorder may increase the emotional, physical, or financial burdens on caregivers. These issues should be addressed to increase the likelihood of success.

Determine

The goal of treating an abnormal mood state or mood syndrome is complete resolution of the problem. This is achievable in the majority of cases but not always. Typically, environmental and psychosocial interventions require the involvement of the caregiver. Measuring success often requires determining if the caregiver is able to carry out the recommended care plan.

If medications are used, 6 to 8 weeks should be allowed for a response. If improvement does not occur, a change in dosage or type of medication should be considered. Electroconvulsive therapy should be considered if the depression is severe or life-threatening or if several medications have failed.

HALLUCINATIONS AND ILLUSIONS

Define and describe

Hallucinations are sensory perceptions without stimuli. Hallucinations can occur in any of the five senses, but visual and auditory hallucinations are most common in dementia. It is essential that hallucinations be distinguished from illusions. *Illusions* are misperceptions of sensory stimuli that are actually present. Illusions are also common in dementia. They differ from hallucinations in that an object is present but is incorrectly perceived. For example, reporting that a chair in a dimly lit room is a person is an illusion, while seeing a person in a clearly lit room when no one is there is a hallucination. The distinction is important because illusions can often be eliminated by environmental changes such as improved lighting or removing confusing objects, while hallucinations infrequently respond to such interventions. Hallucinations should be distinguished from *delusions,* which are false *beliefs.* Hallucinations and delusions sometimes occur together.

Patients with dementia who hallucinate commonly report seeing people in their home or hearing people talk to them. Illusions are almost always visual and are more likely to occur in circumstances of partial sensory deprivation such as low lighting. Both hallucinations and illusions are more likely to occur in patients who have impairments in vision or hearing.

Decode

Cognitive disorder

Hallucinations and illusions become more common as cognitive impairment worsens, probably reflecting the fact that the brain damage is becoming more widespread. The cognitive state may also affect how the patient reacts to a hallucination. Individuals with more severe cognitive impairments, especially those who are unable to communicate their experiences, seem more likely to become explosive, aggressive, or catastrophic in response to a hallucination or an illusion. There are no specific associations between hallucinations and aphasia, agnosia, apraxia, or executive function disturbances.

Psychiatric disorder

Hallucinations and illusions are specific psychiatric symptoms. In addition to dementia, they are seen in delirium, schizophrenia, major depression, mania, and alcohol/drug intoxication/withdrawal.

Medical disorder

Acute brain injury (e.g., stroke), alcohol withdrawal, or seizures can precipitate auditory or visual hallucinations. Any metabolic infections or toxic disorder that causes delirium can induce hallucinations. Impairments in visual acuity or hearing are risk factors for developing hallucinations. Certain classes of drugs, especially benzodiazepines, anticholinergics, steroids, and dopamine agonists (L-dopa and many others), are associated with hallucinations.

Environment

Environments that encourage sensory deprivation, such as poorly lit rooms, may predispose to illusions and hallucinations. Conversely, settings that are very noisy, for example those with loud air conditioners or noisy dining rooms, produce stimuli that can be misperceived .

Caregiver

Caregivers do not cause patients to have hallucinations or delusions, but their response can affect how the patient reacts to these distressing symptoms. Caregivers who are supportive, who attempt to distract the patient, and who are not challenging, scornful, or disdainful are more likely to help patients avoid becoming markedly distressed or upset when they hallucinate.

Devise

If a specific psychiatric syndrome such as delirium, schizophrenia, or mood disorder is present, it should be treated appropriately. Medications that may be causing hallucinations should be discontinued, if possible, or their dose lowered. Medical conditions such as urinary tract infection, pneumonia, and acute stroke should be considered and treated if present. If vision or hearing is impaired, this condition should be corrected as much as possible with glasses or hearing aids or by removing cataracts.

It is important to determine how the hallucination or illusion is affecting the patient. Some individuals find these experiences comforting. One of our patients, for example, had a hallucination of a loving mother talking to her. Often, however, hallucinations are frightening and cause patients to become aggressive or try to get away.

If patients become upset in response to a hallucination, they should be comforted and calmed. The goal is to reduce distress rather than to remove the experience. Sometimes this is all that is needed whenever the patient becomes symptomatic. Reassurance and distraction often help ("Bill, I know you're upset. Can you come over here and help me?").

It is rarely helpful to challenge the person ("I don't see anything. What are you talking about?"). Occasionally, it helps to acknowledge that the person is hallucinating ("I know you see the children, but I don't"), but this approach often upsets the patient more. When possible, modifications to the environment should be made to increase ambient lighting, reduce the number of people around the patient, and reduce the sensory overstimulation associated with loud noises, running children, and television. These interventions are more likely to help diminish illusions than hallucinations.

When hallucinations are troubling to the patient and neither support nor simple environmental modifications relieve the distress, antipsychotic medication should be considered. Low-dose, high-potency *atypical* neuroleptics are less likely to cause side effects. In our experience, these drugs rarely diminish hallucinations and almost never affect illusions. Chapter 10 discusses the use of these medications in greater detail.

Determine

If a specific cause can be found and removed (e.g., an eye problem, a medication, or a bladder infection), then abolishing the symptom is possible. However, for many patients, the primary goal is to reduce or minimize the distress caused by hallucinations and illusions.

Distraction, reassurance, and environmental modification are often effective almost immediately. If pharmacologic treatments are tried, a response should occur within several weeks of starting the medication. Sometimes pharmacotherapy does not abolish the hallucinations but helps the patient by reducing distress. If neither occurs, the medication should be stopped. If the medication has benefited the patient, then the need for continuing it should be reassessed every 2–3 months. After 3–6 months, particularly if the dementia appears to have progressed, the dosage should be reduced gradually and then discontinued if there is no recurrence of the hallucinations.

SUSPICIOUSNESS, PARANOIA, AND DELUSIONS

Define and describe

Patients with dementia develop a range of false or unusual beliefs. They may insist that someone is stealing their belongings, that a spouse is unfaithful, or that food is being poisoned. Some patients are suspicious and misinterpret the motives of others as being directed against them. In some instances, these beliefs are fixed and patients can't be talked out of them, even with evidence to the contrary. Occasionally they will drive patients to behave in predictable ways. For example, those who feel that they are being robbed may hide their belongings so that they are not stolen. Then they may discover that they can't find something they have hidden and believe that others have stolen it. Those who feel persecuted may barricade themselves in their room. Those believing their spouse is unfaithful may become aggressive or even violent toward the spouse. In many instances, these false beliefs are benign and do not lead to distress in the patient. Indeed, in most cases, patients can be talked out of these beliefs or distracted from them through activity and structure.

In as many as 25%–30% of patients, these beliefs become persistent. These are referred to as *delusions,* that is, fixed, false, idiosyncratic (specific to that individual) beliefs. The identification of delusions is important because it indicates that the patient is experiencing a symptom of the dementing disease, gives a name to a problem that may be very distressing to the caregiver, and often implies an avenue for successful treatment.

Decode

Cognitive disorder

Many suspicious, paranoid, or untrue ideas and beliefs that patients develop can be linked directly to the cognitive disorder. For example, amnesia causes patients to forget where they place things and leads to the idea that someone has stolen their belongings. Alternatively, agnosia causes an inability to recognize the environment and leads to the belief that patients are not in their house or room when they are. Aphasia may lead patients to make statements that others misinterpret as bizarre or false. Finally, executive dysfunction can lead patients to be disinhibited, socially inappropriate, and to express what is on their mind before they have had a chance to think it through and form a belief or an opinion.

Psychiatric disorder

Delusions and other false beliefs can be part of a major depression, a manic episode, or delirium. Recent evidence has suggested that delusions unaccompanied by hallucinations are often part of a mood or affective syndrome such as depression. This is important because in this case the suspiciousness or delusions may improve after treatment with antidepressants, which are generally safer than antipsychotics.

Medical disorder

Some medications, in particular steroids, L-dopa, and stimulants, have been associated with the development of delusions in the absence of delirium. Patients with dementia due to PD and stroke are prone to developing delusions. Delusions can be a symptom of a delirium due to any medical problem.

Environment

Environmental contributions to delusions are uncommon, but a cluttered environment may increase the likelihood of misplacing things. An environment that is too loud or too stimulating may lead patients to misinterpret events and develop persecutory beliefs about things going on around them.

Caregiver

Caregivers who speak in half sentences or mutter, or who are irritable and impatient, may give patients the impression that they are trying to hurt them. This may give rise to misinterpretations, false beliefs, or even delusions. Spouse caregivers who are often absent may unknowingly be contributing to the patient's belief of infidelity. Caregivers who do not offer reassurance when patients are confused may also unknowingly be contributing to the development of false beliefs and misinterpretations.

Devise

Some patients are comforted by false beliefs, and aggressive efforts to stop them are not appropriate. If associations are made between distressing delusions and environmental or caregiver approaches, these should be corrected. If delusions or suspiciousness are occurring in the context of a depression, medical disorder, or medication use, appropriate action should be taken, including pharmacologic managment. In the context of depression, careful consideration should be given to whether treatment of both the delusions and the mood syndrome should be pursued simultaneously. However, recent evidence has suggested that antidepressant treatment alone may be beneficial for the treatment of delusions occurring in the context of depression.

When there is no obvious cause and the delusion is chronic, the decision of whether and how to treat is based on the extent to which the delusion or suspiciousness is distressing to the patient or places someone at risk of being harmed. The extent to which the problem burdens the caregiver is a lesser consideration.

If the risk of harm to the patient or others is low, behavioral or psychological interventions should be instituted first. Frequent scheduled activities, distraction, one-on-one attention, removing clutter from the environment, and periodic separation of the person who is the target of the suspicions and the patient can reduce the frequency of misinterpretation and the development of false beliefs.

If patients are clearly delusional, and the delusions are either distressing to patients or leading to behavior that is a threat to the patients or others, pharmacologic treatments should be considered. Randomized, controlled trials show that neuroleptics decrease the severity of delusions. Antipsychotics can be chosen from any group, as discussed in Chapter 10. Patients with dementia who are delusional are more prone to developing the extrapyramidal side effects of antipsychotics than comparably aged nondemented individuals. Therefore, caution should be exercised whenever they are prescribed and an attempt made to find the lowest effective dose, especially given recent evidence of increased mortality associated with antipsychotics.

Determine

If the misinterpretations, false beliefs, or delusions are not distressing or dangerous, a reasonable goal of treatment is to prevent them from causing distress or escalating into dangerous behavior. In cases where there is serious distress or danger and treatment using medications is attempted, noticeable improvement should be observed within 4–6 weeks. If this does not occur, the medication dosage should be adjusted or a new medication tried.

SOCIAL WITHDRAWAL AND APATHY

Define and describe

Apathy is a state characterized by lack of initiative and motivation, as well as lack of interest in activities previously enjoyed. Apathetic individuals are inactive and seem content doing little or nothing. When they participate or follow directions, they do so slowly and after persistent encouragement. Apathy is often present early in the subcortical dementias. It arises late in the cortical dementias. *Social withdrawal* refers to the active avoidance of interaction with others. The apathetic person is almost never active, while the socially withdrawn person may be active when alone. The apathetic individual may attend a day center and appear content to do nothing while the socially withdrawn person is more likely to try to leave or participate only in solitary activities. Ironically, the apathetic person may readily accompany a caregiver to activities and sit quietly for hours.

Apathy is a problem because being active and productive is considered a sign of health. Therefore, families complain when a loved one is inactive. Apathy can lead to frustration and anger in caregivers because the ill person is unresponsive to maximal amounts of encouragement and stimulation, and because caregivers often restrict their own activity to be with the patient. When apathetic patients do respond to stimulation, their activity stops as soon as the encouragement or stimulation stops.

Social withdrawal is problematic for caregivers because there is an element of active resistance. It, too, can lead caregivers to isolate themselves socially. The resistive behavior of the withdrawn person can be socially distressing for the caregiver if publicly displayed.

Apathy and social withdrawal are characterized by a normal level of consciousness and should be distinguished from the drowsy, inattentive state of delirium.

Decode

Cognitive disorder

Social withdrawal can result from cognitive impairment. Patients who are aware that they are unable to remember (amnesia), converse (aphasia), participate in an activity (apraxia), or recognize other people (agnosia) may actively avoid participation in activities or discussion with others because of embarrassment.

Apathy is a defining feature of the frontal-subcortical dementias and of executive disturbance. It is often accompanied by other signs and symptoms of impaired executive function such as slowed thinking, inattentiveness, and difficulty with decision making. Families often describe such patients as "bumps on a log."

Psychiatric disorder

Withdrawal and apathy can be symptoms of major depressive disorder. Depressed patients often complain of being unable to participate, think, or move. They may feel unworthy, hopeless, useless, and responsible for the ills of the world. Depression is a common cause of apathy and withdrawal and should be considered whenever they are present.

Suspicious ideas and delusional beliefs, whatever their cause, can lead to social isolation. Individuals who barricade themselves in their room may be doing so in response to a delusion or hallucination or may be trying to escape from a verbally or physically threatening roommate. Apathy and social withdrawal can be symptoms of schizophrenia, delirium, panic disorder, or agoraphobia (the fear of outdoor spaces).

Medical disorder

Acute and chronic hypoxia caused by pneumonia, chronic lung disease, and other respiratory disorders can cause withdrawal and apathy. Hearing and visual impairments can lead to social withdrawal. Certain cancers, for example pancreatic cancer, can cause paraneoplastic syndromes that include apathy as a symptom. Hypothyroidism, Addison disease, anemia, chronic renal failure, hepatic encephalopathy, diseases of the basal ganglia (PD and HD) and hydrocephalus can cause apathy. Sleep apnea can cause daytime drowsiness and sleeping that mimics social withdrawal and apathy. Medications that cause apathy include antipsychotics, anticholinergics, tricyclic antidepressants, barbiturates, benzodiazepines, long-acting cardiac antiarrhythmics, beta blockers, SSRI antidepressants, and alcohol.

Environment

Overstimulating environments that place excessive demands on patients can lead to social withdrawal. Noise, crowds of people, easily misinterpreted objects like medication carts, and too many activities can be overwhelming. An example is the busy dining room in a nursing home. Noisy, threatening, or physically aggressive residents can cause social withdrawal. Very active small children may overwhelm some individuals. The noise from television and radio may be misinterpreted or may frighten a person with dementia and lead to social isolation. In the home setting, it is important to limit holiday celebrations and pace them slowly.

Conversely, environments that are insufficiently stimulating exaggerate an underlying tendency to be apathetic. Patients who are quiet and inactive may "fall through the cracks" because they are easy to manage and care for. This is an example of the environment's preventing recognition of a potentially treatable problem or condition.

Caregiver

Caregivers who are too demanding or who understimulate patients can contribute to social withdrawal. An incorrect assessment of the patient's capacities may induce social withdrawal. For example, attributing a patient's lack of response to a proposed activity to a lack of interest rather than a lost ability (e.g., an inability to read) prevents the caregiver from assessing inactivity and planning appropriate activities in which even small successes can be achieved. Patients cared for by abusive, critical, and neglectful caregivers can become socially withdrawn.

Devise

Treatable causes of apathy and social withdrawal such as depression, cataracts, deafness, hypothyroidism, or medication intoxication should be ruled out before a purely environmental treatment is initiated. Even when a potential cause is found, the treatment should include both specific and environmental interventions. Education is crucial because it helps the caregiver understand the source of the problem and develop realistic expectations and plans.

The ideal approach provides the amount of environmental stimulation appropriate to the capabilities and prior interests of each individual. A recent randomized trial reported that simple one-on-one hourly activity with a friendly and creative person may be enough to reduce apathy if this activity is sustained several times a week over several weeks. Sometimes patients' prior interests, capabilities, or social status prevent caregivers from trying interventions that may benefit them. Tossing a ball may seem undignified for a person who was a banker but may provide pleasurable stimulation. Because most dementias are progressive, caregivers must continually modify the type and level of stimulation. If the patient becomes repeatedly frustrated when encouraged, the caregiver should stop. Caregivers need to be aware that frustration in patients can demoralize and discourage them and worsen withdrawal.

Stimulation is a double-edged sword and needs to be adjusted to the tolerance of the individual. It is sometimes necessary to stop stimulating patients when they become distressed or do not respond or when the caregiver becomes frustrated.

If environmental stimulation is unsuccessful and the lack of activity is harming ill persons, depriving them of pleasure, or preventing a spouse from maintaining a social life, pharmacologic treatment should be considered. Unfortunately, benefit is uncommon. Drugs that increase brain dopamine or serotonin activity are theoretically beneficial. These include amantadine, the antidepressant medications bupropion and SSRIs, modafinil, and the psychostimulants methylphenidate or dexadrine.

Determine

If apathy or social withdrawal is associated with a specific psychiatric syndrome, medical condition, or medication, the treatment response may take weeks or months. Specific target responses include participating longer in an activity or participating in new activities. Some severely apathetic patients are active as long as they are stimulated but sink into inactivity the instant the stimulation stops. This can place overwhelming demands on caregivers, especially if they are the sole caregivers. Pharmacologic treatments improve apathy within several weeks when they work.

One frustrating element of *environmental activation* is that the patients often forget what they did. When asked, they may say they have done "nothing all day" when they have just completed 45 minutes of exercise. This may be misinterpreted as being ungrateful or the caregiver may question the benefit, and yet the patient's enjoyment while engaged in the activity is obvious. Therefore, family members and staff should check with an involved staff person before concluding that a patient has been inactive.

Unfortunately, attempts to reduce apathy and social withdrawal can induce distress. Apathetic patients are often content to be left alone and become frustrated, angry, and even explosive if pushed or encouraged. If attempts to improve apathy fail, caregivers should be reassured that it is very unlikely that stimulation will alter the course of the illness and more likely that excessive stimulation will adversely affect the patient's quality of life. When apathy is the object of treatment, it is important to keep in mind whether the treatment is for the patient or the caregiver. If there is no evidence that the patient is benefiting from the treatment, it should be stopped.

9

NONCOGNITIVE FUNCTIONAL DISORDERS AND DISTURBANCES IN SLEEPING, EATING, AND SEXUALITY

EATING PROBLEMS AND WEIGHT LOSS

Define and describe

Problems with eating include undereating, overeating, eating nonfoods, forgetting to chew and swallow, choking, food refusal, and weight loss. The average person with AD loses 2–4 pounds of weight per year; the average person over the age of 70 loses 1 pound per year on average. The reasons for this slight, gradual weight loss are not well established, but it is likely that many factors contribute.

The process of ingesting food in humans includes two aspects: food preparation and feeding. Food preparation is a process. It is easy to overestimate a patient's ability to purchase or obtain food, organize and prepare meals, or maintain a well-balanced diet. This is especially problematic for patients with mild dementia who live alone. They may eat only prepared snack foods because these are easy to open and don't require preparation.

Feeding consists of a complex set of steps and behaviors: (1) finding the dining area; (2) sitting comfortably; (3) recognizing food; (4) recognizing and grasping utensils; (5) successfully picking up food with utensils or fingers and bringing it to the mouth; (6) chewing and swallowing; and (7) continuing the process until the meal is finished.

The process of eating can break down at any of these steps. When feeding problems exist, careful observation of the entire process often identifies at which step the problem or problems is occurring. If necessary, a patient

169

with dementia can be safely spoon-fed. A discussion of feeding a patient with end-stage dementia is found in Chapter 12.

Decode

Cognitive disorder

Because of amnesia, patients may forget that they have just eaten and request another meal. Obesity can result. Apraxia leads to gradual loss of the ability to use a knife, fork, and spoon. Patients with severe dementia at times will appear to have "forgotten" how to eat. Sometimes they can be coaxed to eat and drink once the process is started. Late in the course of dementia many patients lose the capacity to chew and swallow. These conditions are sometimes referred to as *apraxias of eating and drinking.* Agnosias result in the inability to recognize the plate, utensils, or food. Some patients recognize individual objects but are unable to perceive that this collection of objects is a meal. Misperception can lead patients to eat or drink nonfood items such as soap or paint, or to eat spoiled or uncooked food. Taking food from others is seen in patients with *stimulus-bound behavior.* Executive dysfunction can lead to rapid eating, even stuffing of the mouth, which can cause choking. *Hyperorality* can lead individuals to place dangerous objects in their mouths.

Psychiatric disorder

Depression commonly causes a lack of appetite. Severely depressed patients may actively resist being fed. In patients without dementia, major depression sometimes causes overeating, but this rarely occurs in patients with dementia. Suspiciousness and delusions, such as the belief that food is being poisoned, can lead to refusal to eat. Mania can cause both physical overactivity and an inability to attend to eating, resulting in malnutrition and dehydration.

Medical disorder

Dental caries, gum inflammation, malfitting dentures, or a sore throat can cause resistance to eating. Visual impairment may interfere with the eating process. Constipation, cancer, reflux esophagitis, peptic ulcer, hyperthyroidism, renal failure, and liver disease are among the medical causes of diminished eating. Stroke and amyotrophic lateral sclerosis are neurologic disorders that impair the eating and swallowing process.

Acute food refusal can be caused by the need to void or defecate. Clues to this are resistance to sitting at the table or constant tugging at clothing.

Patients with HD and other movement disorders have high caloric needs because of their constant choreiform movements and may lose weight on a standard diet. Toxicity from many medications can cause apathy and sedation that interfere with eating. The extrapyramidal side effects of neuroleptic drugs can interfere with the ability to feed oneself and cause swallowing difficulties. Some medications cause a loss of the ability to taste and smell, impairing appetite as a result.

Environment

Noise, activity, dining area clutter, and television can interfere with meal preparation and eating.

Caregiver

Some caregivers provide inadequate supervision in the preparation or consumption of meals. Others rush patients and do not allow enough time to chew and swallow. They may remove a dinner plate prematurely, assuming that the patient is not hungry, when what the patient needs is encouragement and assistance to initiate eating.

Devise

Optimizing the nutritional intake of patients with dementia often requires a variety of approaches. The ability to eat in as normal a manner as possible should be maximized, but the maintenance of adequate caloric intake is the primary goal. A calm, quiet dining area and an unrushed atmosphere encourage patients to eat on their own.

Finely chopping or pureeing food can help patients who have difficulty chewing because of lack of teeth or ill-fitting dentures.

If patients can still use utensils but have trouble manipulating them, foam handles may facilitate grasping. Utensils that patients can no longer use should be removed. If necessary, food should be cut ahead of time out of the patient's sight. Patients who cannot use a spoon may be able to drink soup from a cup. Rubberized placemats that contrast with the color of the plate will increase the ability to see the plate and prevent it from slipping. Plate guards help the patient pick up food by providing a "wall" against which food can be pushed onto a utensil.

Patients who are distracted by others or who take food from the plates of others sometimes eat adequately when fed alone. While some might view this as isolation or punishment, we believe it can increase the well-being and health of ill persons by enabling them to feed themselves, improving nutrition and providing a less stressful environment.

Patients who put food in their mouths and forget to swallow can sometimes be cued to do so by gently stroking the sides or front of their neck. If they have a small amount of food in their mouth, fluids can often safely stimulate their swallowing reflex. Commercially available thickeners enable some patients to swallow without choking.

Some patients do not open their mouths when food is presented. Offering a favorite food or a sweet item may start the process. Placing a small amount of food on the lips or inside the lower lip can start the eating process. Some patients who refuse or are unable to open their mouths or allow feeding by someone else will use a straw.

When assisting a patient who must be fed, the care provider should be seated at eye level with the patient. Cuing helps many feeding-impaired individuals. Cues include putting a utensil in the hand, putting food on the fork or spoon, and moving the utensil toward the mouth. Patients who lose the ability to use utensils can often eat "finger foods" that can be picked up by hand.

Some patients eat very rapidly and risk choking because they do not stop to chew before they swallow. Their food should be offered in small amounts, adding more food only after they swallow. Keeping food and nonedible objects that look like food out of sight may be necessary since some patients will try to eat whatever they see.

Patients should be offered fluids throughout the day. Many elderly individuals lose the ability to monitor thirst. This compounds the difficulties that patients with dementia have in finding appropriate things to drink. Inadequate fluid intake is a common cause of dehydration and constipation.

Family members and professional caregivers should be taught the Heimlich maneuver to assist a choking patient. If recurring constipation is a problem, the caregiver should keep a record of bowel elimination. No bowel movement in 3–5 days signals a problem.

Liquid supplements should be used if adequate weight cannot be maintained with solid or pureed food. Commercially available supplements have the benefits of concentrated calories (most commonly 250 calories in 8 ounces), protein, minerals, and vitamins. They are often sweet and well accepted by patients.

Determine

Weight should be used as the measure of adequate food intake. Charts that list ideal weight by height and body build are widely available and should be used.

BATHING

Define and describe

Bathing involves numerous steps and can break down at any point. A careful description of when the patient becomes upset and what specific portion of the task is being done when the problem develops is crucial. It is important to determine whether there is a pattern to the occurrence in the time of day, setting, or caregiver involved.

Steps involved in helping patients bathe include (1) approaching, greeting them socially, and telling them it is time to bathe; (2) gaining cooperation and inviting them to the bathroom; (3) having them disrobe or helping them undress; (4) entering the bathroom, shower room, or tub room; (5) transferring into the tub or shower; (6) washing the body and hair; (7) transferring out of the tub or shower; (8) drying the body and hair; (9) putting on clothing; and (10) leaving the bathroom. Problems at any of these steps include resistance, aggression, passivity, and an inability to perform.

Decode

Cognitive disorder

Amnesia may lead patients to forget when they last bathed or that it is time to bathe. Aphasia may lead to trouble understanding verbal or nonverbal directions at any one of the bathing steps. It may also limit the patient's ability to communicate his or her wishes regarding how and when to bathe or to communicate discomfort during bathing. Apraxia may affect the patient's ability to get to the bathroom (gait apraxia), enter the tub or shower stall, or perform any of the motor tasks involved. Agnosia may limit recognition of the person attempting to assist, of the bathroom, of the tub, or of soap, sponges, shampoo bottles, and other bathing wares. Any or all of these can cause a patient to fail to understand what is going on and induce fearfulness, lashing out, or hitting.

Psychiatric disorder

Patients may resist care because of depression. If diurnal mood variation is present, patients may have greater difficulty bathing in the morning. Patients who are delusional may believe that the caregiver is trying to harm them. Visual hallucinations may be frightening and cause distress. Patients commonly misperceive their reflection in the mirror or have other illusions.

Medical problems

A rash that burns on contact with soap and water may lead to resistance in bathing. Removal of hearing aids and glasses may worsen perception and increase behavioral problems. If possible, remove them only to wash the face and hair. Pain and shortness of breath secondary to medical problems may worsen during transfer or movement.

Environment

Cold, noisy, brightly lighted, or institutional appearing bathrooms may contribute to patient distress.

Approach of the caregiver

The patient may have difficulty understanding verbal instructions or may be receiving instructions from several caregivers simultaneously. The caregiver may be rushing the patient or may be unfamiliar with new bathing routines. A care provider of the opposite sex who is perceived as a stranger is more likely to induce problems.

Devise

Depression, delusions, hallucinations, and executive dysfunction should be addressed as reviewed in Chapter 8, as should a medical condition causing unsteadiness or a wound that is painful. Caregivers may have to be educated in how to develop and follow a routine tailored to each specific patient. Caregivers who are familiar to the ill person, whether they are professional or family, are usually more successful.

Bathing goes best if the process is planned ahead of time. Bathing should be provided in as consistent a manner as possible. It should be done at the time of day determined to be best for the patient, not when it is most convenient for the staff. It is important to be flexible and to allow patients to bathe less frequently or to bathe at different times of the day if this is their wish. Being prepared means laying out supplies ahead of time. Before bathing, be casual and social. Smiling and using nonconfrontative body language can diminish the patient's feeling of being threatened or cornered. Nonthreatening statements such as "I'd like to help you freshen up before your visitors come" may be more successful than arguing with patients who maintain that they have just bathed and do not need the assistance of anyone. If they are adamant that they have just bathed, it may help to ask them whether they enjoyed the experience, all the while accompanying them to the bathroom. It is often impossible to convince patients that they have not bathed for several days. Caregivers should not have to leave to gather towels or soap since this could place ill persons in danger, be upsetting, precipitate wandering, or frighten them. We recommend not having clothes visible since they can become a cue for the patient to dress before entering the tub. Allowing sufficient time to bathe provides a calmer and less hectic environment.

For many patients, being in a strange bathroom with many echoes and confusing sounds is overwhelming. Getting patients undressed and into a robe in their own room can be helpful. Clothing, once taken off, should be put out of sight if possible. Showing a robe and slippers to a patient indicates that the process of undressing is about to begin. The patient should be assisted only as much as is necessary. Unnecessary dressing and undressing should be eliminated.

Ideally, the bathing area should look like a bathroom. Home-like cues such as attractive towels or bath mats can help. A chair should be available to help patients sit down and take off footwear.

The temperature of the shower, tub room, or bathroom should be comfortable, and patients should be kept in a robe until immediately before the bathing process begins. If possible and safe, the bath water should be drawn and the faucet turned off before the patient enters the room to eliminate confusing sounds. Guiding patients' hands to touch the water before they step in and using bubble bath can help patients who are frightened of stepping into the tub. A hand-held showerhead on a flexible extension helps avoid getting water in patients' faces. If they can hold the nozzle, they may feel in control of the process.

A colorful floor mat at the entrance of the tub or shower can make stepping into the tub or shower easier. The patient can be invited to "step onto the yellow square" rather than to get into the shower. For patients who are unsteady on their feet or seem afraid of falling, a tub bench or shower bench can provide security. Patients often misperceive these benches since these are almost white or the same color as the shower. Draping the bench with a colorful towel will give the patient a target and provide warmth and comfort. Handrails can also assist in guiding the patient into the tub or shower.

It is often helpful to offer patients a washcloth and begin the motions of washing so that they can participate in the task. For patients who resist soap or are frightened by it, bathing lotions that can be put in tub water are helpful. Ideally, only one caregiver will talk to the patient and do the bathing. Hair should be washed with nonstinging shampoos like those used with children. Since the process of hair washing is often frightening to patients, shampooing in a setting that looks like a barbershop or beauty shop may be helpful. Plastic hoods that direct water away from the eyes can be purchased.

Before transferring patients out of the tub, be sure to have the patients' attention and to turn off the water. Patients should be assisted out of the tub or shower one step at a time. A nearby robe will allow the patient to be covered quickly. A nearby chair will help the patient feel comfortable while the drying process is completed. Grooming aids (combs, brushes, toothbrushes) that are immediately available can be used to occupy patients until the process is over.

For some patients, a bed bath is less threatening than a tub bath. With an appropriate room temperature and a calm caregiver, it can also be very soothing. It is sometimes best to keep the patient covered with a bath blanket or flannel sheet and only uncover the limb or body part that is being washed. If this is comfortable for the patient, each body part should be washed and then covered before moving to the next body part.

Occasionally, patients will respond better to instructions to bathe from an unfamiliar caregiver rather than their usual companion. This is most often the case when a child must bathe a parent of the opposite sex. Sometimes a nursing assistant or male aide can be more directive with patients than their own family. A nursing assistant who can come in several times a week to take over this very challenging task can eliminate an emotional and physical struggle for the patient and provide respite for the caregiver.

Determine

Realistic goals must be set regarding bathing. For example, the goal may be for the patient to bathe three times per week without incident. To achieve this goal, the caregivers require instructions on how to bathe the patient. Classroom teaching may be adequate, but if this does not succeed, observation may be necessary. At first, another caregiver may be the observer. For those residing at home, an in-house occupational therapy evaluation may be used to observe and offer advice on bathing. Alternatively, the interaction could be videotaped and reviewed by an expert dementia-care clinician. Typically, interventions to improve bathing problems are successful within 1–2 weeks. If this is not the case, alternative interventions should be planned and attempted.

INCONTINENCE — PROBLEMS WITH TOILETING

Define and describe

Incontinence is the discharge of urine or stool (or both) in an inappropriate place, that is, not in a toilet. It is a distressing symptom to the caregiver and often to the patient. It can be a source of discomfort (to the patient), danger (slipping in urine), skin infection, and embarrassment. It also increases the likelihood of institutionalization. A helpful description includes what happens (e.g., dribbling of urine, sudden loss of urine), where it happens (e.g., on the way to the bathroom), how often it happens (e.g., several times daily or infrequently), and when it occurs (e.g., only at night). Urinary and fecal incontinence are often due to different factors and should be considered separately. Some patients, almost always men, will urinate in an inappropriate place, such as in wastebaskets. Some caregivers interpret this as a defiant gesture but, as discussed below, this behavior almost always results from some aspect of the dementing disease.

A good understanding of a patient's ability to proceed with the usual toileting is also needed. If possible, the clinician should seek to personally observe (or have a caregiver report on) the patient's performance at each of the steps involved in toileting. Are they able to recognize an internal signal of the need to toilet? If not, how do they respond to a regular reminder of a need to toilet? Can they distinguish a bathroom from inappropriate places to void? Can they identify a toilet bowl? Can they move swiftly enough to the toilet? Can they position themselves properly to toilet? Can they lift the lid? Can they manipulate and remove their clothing? Can they sit properly? Can they toilet and wipe? What do they do afterward, that is, can they put their clothes back on, wash their hands, and find their way out of the bathroom?

Decode

Cognitive disorder

Amnesia and visuospatial misperception may prevent the patient from finding the bathroom. Aphasia can interfere with the ability to communicate the need to go to the bathroom. Apraxia can cause an inability to lower a zipper, remove clothing, or sit down on the toilet. Visuospatial impairment (agnosia) may cause misperception of the toilet and result in urinating on the floor rather than into the toilet or being unable to sit on the toilet without help. In many dementias, particularly in later stages, brain (*neural*) control of urination becomes impaired because the brain pathways that control continence are destroyed. Marked apathy may cause some patients to ignore the signals to toilet. Some very agnosic patients do not recognize feces and may play with it or carry it around. In addition, some patients become frightened when seeing their reflection in the bathroom mirror and resist entering the bathroom. Not cleaning the perineal area after toileting due to amnesia, apraxia, or apathy places women at increased risk of infection.

Psychiatric disorder

If demented patients are suspicious or delusional, they may resist help with toileting. Severe depression can lead to or worsen apathy and prevent the patient from using the toilet. Hallucinations can frighten individuals so that they will not go into the bathroom.

Medical disorder

Whenever urinary incontinence begins abruptly, a urinary tract infection should be the first consideration. Such infections are especially common in elderly women. Often, incontinence or irritability will be the only signs of an infection. Patients with dementia infrequently complain of the usual signs of a urinary tract infection, that is, pain or burning on urination.

Incontinence of stool may be due to diarrhea (such as with gastroenteritis) or, paradoxically, constipation and stool retention. Colon cancer, especially in the rectum, occasionally presents with incontinence.

Diet and fluid intake can lead to incontinence. For example, urinary incontinence that occurs only at night suggests heavy evening fluid intake or diuretic medications taken late in the day. Sedative medicines can make some patients too drowsy to awaken and void in the bathroom.

Prostate problems in men can cause urinating frequency, dribbling, and retention. A prolapse of the uterus and/or bladder in a woman can cause urinary incontinence.

Conditions that cause weakness or slowness, such as stroke or PD, can impair access to the bathroom. Patients who are able to respond to the cue to void but are weak or slow can become incontinent if they become unable to manipulate their clothing rapidly enough to avoid soiling.

Environment

Bathroom areas that are not clearly marked can result in incontinence. Bathrooms in which everything is a single color—for example, a white toilet, white sink, white tub, white floor and walls—make recognition more difficult for patients with visuospatial impairments. Inadequate lighting, especially at night, can exacerbate incontinence. As stated earlier, mirrors can be upsetting to some patients. It is common for patients who are moved from a familiar home environment to a setting to have difficulty with toileting.

Caregivers

Caregivers should not assume that incontinence is untreatable, is an inevitable part of dementia, or is used to frustrate them. Caregivers should recognize that incontinence is frustrating and demands time and energy. While the caregiver's distress may make addressing the problem of incontinence difficult, it is rarely a cause.

Devise

A urine specimen should be obtained when a patient abruptly becomes incontinent of urine or undergoes a sudden change in behavior. Putting a collecting device (a *hat* or *nun's cap*) in the toilet is one means of obtaining a sample. Though sometimes difficult, gynecologic exams should be carried out annually to detect vaginal, uterine, or bladder pathology. Operations such as bladder suspension surgery can eliminate incontinence in some women and decrease the burden of care. Men suspected of having prostate problems should undergo a digital rectal exam and/or be referred to a urologist.

Depression should be treated. An environmental assessment should examine signage, lighting, ease of identifying the bathroom and toilet, and ease of access to the toilet.

If no specific cause of incontinence is found, the incontinence is likely secondary to the progression of the cognitive disorder or dementing disease. When this is the case, the patient's performance at each step of the toileting sequence should be assessed to see where the problem lies. Efforts should be made to identify the earliest step in the sequence that the patient can perform since performance usually breaks down at earlier steps first. This method of *backward training* is helpful in identifying how much assistance and supervision the patient needs. Backward training should be repeated periodically as the dementia progresses.

For many patients, a *schedule* that encourages them or reminds the caregiver to bring them to the bathroom is all that is needed to keep them dry, especially when the dementia is relatively mild. We recommend doing this "by the clock" every 2 hours (e.g., 10 A.M., noon, 2 P.M., etc.). The most common error is not keeping to the schedule. Schedules rarely help with nighttime incontinence, however, so diapers and/or plastic/absorbent sheeting are often needed when incontinence occurs after bedtime.

Caregivers should assume that patients need assistance with toileting. Some will need assistance only with remembering, but others will need to be guided through the task. When accidents happen, caregivers must recognize that criticism is not helpful. Caregivers need to learn to be sensitive to the cues indicating that an individual needs to void or defecate and to initiate toileting as soon as possible. This provides enough time to assist the patient and avoid embarrassment. In addition, caregivers should be trained how to do perineal care. Many men are not aware that it is essential to wipe the woman from front to back to avoid contaminating the urethra and predisposing to urinary tract infections.

For those whose gait is slow or who tend to dribble urine on the way to the bathroom, several solutions can be tried. Laying newspaper on the floor between the bed and the bathroom at night can accomplish two things. First, the noise of a person walking on the newspaper can alert and awaken caregivers and allow them time to assist the patient; second, the newspaper will absorb urine and avoid soiling the carpet or floor. Putting a piece of plastic artificial grass next to the bed can remind patients to stay in bed and call for help or can slow them down and give the caregiver time to come to their aid. A motion sensor by the side of the bed can alert caregivers that someone is getting out of bed and needs help. Sound amplifiers such as those used to monitor infants can be placed at the bedsides of patients and caregivers for the same purpose.

Modifying clothing can enhance the ability to toilet independently. For men, the fly and button closure on a pair of pants can be replaced with Velcro. Sweatpants with an elastic waist can be pulled down easily for voiding and defecating. The use of suspenders can make it easier to undress. Women should avoid complicated undergarments such as panty hose and girdles. Dressing men in overalls may increase the likelihood that they will tug at them as a sign that they need to be taken to the bathroom.

When patients are apractic for toileting, it is useful to have grab bars installed on both sides of the toilet and to slide a bedside commode with the container removed over the toilet so that it simulates a chair. These can make it easier to move patients in front of the toilet, for patients to reach their hands back to grasp the arms or bars, and to sit down in a reflex manner. An extender or commode on top of the toilet lessens the distance needed to sit down but must be securely attached.

Some patients become frightened as they grow more impaired because they do not understand what is going on. They may play with feces or wrap it in paper and hide it because they no longer recognize what it is. When this occurs, the patient needs to be accompanied to the bathroom and assisted.

Maintaining continence when one is away from home is a challenge for caregivers. Unisex or family bathrooms are becoming more common in public places but are still rare. When they are not available and a person of the opposite sex must be helped, family members should ask someone to go into the bathroom to check to see that no one is there and then proceed to take their relative in. Some caregivers carry signs with them saying "Out of Order" or "Helping a family member with Alzheimer disease" with plastic suction cups attached to the back for easy attachment to the door of a restroom.

Trips should be planned to provide a stop approximately every 2 hours for toileting if the patient is on a schedule. A simple urinal can be made from a plastic milk jug, with an opening cut with a pair of scissors. For patients who have frequent incontinent episodes, it is best to put a flannel-backed tablecloth on the car seat. It will remain in place and protect the upholstery.

It is important to have discussions with caregivers early on about how they feel about providing toileting care for the patient. For example, sons caring for a mother who has dementia may feel uncomfortable providing personal care. In such a case, it is important to help the family to plan ahead so that they can find someone who will perform the task. For some families, that is the point at which they consider institutional care.

Determine

Depending on the results of the decoding and the patient's toileting assessment, realistic goals for a specific patient should be set. For some patients, the goal may be no incontinence. For others, the goal may be no daytime or no stool incontinence. Sometimes the best achievable goals are no urinary tract infections due to incontinence and the patient's acceptance of the use of diapers. It is important to remind caregivers that continence goals usually change over time. If patients meet a goal and maintain it over time but then fail to reach the goal 6 months later, a reassessment should be conducted and the goal reassessed.

DRESSING

Define and describe

A wide variety of problems can occur with dressing, but they fall into three general categories: difficulty with what is put on, impairments in how it is put on, and problems with when or where clothes are changed or refused to be changed. Patients with dementia may lose the ability to select clothing, so that inappropriate items are worn or colors are uncoordinated. Clothes may be inappropriate for the weather or the occasion. Many families complain that their relative is not as meticulous as before and wears soiled or wrinkled clothing.

As dementia progresses, clothing is often put on inside-out or backward. Multiple layers of clothing and undergarments may be put on and multiple undergarments put on over a dress or pants. Some patients refuse to change their clothing for days or insist that they have just changed. Others refuse to change into night clothes to go to bed. Other challenging behaviors include repeatedly disrobing in public. This is not a common behavior but it is distressing to caregivers, both professional and family. Disrobing may be perceived as sexual or deliberately seductive, although this is rare in our experience.

Some patients want to change their clothing many times a day. Others awaken at night, get dressed, and attempt to leave the home or nursing home. Wearing clothing inappropriate for the weather—for example, going out in the winter without shoes or a coat—places an individual at serious risk. Grooming and dressing behaviors are long-term habits and are often hard to change. For example, women who always wear dresses or uniforms and men who always wear coat and ties or uniforms, can have greater problems because they are less flexible.

Decode

Cognitive disorder

Most difficulties with dressing are the result of cognitive impairment. Amnesia prevents patients from remembering what is suitable attire for an occasion. Disorientation to season and weather may result in putting on inappropriate clothing. Inability to comprehend complex multistage verbal instructions to dress can result from aphasia.

Apraxia interferes with the correct putting on of clothing and can result in clothing that is put on backward or upside down. Shirts may be buttoned in an awkward manner or not at all. Complicated clothing such as brassieres, girdles, panty hose, neckties, zippers, and belts can be especially challenging for the person with dementia who is apractic. Dresses that must be pulled on over the head and secured in the back with zippers or hooks and eyes are also difficult.

Visual agnosias disrupt the ability to recognize what particular items of clothing are and interfere with the accurate perception of clothing. Cognitive impairment also interferes with the realization that clothing is soiled, worn, or inside out.

Psychiatric disorders

Depressed persons with dementia may neglect their appearance, dress in the same clothing day after day, or seem unconcerned that they are dressed inappropriately. Patients who develop mania may wear too much clothing or clothing inappropriate to the patient's age or situation. Such was the case with a dementia patient who walked about the nursing home in a bikini with a rose in her teeth.

Delusions also influence attire. A patient who is convinced that he or she must go home may constantly wear a hat and coat and carry an umbrella. Patients who are convinced that someone will steal their belongings may wear many layers of clothing to keep themselves safe. Those who believe they must go to work will dress accordingly. A patient who is having visual hallucinations may refuse to undress in front of those "strangers" he or she sees in the room. When the ability to dress declines abruptly, an underlying physical cause such as delirium is likely to be present.

Medical disorder

Disrobing is often a reaction to discomfort. This can be present when a rash develops, when clothing no longer fits due to weight gain, or when it is put on in a way that produces discomfort. Abdominal pain related to constipation may lead to attempts to disrobe to relieve pressure on the abdomen.

Tugging at or removing clothing can also be a sign that the person needs to void or defecate.

Environment

Many patients cannot make choices from a large array of options, usually because of agnosia or apraxia. Thus, patients who are left in front of a full closet to select clothing will have difficulty. Cues from the environment can be powerful stimuli to dressing. For example, the patient who awakens at night and sees a hat or coat will be cued to dress and leave. Patients who constantly dress and undress often are responding to similar cues in the environment.

Caregiver

Conflicts over dressing can arise from caregivers' unrealistic expectations of patient's abilities and their insistence on patients' dressing as they did before developing dementia. Caregivers who offer too many choices, or who lay clothing out and expect the patient to select the clothing and put it on the proper sequence, may be frustrated when the patient is unable to do so. Patient frustration may also result from a lack of assistance from the caregiver. Insisting that the patient dress in the same meticulous and color-coordinated manner as before the onset of dementia can result in tension and conflict.

Devise

A plan to address dressing includes an assessment of what the patient is able to do and what is truly important to the patient's welfare. Choices should be limited and clothing laid out for patients who are able to dress themselves. Many families clear out one closet or drawer and put in a single coordinated group of clothing for the patient to retrieve; this increases the opportunity for success. When patients need assistance to dress, clothing should be laid out in the sequence in which it is put on. To promote improvement, a solid bedspread is used to facilitate perception of the items of clothing.

When patients insist on wearing the same clothing repeatedly, identical sets of clothing can be obtained. When the patient is in the shower, a clean set can be placed where the dirty clothes were.

Careful assessment for sources of discomfort should be made if the patient is constantly disrobing. Clothing such as hats and coats should be kept from view to eliminate their functioning as cues to dress and leave. It is often best if clean clothing is not brought into the shower room, as patients may be cued to redress as soon as they are undressed before showering.

If persistent disrobing or tugging is the primary signal or the person needs to use the bathroom often, a toileting schedule should be developed and the patient assisted to the bathroom.

In general, clothing should be simplified to decrease frustration in the dressing process. This can present difficulties for families and patients who resist change. Clip-on ties can be substituted for neckties, knee-high stockings for panty hose or stockings. Brassieres that hook in front are preferred. Velcro can replace zippers on men's pants or snaps and buttons on shirts and dresses.

To prevent layering, only those items of clothing that are needed should be available to the patient. Assistance should be provided one step at a time to ensure that clothing goes on in the correct order. If necessary, closets and drawers should be locked to prevent constant dressing and undressing. In nursing homes and other long-term settings, each piece of clothing should be clearly labeled for easy identification. This includes eyeglasses, hearing aids, and dentures. In some nursing homes, when glasses, hearing aids, and dentures are removed for the night, they are secured in a designated drawer or a medicine cart that is locked.

When patients refuse to change into night clothes to get into bed, we suggest that they be allowed to sleep in regular clothes, followed by an attempt to change them in the morning.

Determine

Determining if a dressing plan has been successful usually requires compromise in defining success. It may not be worth the struggle to have patients dressed the way they dressed in the past. This is often more upsetting for families than for patients. For example, it can be upsetting for the family of a prominent businessman to see him in a sweat suit even if he is quite comfortable. Sometimes the most practical goal is to decrease the frequency of problematic dressing behavior, such as disrobing, rather than totally stopping the behavior.

SLEEP PROBLEMS

Define and describe

The aging process is often accompanied by fragmentation of sleep. Cognitively normal elders have more nighttime awakenings, more light sleep, and less deep sleep than younger individuals. The average older person spends more time in bed but sleeps about the same number of hours as when younger. Some individuals need naps as they age.

Sleep problems in dementia include too much sleep, too little sleep, and a reversal of the sleep/wake cycle, that is, staying up at night and sleeping during the day. When a complaint of too little sleep is investigated further, it often turns out that the person sleeps intermittently throughout the day and night. Therefore, when problems with sleep occur, it is important to document when persons go to sleep, when they awaken, and how many hours they have slept per 24 hours. A chart that records any sleep, day or night, is essential for establishing the existence of a sleep problem and its pattern. Aides and family members must often be convinced of the importance of such documentation.

The assessment of a sleep disorder requires vigilance on the caregiver's part. In a long-term care facility it requires cooperation among all shifts so that every period of sleep, no matter how short, can be accurately recorded. In patients who have a reversed sleep/wake cycle (sleeping during the day and awake at night), it should be determined whether this is a lifelong pattern in someone who worked the night shift or a rotating shift.

Decode

Cognitive disorder

In AD there can be destruction of the suprachiasmatic nucleus, a group of cells that controls the normal sleep/wake cycle. Amnesia may not allow persons to remember that they have moved to a new residence and lead to the feeling that they are being asked to sleep in a new and unfamiliar place. Agnosia may prevent the patient from becoming familiar with and recognizing the bedroom.

Psychiatric disorder

Psychiatric disorders and symptoms causing sleep disorder include depression, mania, anxiety, delusions, and hallucinations. Patients who are suspicious can become fearful and be unable to sleep.

Medical disorder

Patients with dementia who have certain coexisting medical conditions such as congestive heart failure, sleep apnea, or prostatic hypertrophy often have trouble sleeping because of shortness of breath, snoring, or awakening to urinate. Medications such as beta blockers, antidepressants, and antiparkinsonian drugs can cause nightmares that awaken and frighten them; because of amnesia or aphasia, patients may be unable to report or remember the dream, however. Leg cramps or pain in the evening are also difficult to diagnose.

Urinary tract infections are common in patients with dementia, especially women, and can lead to sleep disorder. Medications and other substances that increase the amount of urine or act as stimulants, such as diuretics, antidepressants, alcohol, or caffeine, as well as stimulants, can interfere with sleep. Chronic use of benzodiazepines can disrupt the sleep/wake cycle.

Diseases that cause visual impairment may alter a person's ability to respond to the cues of light and dark. These cues play an important role in regulating the normal sleep/wake cycle.

Environment

Noise, bright lights, and uncomfortable or unfamiliar beds, sheets, pillows, and rooms can contribute to difficulty sleeping. For many people, sleep is a behavior that is promoted by a routine—going to bed at the same time, following the same procedures, having the same person with them, using the same pillow, and so on. Alterations in any of these can interfere with the ability to fall and stay asleep. Having other patients in the room can cause many of the problems listed in this paragraph. Levels of daytime stimulation and activity may encourage daytime napping and diminish the need for nighttime sleep or alter the usual sleep/wake cycle.

Caregiver

Spouse caregivers who have slept with the patient in the past may want to go to bed later (to have free time for themselves) or may no longer want to sleep with the ill person. Such changes in routine can interfere with the usual sleep process. The professional caregiver may put the patient to bed early to lessen work or because of other responsibilities. This can lead to early awakening that is then labeled a problem.

Devise

A sleep disorder should be treated when it is causing difficulties for the patient, the caregiver, or other residents of a long-term care facility. As with the other conditions addressed in this chapter, treatable psychiatric or medical conditions should be identified and treated. Environmental and other non-pharmacologic management strategies, referred to as *sleep hygiene,* are recommended even if a psychiatric or medical cause is found. Often such interventions eliminate the sleep problem. If persons are getting between 5 and 8 hours of sleep with a combination of daytime naps and nighttime sleep, an attempt should be made to keep them busier and more active throughout the day. Patients with sleep disorder who are home during the day can benefit from attending an adult day-care center. Going to bed at a later time or disallowing daytime naps should be considered

If a diuretic medication is prescribed, it should be given early in the morning. Caffeine should be avoided after early evening and the medication list reviewed for the presence of agents that can cause restlessness. Restless leg syndrome should be treated in the customary manner (with levodopa or benzodiazepines).

A bedtime routine should be established and maintained when this is realistic. It should include getting undressed, washing, brushing the teeth, and saying prayers. It often requires the assistance of a caregiver. Some patients sleep better after a warm bath, a glass of milk, or a small amount of food.

For patients who need to use the bathroom during the night, consideration should be given to limiting fluid intake after dinner and to encouraging them to use the bathroom before going to bed. They should be assisted safely to the bathroom and returned to bed when they get up to void; otherwise, they may become confused and fall. The use of inexpensive motion sensors can alert a caregiver that the ill person is getting up. Putting a mat made of artificial turf at the side where the patient gets out of bed will be uncomfortable for some patients and slow down their exit from the bed, giving the caregiver time to reach them and assist them.

For patients who awaken at night and insist that it is time to go somewhere, the caregiver should try distraction, such as saying "We will leave as soon as we've had breakfast" or "It's Saturday, so we can sleep late." A snack given in a dimly lit room may distract the patient and allow a return to bed. Environments that are stimulating during the day and quiet at night help regulate sleep. Structured activity in the evening may prevent patients from going to bed early for lack of something else to do. If patients are unable to adjust the heat or air conditioning in their bedroom, the temperature should be regulated appropriately. Some individuals with dementia benefit from an afternoon nap. This should be determined by trial and error. It is best to limit the duration of afternoon naps.

If environmental interventions fail and the sleep disorder is causing distress to the patient or the family caregiver, a pharmacologic treatment specifically targeting sleep may be tried. We recommend using sedating medications only when there is a clear potential benefit for the patient or the caregiver and minimal risk to the patient. Unfortunately, few studies are available to guide clinicians' choice of medication when the only goal is to improve sleep. We do *not* recommend regular use of antihistamines such as diphenhydramine (Benadryl, Nytol, Tylenol PM) since these have significant anticholinergic activity and can worsen memory. Some clinicians recommend the sedating antidepressant drug trazodone, starting with 25 mg at bedtime and increasing to 100–150 mg at bedtime to help with sleep. Others prescribe zolpidem (Ambien) or zalpelon (Sonata), 5 or 10 mg. In the past, the sedating barbiturate derivative chloral hydrate was used; we occasionally prescribe it in doses ranging from 250 to 1000 mg. We very rarely use benzodiazepines for sleep.

If depression is present, the primary treatment is often pharmacologic. The use of antidepressant medications for depression and the use of neuroleptic medications for hallucinations, delusions, or mania are discussed in Chapter 10. If a neuroleptic is being prescribed for other symptoms, it can be given at bedtime to help the patient sleep. More sedating antidepressant medicines such as trazadone, or one of the tricyclics, may be used to treat a depression if there is an associated sleep disorder.

Some studies suggest that *bright light therapy* may improve daytime and nighttime behavior and possibly lead to improved sleep. This therapy consists of exposing individuals to bright lights (a brightness of 10,000 lumens is recommended). This is equivalent to a bank of several fluorescent light tubes. Further study is needed before this can be recommended as a first-line treatment for nighttime sleep disorder. Daytime sleepiness can be very difficult to address. Sometimes daytime activity programs help. Nighttime sedation rarely helps. Very rarely, stimulant medication in the morning reduces severe daytime drowsiness if apathy is present.

Determine

Treatment response is best determined by measuring how many hours and when the person sleeps. If medication is used, careful attention should be given to toxicity. If the desired response is not occurring, then the medicine should either be increased or discontinued. If an antidepressant medication is used to treat both depression and sleep disorder, and it is effective, then the drug should be continued for at least 6 months and probably for 1 year or longer.

FALLING AND DIFFICULTY WALKING OR TRANSFERRING

Define

As many as 30% of patients with early-stage dementia and as many as 70%–75% of patients who are institutionalized experience a fall during a 1-year period. The majority of these falls have relatively minor consequences—bruising, pain, or abrasions—but major injuries such as hip, wrist, or arm fractures and subdural hematomas are common. Falls are particularly common at night and are more likely to occur in the bedroom, bathroom, or stairway. Patients who are at highest risk of falling are those with multiple medical problems, advanced dementia, and significant functional impairments. Those who wander and are in good health are also at higher risk of falling.

Impairment in gait (walking) develops in most dementias and is often accompanied by poor balance. Patients with gait disorder cannot move their feet to correct a stumble and cannot use their arms to steady themselves or prevent falling. Sometimes it is hard to distinguish a true fall from an apparent fall because patients can sit down on the floor and be found there by staff.

The term *transferring* refers to moving from one position to another—for example, in and out of a chair, tub, automobile, or bed. Difficulty in transferring becomes more common as the dementia progresses and can result in appearing fearful of or being unable to sit on a toilet seat or in a chair. Difficulty transferring can lead patients to sit on the floor rather than where they meant to sit ("missing the seat").

Decode

Cognitive disorder

In general, the likelihood of falling and difficulties in transferring and walking increase as dementia becomes more severe. Cortical dementias are characterized by apraxias and agnosias that impair the ability to know how to walk, to cross thresholds, to go up steps, or to perceive objects in the environment that can cause tripping such as loose rugs, low tables, cords, small animals, or children. Eventually, the cortical dementias impair the ability to know where to look when walking. Subcortical dementias impair reaction time, the planning of motor action, and the response to minor imbalance. Ultimately, all progressive dementias lead to physical inactivity, which in turn places patients further at risk of falls because of muscle weakness and bone demineralization.

Psychiatric disorder

Depression often results in social isolation and a decreased activity level that exacerbates muscle weakness and deconditioning. Patients who are suspicious or manic may try to move quickly or spend more time on their feet and thereby be at increased risk for falls. Patients who wander about are also more likely to fall. Delirium increases the risk of falling due to worsened cognition and to the ataxia and weakness that accompany it.

Medical disorder

Visual or auditory impairments, gait or balance disorder due to arthritis, neurologic disease, muscle weakness, or physical dependence increase the risk of falls. Many medications, especially psychotropic medications, and any medical condition that causes frailty increases the risk of falling. These should be regularly reassessed, especially in patients who have had a fall. Shuffling gait can be due to PD or parkinsonian side effects of neuroleptic medications. Orthostatic hypotension, a drop in blood pressure that occurs when moving from lying or sitting or from sitting to standing, can be caused by many medications, dehydration, and some medical disorders. Weakness, paralysis, impaired sensation (peripheral neuropathy), and coordination can lead to falls. Deconditioning, weakness due to lack of use of muscles, can be caused by restraints, being confined, or lack of exercise and predisposes to falling.

Environment

Furniture, throw rugs, clutter, slippery floors, raised thresholds, staircases, bathtubs, narrow passageways, dim lighting, and loud noises increase the risk of falls associated with dementia.

Caregiver

Caregivers may not know the correct way to help a person get up and down from a chair or bed, transfer into a bathtub, or supervise dressing or bathing and thus may increase the risk of a fall. Patients who are at significant risk of falling should not be left alone. Caregivers who do not appreciate fall risks are much less likely to act to prevent falls. In a patient with dementia who is falling frequently, caregiver abuse or neglect should be considered.

Devise

The ideal approach to falls in dementia patients is to prevent them. This requires an appreciation of the risk factors for falls discussed above and of the interventions that will address them. Since the fall risk increases as dementia progresses, more attention should be paid to fall prevention over time. A MMSE score in the 0–10 range identifies a very-high-risk patient. Patients who are experiencing agnosia or apraxia early in the course of dementias are at high risk much earlier. Psychiatric disorders that lead patients to move around rapidly, such as affective disorders, agitation, delusions, hallucinations, or akathisia, should be treated to prevent falls. Medication regimens should be simplified as much as possible, and visual and hearing impairments should be corrected if possible to assess for orthostatic hypotension. Blood pressure should be measured in two positions, lying and sitting or sitting and standing. The second measurement should be performed after a 2-minute wait in the second position. Measurements should be obtained *before* giving medications and afterword to monitor for change. A medical reassessment should be undertaken whenever falls occur without an identifying etiology.

Environmental modifications should address the items listed under "environment." For example, low tables should be moved, throw rugs eliminated, and exposed cords made safe. Gates or stairwells can be dangerous, as they may cause falls. Doors to stairwells should be locked. Proper lighting should eliminate glare and minimize shadows. A home occupational therapy assessment can identify potential environmental hazards and suggest practical solutions. Specific devices reimbursed by Medicare if ordered by a physician. Caregivers should be taught how to help the unsteady individual in a manner that both prevents falls and protects the caregiver from harm. A physical therapy evaluation can also provide useful guidance. It can develop exercise or actions plans to strengthen muscles and improve balance. Assisted walking devices such as canes and walkers may be helpful, but many dementia patients forget to use them or develop apraxias that make them unsafe. Occasionally a reminding device can help. For example, on occasion, we have used a device to sound a signal when the person is more than a few feet from the walker. Motion sensors can alert caregivers that a patient is attempting to stand and signal the caregiver to assist the patients. When patients fall at night, it may be necessary to place their mattress on the floor. Very rarely, a chest or waist restraint has to be used to prevent patients who are too weak to support their weight from arising without supervision. However, patients can fall even when watched very closely or restrained. Furthermore, restraints can cause harm or death and are conceptually repugnant. Finally, special underwear with hip pads that look like boxer underwear and contain shock-absorbent gels in their sides should be used to prevent hip fracture from falls. Such underwear is inexpensive, machine washable, and very acceptable to both male and female patients. It has been shown in randomized, controlled trials to prevent hip fracture after a fall in the great majority of older patients who are at risk for a fall.

Determine

It is impossible to reduce the fall rate role to zero without unacceptably impairing the quality of life. For many patients and families, a certain aamount of falling, even if it may lead to serious injury, is acceptable if the patient is allowed a certain amount of freedom and independence. Therefore, the goal of the treatment for falls should be to reduce the risk of falling to an acceptable level that does not unduly compromise the patient's quality of life. Using hip-padded underwear often helps reassure caregivers that if a fall occurs, an injury is less likely.

A surveillance system, perhaps a semiannual check by a clinician, that assesses a patient's gait regularly and determines when, where, and how often falls are occurring is a must since it provides a warning that falls are likely to become problematic. Any environmental modifications should be given sufficient time to determine if they are effective. Typically, 7–10 days should be adequate to determine if an intervention is working.

DRIVING

Define and describe

Even when problems are not obvious, driving by patients with dementia can be dangerous. First, situations may arise in which a patient is unable to react quickly to an emergency or to make the decision needed to avoid an accident. Another challenge is that most dementias are progressive. Even when patients with early dementia are driving safely, a time will come when they will be at high risk for accidents. Unfortunately, it is impossible, at present, to predict when driving will become risky. Therefore, we recommend that driving should be discouraged soon after a diagnosis has been made.

Dementia is associated with problems such as getting lost, forgetting where the car is parked, sideswiping cars, leaving the scene of an accident, and running others off the road. Thus, during the assessment, it is important to ask direct questions of patients and their caregivers about driving. Include a query about unexplained dents and scrapes on the car. Patients often are confident of their driving ability and may forget incidents.

Driving is presented in this book as a functioning problem because it is a capacity that clinicians should address and because the approaches taken to stop it are often behavioral. However, driving prohibitions cause practical problems because they change the lives of patients and their spouses, especially if the spouse does not drive. Stopping the ill person from driving can be a major source of difficulty for the family because many patients feel that their driving is fine and that they should be allowed to drive even when it is clear to others that their driving is dangerous.

One reason driving is difficult to address is that it has powerful social meanings. For many individuals, driving is equated with being an adult and having the freedom to go where one wants to go. Losing the privilege to drive, therefore, means a loss of freedom and becomes a frequent reminder that the person is ill. Since caregivers must often repeatedly stop ill individuals from driving, they can become the target of angry outbursts from patients who feel confident that they can drive safely.

All patients with a progressive dementia eventually have to give up driving. This may also be necessary in patients with nonprogressive dementias.

There are several ways to determine if a patient should stop driving: (1) Ask family and friends about the patient's driving performance. They have often observed dangerous driving behavior caused by the dementia. Asking patients' children if they would let the patient drive their own children alone is a useful question. If the answer is "No" (referred to as the *grandchild sign*), the patient should probably not be driving. (2) Find out if there have been accidents or if the patient has been lost while driving since the onset of dementia. If these have occurred, the patient probably should not be driving. (3) Estimate cognitive capacity: patients with moderate or severe dementia (an MMSE score <18) probably should not be driving. (4) Have the patient take a formal driving test at a driving school or a clinical center. Some occupational therapists provide specific driving evaluations. At Johns Hopkins, a dementia-specific driving evaluation program has been developed and has been very helpful. About one-third of the people with dementia referred to this program are able to continue driving safely for several months longer with close monitoring.

Decode

Cognitive disorder

Driving depends on many cognitive capacities. An impairment in any one of them can adversely affect driving. Those capacities relevant to driving include visuospatial function, praxis, mental flexibility, and judgment. The motor impairments and slowed reaction times that accompany most subcortical dementias are other sources of driving impairment. These include bradykinesia, rigidity, and tremor. Driving is an overlearned or automatic behavior. Much of it can be done without thinking about it. Therefore, mistakes are few early in dementia, even when the capacities that underlie driving have begun to fail.

Psychiatric disorder

We are not aware of specific syndromes that have been consistently associated with impaired driving. Rarely, a manic syndrome with grandiosity may lead patients to overestimate their capabilities and to drive aggressively.

Medical disorder

Medical disorders and medications can affect cognition, and may further impair a patient's decision-making and driving capacities. Sedating medications can be especially hazardous. Impairments in vision and hearing can magnify existing cognitive impairments.

Environment

For many Americans, the ability to drive allows them to remain independent, go shopping, and engage in social activities. Alternatives to driving, such as public transportation, mobility services, family members, friends, social agencies, and other caregivers, can be a source of help. The lack of these resources can result in driving after it has become unsafe.

Caregiver

Caregivers often find the recommendation that the patient not drive very awkward, since the caregiver is usually the person who has to remind the patient not to drive. Even when caregivers appreciate the problems and dangers associated with driving, patients often resist or refuse to stop. Sometimes, however, caregivers do not accept the recommendation to stop driving, perhaps because it will adversely affect their lives. This is particularly true when the caregiver does not know how to drive or is too frail to drive. Thus, it is important to assess the understanding of caregivers regarding a driving prohibition and to help them accept the need for the prohibition. This is particularly difficult when the patient's condition appears to be mild and the caregiver has not observed difficulties in driving. The issue can be further complicated if there are different points of view within the family. Protests such as "She only drives to the beauty shop" or "He's driven around town all his life" are common. Families should be reminded that most accidents occur close to home and that even a minor unexpected event, such as a car pulling out, can unmask deficits and place the driver, passengers, and others at risk.

Devise

The main purpose of a recommendation to stop driving is to prevent the dangers of automobile accidents, getting lost, being victimized, and placing others at risk. The first goal is to persuade the patient to stop driving completely. Some patients accept the recommendation willingly. Often the family needs help persuading patients that they should not drive and enforcing the prohibition.

In some states, it is permissible for the physician to breach confidentiality and report to the Motor Vehicle Administration that a medical condition exists that makes driving dangerous. In other states, reporting is required; in still others, it is not legally sanctioned. When the last is true, the spouse or other family members should be encouraged to write to the Motor Vehicle Administration and report that a spouse or parent has been advised to stop driving. All jurisdictions have individuals or medical advisory boards that will review the recommendations. On-road tests are sometimes conducted to decide whether the person should be allowed to continue driving. Many impaired individuals can pass a simple vision test because it does not assess for cognitive impairment.

The decision to involve the motor vehicle authorities is complex. It should always be pursued when the clinician has a high concern that continued driving may be dangerous. If the patient has been having accidents, refuses to stop driving, and caregivers are unable to enforce the prohibition, it is appropriate for the clinician to consider legal advice. We are aware of one instance in which a patient was driving in spite of a medical prohibition and had a serious accident, and was then told by the insurance company that he was not covered for the accident because he had been driving against medical advice. Of course, it is hard for an insurance company to find out that a patient has been driving against medical advice, but in instances of accidents, as above, medical records may be available through court actions. Advising patients and their families of this example can encourage the patient to stop driving.

Making changes in daily life so that patients and spouses can maintain their activities and independence without driving is a critical part of any intervention. The use of public or family resources is the most common method of accomplishing this. However, for some patients, a prohibition on driving means moving to a different residential situation. This has serious emotional and practical implications.

Helping caregivers enforce a driving prohibition is important. Clinicians may suggest that caregivers remove vehicles from the home or incapacitate them. Caregivers may "lose the keys" or keep the cars "in the shop," or always offer to drive when the patient wants to use the car. The gender of the patient and the caregiver is an important issue in our experience. It is typically much harder for men to accept a recommendation to stop driving than for women. We strongly recommend that the spouse repeatedly identify the physician as the source of the prohibition. "Dr. X says you shouldn't drive. At your next appointment, you should talk to her and tell her you disagree." While the health professional can have empathy with the situation, he or she has a responsibility to disagree with a patient who wants to drive and to make every effort to keep the patient from driving. Sending the patient a written notice or writing on a signed prescription form, "Do Not Drive" may help. Caregivers can use them to remind patients of the medical prohibition and take the onus of the recommendation off of themselves.

Determine

After a recommendation not to drive has been made, it is important to document this in the medical record (for medical-legal purposes) and to ask at the next appointment if the recommendation has been followed. When driving is deemed safe (or at least if there is no basis on which to recommend that the patient stop driving), the clinician should tell the patient and family that the patient's driving ability is likely to become impaired in the future, and needs to be monitored by them and reassessed by the clinician. We recommend a reassessment every 6 months.

SEXUAL PROBLEMS

Define and describe

Complaints about sexual behavior are uncommon in dementia. While this might relate to the reluctance of care providers to discuss sexual intimacy or the reluctance of clinicians to inquire about it, no studies have found a high prevalence of problems related to sexual behavior in persons with dementias. The most common complaint related to sexual behavior is a lessening of desire for sexual intimacy in the spouse caregiver without a corresponding decline in the patient. Another common complaint is that the patient forgets that there has been recent sexual intimacy and requests it frequently.

In the long-term care setting, and at times at home in the community, complaints revolve around heightened sexual desire, public masturbation, and inappropriate touching of other residents and staff. Although intimate sexual relationships between long-term care residents are rare, they create significant anxiety and concern in family members and staff when they occur.

Because exposing or touching one's own genitals or those of someone else is upsetting to many people, a careful description of the behavior is crucial. This often clarifies the goal of the behavior and suggests an appropriate intervention. For example, a male patient who is forgetful and apractic may appropriately find the bathroom but then walk back out without closing his fly. Patients may disrobe because they believe they are in their bedroom or bathroom or because they have a skin rash that makes their clothing uncomfortable. It is important that the characteristics of the behavior be thoroughly explored before someone is "reported" for sexual deviance.

Decode

Cognitive disorder

Amnesia may lead to forgetting when sexual activity last occurred or what common sexual practices were used with the patient's partner. Aphasia may lead to inability to understand the intimate expressions of a partner or to difficulty expressing sexual desires verbally. Agnosia may lead to lack of recognition of a sexual partner or to misidentification of others as one's partner, leading to unwanted advances. Apraxia may impair the ability to perform movements necessary to sexual interaction. Disturbances of executive function may lead to disinhibition of sexual drives or to attempts to have physical contact with others that is not sexual in intent (e.g., hugging, kissing, holding hands, or sitting in someone's lap) but that is interpreted as such.

Psychiatric disorder

Mania may lead to hypersexual behavior, while depression can greatly reduce sexual drive. Delusions or hallucinations can lead to suspiciousness or avoidance of one's sexual partner. Delirium may reduce awareness of the surroundings and reduce sexual interest.

Medical disorders

Many medications have been associated with reduced sexual desire or functioning. These include beta blockers, psychotropics (e.g., antidepressants, neuroleptics), digitalis, anticancer agents, antihypertensives, sedatives, and antihistamines. Diabetes, hypertension, arthritis, cancer, anemia, and many chronic diseases are associated with a reduced sexual drive or the inability to perform sexually. Pain, constipation, stroke, prostatic hypertrophy, and gynecologic disorders (such as prolapsed uterus, diminished vaginal secretions, vaginocele, and perineal rashes), can adversely affect sexuality in dementia patients.

Environment

Patients who no longer live at home may have fewer cues to remind them of their sexual life. Others may be stimulated sexually by other patients who are disinhibited. Elderly men (and at times women) who are receiving one-on-one care by younger women (men) may misinterpret the situation, become stimulated sexually, and touch or grab the care provider.

Caregivers

The sexual partners of dementia patients may assume that the sexual life of their loved one is unaffected and seek to maintain it when the patient is no longer interested or is unable to perform. Nonfamily caregivers who behave in an overly familiar manner (e.g., calling patients "sweetie" or kissing patients on the cheek) may provoke unwanted sexual advances in a disinhibited or agnosic patient.

Devise

When complaints about sexual behavior arise, there is almost always distress on someone's part. Therefore, a treatment plan is almost always appropriate. When family caregivers report a disparity between their interest in sex and the desires of the patient, a careful history is the first step. Information should be gathered about the nature and frequency of sexual relations prior to the illness and how these have changed. It is important to explore the caregiver's emotional relationship with the ill person. The caregiving role often leads to a change in the roles of patient and caregiver, and this can diminish interest in sexual activity. Some caregivers report a total loss of interest in sexual relations, while others report a diminution. Exploring these issues in an open, supportive way is an important aspect of helping the caregiver.

If the genesis of the complaint appears to be the patient's forgetting that there had been recent sexual relations and a request for repeated relations, the caregiver can be instructed how to gently remind the patient of this. Caregivers may offer a stalling tactic such as saying "We'll be alone soon, but first let's go out for a walk." Substituting another pleasurable activity may distract the patient. This is one issue about which caregivers must sometimes lie to the patient if they feel they are no longer able to engage in an intimate sexual relationship. It is important to explore the meaning of other forms of intimacy such as hugging and kissing. For some individuals this can substitute for sexual intimacy, but this is not always the case.

Public masturbation is intrusive to other individuals and is most appropriately handled by redirecting the person to a private place. Most patients respond to this redirection, but an occasional patient becomes upset by it. One impediment to redirection is the discomfort that staff and other residents experience in the presence of a public display of sexuality. Often a staff person can identify very early manifestations of public masturbation, such as tugging on the crotch of pants or unzipping the fly, and move the patient to a private place before masturbation begins. Moving the patient quietly and quickly without criticism can sometimes avoid the development of a catastrophic reaction. More intrusive behaviors, such as touching the breasts or crotch of caregivers during care or touching other residents in day-care centers or institutions, is a sensitive and important issue. If the person being touched or propositioned is also cognitively impaired, he or she may have diminished capacity to resist or avoid the initiator. The latter problem should always be addressed. It may mean seating the two individuals in separate areas of the dining room, not allowing a male resident to attend groups with women (or the woman who is the object of the sexual behavior), or moving one person's room to the other end of the hallway or to a different floor.

Sexual touching of nursing staff in institutions (or hospitals) and adult day-care centers is distressing as well. Staff should be aware that behavior they think of as affectionate may be misinterpreted as a sexual advance by an impaired person or that not all touching has a sexual agenda. However, grabbing and touching can have a sexual purpose or be upsetting to the staff member. It is rare, in our experience, that a spouse will ask for privacy with an ill person in a nursing home. This should be provided when appropriate.

On several occasions, questions have arisen about supporting sexual intimacy between two unrelated patients who are cognitively impaired but appear to be consenting. The fact that people suffer from dementia should not be used to deprive them of the intimacy of relationships with others or of the ability to establish new relationships. When a question arises on this issue, we believe an expert should assess the capacity of the two individuals to consent. Such a situation requires the inclusion of family members and legal representatives if patients are found to be incapable of consenting to sexual interaction. In general, interactions between assenting demented patients may be acceptable if stopping them would adversely affect their quality of life and if family members are in agreement after a meeting with the clinicians in which the situation has been discussed.

Nonsexual intimacy such as holding hands occurs much more frequently than sexual intimacy. This behavior provides a means of displaying affection even when the ability to communicate verbally is diminished. Often this reflects a friendship that has developed between individuals. There is always concern that one individual may be exploiting another. It is important to openly discuss any concerns about this type of behavior with the family and to assess whether exploitation is occurring. Rarely, pharmacologic treatment of sexually inappropriate behavior is necessary. Indications include an inability to stop the repetitive touching of residents or persistent seeking of sexual relationships with other residents. There are no adequate studies of pharmacologic treatment, and none is likely to be carried out because of the infrequency of this problem. Case reports and our experience support the occasional use of oral hydroxyprogesterone (Provera) in men, beginning at 5 mg per day and increasing by 5 mg per week up to 15 mg/day. Alternatively, injectable, long-acting hydroxyprogesterone (Depo-Provera), 100 mg intramuscularly (IM) every 4 weeks, or leuprolide 7.5, mg IM every 4 weeks, may be used. Antipsychotic drugs are sometimes prescribed, but their efficacy is unclear. The SSRI antidepressants can impair erection in men and are occasionally used for this reason. Pharmacologic treatment of mania can lead to resolution of inappropriate sexual behavior if it is a symptom.

Determine

Clear goals must be set regarding sexual disturbances. If the problem is reduced sexual desire on the part of the patient or the spouse caregiver, a reasonable goal may be the establishment of a new pattern of sexual relations. This may include less frequent encounters or encounters that do not include intercourse. Such a new relationship may necessitate careful planning, emotional support on the part of the clinician, and several months to establish.

If the problem is excessive or inappropriate sexual behavior on the part of the patient, then elimination of the behavior may be the primary goal. Behavioral modification techniques, changes in caregiver approach, consistent limits on the behaviors, environmental modification, and pharmacologic treatment may be tried alone or in combination. Responses typically occur within 4–6 weeks. Alternative interventions should be tried if a response does not occur. The rapidity with which treatments are changed and the invasiveness of the treatment depend on how intrusive the behavior is. The more intrusive the behavior, the more aggressive the therapy should be.

Open discussion of the discomfort some individuals experience when discussing or confronting sexual issues can relieve the awkwardness they experience in discussing and assessing the frequency of inappropriate sexual behavior.

10

Pharmacologic and Other Biologic Treatments in Dementia

The medications useful to treat dementia modify the mechanisms through which brain diseases cause neuropsychiatric mental symptoms, both cognitive and noncognitive. Most currently available medications act by compensating for the damage produced by a disease. Their effectiveness is known from clinical experience or well-designed clinical trails, but their mechanisms of action are not well understood. It is likely that in the future new medicines will be available that will prevent, reverse, or slow down the damage caused by dementia-causing disease, trauma, or toxin exposure. This is especially true regarding AD, in which advances in understanding its etiopathogenesis are leading to the development of medications that may effectively tackle the underlying mechanism of brain damage. This chapter discusses the principles of medication use, individual medicines, and other biologic treatments, electroconvulsive therapy, bright light therapy, and brain surgery.

Principles of Rational Pharmacologic Management of Dementia-Related Symptoms

Medicines should be used only after careful consideration of the purpose for which they are being used, the alternative treatments that are available—including nonmedication approaches—and the risks of their use. If their mechanism of action is targeted against a specific disease or biologic abnormality, accurate diagnosis is necessary to confirm that they are indicated. However, in dementia care, disease therapies often are not available, so decisions are based on careful appreciation of the clinical picture. This is especially true when behavioral symptoms are the target of therapy. Clinicians should develop hypotheses about the causes and mechanisms of symptoms and use them to guide their choice of medicine. For example, if the clinician believes that depression underlies a behavior problem, then an antidepressant should be considered. If delusions are the most likely cause, then an antipsychotic may be indicated. When available, published studies should guide the practitioner's choice of the most effective medication for the symptom being treated.

Before prescribing a medicine for a dementia-related symptom, the clinician should carefully decode its possible causes, as articulated in Chapters 8 and 9. It is especially important to consider whether there is an underlying medical condition or environmental problem causing the symptoms. A common example is the development of aggression due to a urinary tract infection. Sometimes aggression is the *only* symptom of a urinary tract infection and the problem resolves within a few day of the initiation of antibiotics. Another example is the patient who becomes explosive at a particular time of day and only in a specific circumstance because a caregiver is approaching him inappropriately, because he is hungry, or because he is sleepy. Solving the environmental problem typically will lead to resolution of the explosiveness.

Symptoms such as delusions or hallucinations that cause neither distress to the patient nor harm to others usually do not require an antipsychotic agent. The underlying principle is that a treatment should be used only if the benefits outweigh the risks, particularly after a careful weighing of risks in frail patients with dementia. Even if there is some resulting distress, environmental interventions may lead to sufficient reduction of the distress without necessarily eliminating the symptom. We cared for one patient who got very upset whenever a caregiver sat next to her. This led to anger, yelling, and occasional hitting. Careful investigation revealed that the patient believed that her mother was sitting next to her and that the caregiver was sitting next to her mother. The solution to the problem was for the caregiver to approach the patient and ask if her mother was sitting next to her. If the patient answered "yes," the caregiver avoided using the chair in which the mother was "sitting." As a result, the patient no longer became distressed, although she remained delusional about her mother's presence.

Specific classes of medicines are appropriate for specific symptoms. Within each class of drugs, medicines differ by side effect profiles. Therefore, the decision on which drug to use sometimes depends on identifying side effects that can be beneficial to the patient. For example, if a depressed patient is not sleeping well, a sedating antidepressant may be chosen to treat the depression and to improve sleep. On the other hand, potential side effects may direct the clinician away from certain drugs. Antidepressants that cause a drop in blood pressure are usually not the first choice to treat patients who are at high risk of falling or are prone to orthostatic hypotension—for example, those with PD.

Once the choice of a target symptom and a medication has been made, the clinician needs a method of deciding if the medication is actually alleviating the symptom and how long to wait before deciding that the medication is not working.

Once a benefit has been established, it is necessary to decide how long the patient should remain on the medication. Few studies help clinicians decide when to decrease or discontinue a medication that has helped a patient. A general guideline is that a trial off a medication should be attempted 6 months after remission of the symptoms for which it was started. However, the progression of the brain disease that is causing the dementia, the development of other illnesses, and the possibility of adverse effects suggest that clinicians should regularly reconsider whether a medication that has previously helped should be continued.

INDICATIONS FOR THE USE OF MEDICATIONS IN DEMENTIA PATIENTS

Medications are indicated for one of three reasons:

1. *For reversal or stabilization of the underlying disease.* This includes complete reversal of the disease and its symptoms ("cure") or the arrest of disease progression without reversal of the damage that has already occurred. These therapies generally require an understanding of the pathophysiology of the disease causing the dementia. Treatments that stop the spread or amplification of the disease—for example, those that block inflammation and excitotoxicity—are included in this category.
2. *To improve cognitive symptomatology.* This requires an understanding of how cognitive symptoms arise and currently involves manipulation of neurotransmitter systems.
3. *As treatments for noncognitive neuropsychiatric symptoms associated with dementia.* This includes treatments for these symptoms, most of which have been developed without a clear understanding of their pathophysiology.

TREATING THE UNDERLYING DISEASE

The development of disease treatments depends upon the identification of the primary or contributing cause of the dementia syndrome. The ideal treatment would arrest the disease and lead to a full recovery. Examples include the use of vitamin B_{12} to eliminate this deficiency, the replacement of thyroxine in hypothyroidism, and the antibiotic treatment of a chronic central nervous system infection. When significant neuronal damage has occurred, however, treatments often arrest the underlying pathophysiology but do not reverse the dementia. Replacing vitamin B_{12} in pernicious anemia, surgically removing a subdural hematoma, or placing a shunt to reduce intercranial pressure for NPH are common examples of therapies that often lead to partial recovery.

It is important for clinicians to search for such underlying causes of dementia, which in the past were referred to as the *treatable* dementias. However, such underlying causes are rarely discovered, and most of the time they co-occur with another cause of dementia and are often a consequence of the other dementia. For example, in our experience, most dementia patients with mild hypothyroidism or mild vitamin B_{12} deficiency actually have AD and have not been eating well or taking previously prescribed thyroid supplements. Correction of the metabolic deficit is necessary and may help ameliorate some symptoms, but it is unlikely to significantly improve the cognitive symptoms of dementia. It is extremely uncommon to come across a case of dementia caused entirely by such a treatable cause, and even then, full reversal of the dementia is not likely after significant brain damage has occurred, even if stabilization is possible. Thus, the term *treatable dementia* is almost never appropriate.

Reduction of risk factors is another strategy that can slow the progression of the disease but not necessarily reverse it. The best example of this is stroke, where the presumed pathophysiology involves loss of the blood supply to select areas of the brain. Improving the blood supply to the brain by stabilizing atrial fibrillation, reducing serum cholesterol, surgically removing sources of emboli by carotid endarterectomy, or lessening the risk of blood clot formations by anticoagulation with warfarin or aspirin slows the progression of vascular dementia. Presumably, these treatments reduce the progression (or development) of multi-infarct dementia. Some early clinical trial data also suggest that cholinesterase inhibitors, if introduced after stroke, may reduce the likelihood that cognitive decline will develop or worsen in the future. We consider this evidence preliminary. Similarly, there appears to be an increased risk of cognitive decline many years after coronary artery bypass surgery. The mechanisms of this decline are not well understood but may well involve brain vascular disease. At present, there are no good preventive treatments for this condition, even though cholinesterase inhibitors and other "anti-dementia" drugs are being studied for that purpose.

Disease treatments for Alzheimer dementia

Figure 10.1 presents a conceptual model of our current understanding of the pathophysiology of AD. This is presented to set the context for the use of current treatments for AD and also for efforts to develop new treatments. As articulated in Chapter 3, the processing of APP via the beta secretase pathway is more likely to lead to monomers of beta-amyloid 1–42. These are more likely to oligomerize and form insoluble deposits referred to as *beta-amyloid plaques*. Both the oligomers and the plaques, through mechanisms that probably involve microglial activation and other unknown processes, lead to synaptic failure, neuronal injury, and apoptotic neuronal death. The loss of neuronal systems leads to the loss of multiple neurotransmitters, which in turn lead to the emergence of the cognitive, functional, and neuropsychiatric symptoms of the disease. This process occurs over years, perhaps even decades, before the onset of symptoms.

If the amyloid hypothesis is correct, the ideal therapy for AD would be one that either prevents the deposition of beta-amyloid 1–42 or that prevents the synaptic and neuronal damage caused by amyloid. Several treatments along these lines are in development, some in early human trial phases. The most promising are medications that diminish the production of the toxic, insoluble forms of beta-amyloid (see Chapter 3), including inhibitors of beta or gamma secretase, and *immunotherapies,* both passive and active, that are intended to remove beta-amyloid from the brain. One effort at active immunotherapy with a beta-amyloid "vaccine" showed good evidence of efficacy in transgenic mouse models of AD, and some evidence of efficacy in early human trials, before it was stopped because of the development of encephalitis in 5% of patients treated, likely due to immune cross-reactivity with parts of the vaccine molecule. Nevertheless, immunotherapy continues to have promise and to be tested. Ultimately, the best test of the amyloid hypothesis will be in patients with AD. One of the possible outcomes is that amyloid therapies will succeed in clearing brain amyloid but that this may not lead to clinical improvement, either because the therapy is delivered when neuronal damage is irreversible or because the hypothesis is incorrect.

In addition to directly targeting amyloid deposition or clearance, several factors have been identified as accelerators of the Alzheimer cascade, some of which are being considered as targets of therapy:

- Postmenopausal loss of estrogen
- Inflammatory response
- Oxidative free radicals

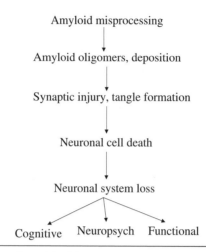

FIGURE 10.1 Conceptual model of the etiopathogenesis of Alzheimer disease.

- Vascular disease
- Glutamate excitoxocity
- Late-life depression

Estrogen replacement, with and without progesterone, has been studied extensively as a treatment for or preventive of Alzheimer dementia. While epidemiologic studies and early clinical trials were promising, several definitive trials have concluded that estrogen replacement does not attenuate dementia progression and in fact may increase the risk of dementia *if it is started* after age 65. There is some suggestion from epidemiologic studies that estrogen replacement for a 5- to 10-year period soon after menopause may delay or prevent the onset of Alzheimer dementia decades later, but this hypothesis will be very difficult to test. For now, estrogen is not an appropriate therapy for AD.

The association of brain inflammation with AD has led to several tests of the hypothesis that *anti-inflammatory treatment* may delay the progression of Alzheimer dementia. Nonsteroidal anti-inflammatory agents (NSAIDs) such as ibuprofen and indomethacin have been associated with a lower risk of developing AD in several epidemiologic studies. However, there is a long-term risk of gastrointestinal bleeding and renal disease, and more recently there is evidence that NSAIDs are associated with uncommon cardiovascular toxicity, such as heart attack and stroke. Also, the proper dosing of these agents for AD is not known. Thus far, trials of prednisone and several NSAIDs have conclusively shown that after the onset of dementia and in the context of MCI (see Chapter 11), anti-inflammatory treatments are not effective. At present, these agents are not recommended for the treatment of AD and should not be used for this purpose. This also applies to the newer Cox-2 inhibitors in this class, such as celecoxib. There continues to be reason to believe that NSAIDs may have a role in the prevention of AD dementia by treating the brain disease before enough damage has occurred to lead to symptoms, but a large-scale National Institutes of Health (NIH)–funded clinical trial studying their use for the prevention of AD was discontinued because of safety concerns.

The association of oxygen free radicals with AD dementia has raised the question of whether *antioxidant therapy* in AD is warranted. The epidemiologic evidence now supports the concept that vitamin E in doses of about 400 IU/day, perhaps in combination with vitamin C at 500 mg/day, may prevent AD. In addition, one randomized trial suggests that high-dose vitamin E, 2000 IU/day, might delay the progression of functional decline in the disease. The trial, however, had methodologic weaknesses that made its findings less compelling. The use of vitamin E is tempered by recent findings that vitamin E therapy did not delay progression of MCI, a putative clinical precursor of Alzheimer dementia (see Chapter 11), and by findings from a meta-analysis, with its own methodologic weaknesses, that vitamin E in very high doses increased mortality in older people. From our point of view, vitamin E is still an option to be considered in doses on the order of 1000 IU/day with the appropriate cautions and disclosures regarding a possible increase in mortality risk. Similarly, the over-the-counter antioxidant ginkgo biloba, and its putative active form, EGB, in doses of 120 mg/day or higher, may have some efficacy in treating dementia, as some trials suggest. However, the effect is likely to be small, and safety concerns have been raised about the use of over-the-counter substances for long time periods in the absence of extensive testing or careful manufacturing oversight for purity. Therefore, in general, we do not recommend the use of ginkgo biloba, but at the same time do not strongly discourage patients who wish to take it.

There is now strong evidence that *brain vascular disease* plays a role in the progression of Alzheimer dementia in two ways. First, brain vascular disease may add to the cognitive impairment of dementia for a given amount of Alzheimer pathology in the brain. This should be no surprise since two pathologic processes would be expected to worsen the clinical syndrome of dementia. Second, brain vascular disease has been implicated as a factor in the development of the Alzheimer pathology, perhaps by accelerating amyloid deposition and by increasing amyloid toxicity to synapses or neurons. Therefore, the management of vascular brain disease and its associated risk factors is now part of the disease treatment for AD in certain groups of patients. Control of blood pressure, especially maintaining systolic pressure below 140 mmHg, has been shown in one clinical trial to be associated with less rapid dementia progression. Treatment of hypercholesterolemia, homo-cysteinemia, and hyperglycemia are other aspects of this approach. There-fore, the treatment of dementia patients should include monitoring of blood pressure, glucose, cholesterol, and homocysteine and the initiation or modi-fication of appropriate interventions when indicated.

Glutamate excitotoxicity has been implicated in the etiopathogenesis of AD. Under certain conditions, injured or dying glutamate-producing neurons will release large amounts of glutamate in their synaptic clefts, leading to toxicity and death in the downstream neurons of their synaptic connections. This process is believed to involve the activation of calcium channels by glu-tamate followed by rapid influx of calcium into the downstream neurons. The hypothesis here is that this mechanism is involved in the progression of AD pathology, particularly its spread through the brain into geographically disparate but synaptically connected regions. Medications that interfere with glutamate effects on its receptors are being tested as ways of delaying the progression of AD. One medication whose putative memantibe of action targets the glutamatergic system is memantine (Namenda), now approved for marketing in the United States for the treatment of moderate to severe AD. Memantine exerts its effects at N-methye-D-aspartate (NMDA) recep-tors of glutamate through uncompetitive blockade: the binding site is acces-sible only if the receptor is activated. Memantine blocks glutamate-activated ions, including calcium currents through the NMDA receptor, which itself is an ion channel. Several clinical trials have reported that memantine slightly delays the progression of Alzheimer dementia, primarily with effects on cog-nition and functioning. There is also evidence that memantine reduces care-giving time in more advanced dementia. Safety data so far are very good, with the most common side effects being dizziness, headaches, and agitation in about 5% of patients. There is also clinical trial evidence to suggest that memantine can be administered safely with cholinesterase inhibitors such as donepezil (discussed later in this chapter).

Most memory experts now recommend memantine to their patients and their families, especially in moderate to severe dementia. It is often used in combination with cholinesterase inhibitors and sometimes with vitamin E. The starting dose is 5 mg in the morning; this is increased by 5 mg/week to a full dose of 10 mg bid after about a month if it is well tolerated. The titration is facilitated by a titration pack made available by the manufacturer through local pharmacists. Once memantine is started, and assuming that it is well tolerated, clinicians often face the problem of deciding whether it is helpful to a given patient. Clinical trial data suggest that about 15% of patients will show improvement on memantine, with most of this improvement being above and beyond a placebo response; 85% of patients do not improve, but may show a reduction in cognitive or functional decline. Physicians and other clinicians must be prepared for this quandary and must also prepare patients and families for it. The decision to continue or stop memantine should be tailored to each patient's situation. A discontinuation trial is often a good idea to help determine if there is continued benefit from this treatment.

Late-life depression, particularly the nonclassic depressive syndrome sometimes referred to as *depression without sadness*, where anhedonia and irritability are prominent, has been associated with a higher risk of cognitive decline and dementia. Patients with late-life depression who have no current cognitive symptoms have a 10% risk of developing dementia in the next 3 years in one study; this risk increases to over 30% if they have some cognitive symptoms. The mechanisms underlying this association are actively being investigated, but a detailed discussion is beyond the purview of this chapter. Treatment of depression in late life with antidepressants, a major public health priority in its own right, has been shown to reduce symptoms of depression, but it is less effective in treating cognitive symptoms or in alleviating the dementia risk years later. However, such treatment may reduce functional decline after the onset of dementia. The identification and treatment of depression in dementia is an important part of dementia care and may in fact be part of disease treatment.

TREATMENT OF COGNITIVE SYMPTOMATOLOGY

Agents that increase levels of the brain neurotransmitter acetylcholine (ACh) improve memory and other cognitive symptoms. They may also stabilize or prevent the onset of milder noncognitive neuropsychiatric or behavioral symptoms, although their use as exclusive agents for the more severe forms of the latter symptoms is not supported by data and is not recommended. Several lines of evidence suggest that (ACh) neurotransmission is important to the normal functioning of memory. Inhibitors of ACh, such as atropine, or diseases that reduce ACh levels, such as AD, lead to memory loss.

Approaches taken to increase ACh levels in diseased brains include increasing production by providing the building blocks, or chemical precursors, directly stimulating the ACh receptor, and delaying breakdown of the ACh that is naturally produced. It is not possible to give ACh choline directly because it is very short-lived.

Acetylcholine precursors, such as choline and lecithin, are taken up by brain neurons to make more ACh. They are not effective in the treatment of memory disorder or AD, however. Direct stimulation of cholinergic postsynaptic receptors (through nicotinic and muscarinic agonists) is still under investigation but does not appear too promising, due both to safety concerns and to limited efficacy.

The most successful approach has been to reduce the naturally occurring degradation (breakdown) of ACh. Acetylcholine is normally degraded through an enzyme known as *acetylcholinesterase* (AChE), which floats outside neuronal cells in brain tissue. Inhibition of AChE results in increased ACh levels because of reduced degradation.

Four drugs—tacrine (Cognex), donepezil (Aricept), rivastigmine (Excelon), and galantamine (Razadyne)—have been approved by the Food and Drug Administration (FDA) for the treatment of AD. In addition, huperzine-A, an over-the-counter *nutriceutical,* has been shown to have cholinesterase activity and has efficacy as a treatment of the cognitive symptoms of AD in some clinical trials. However, huperzine-A has not been adequately tested for this purpose and, given the availability of alternative agents, is not high on the list of possible treatments.

Of the four FDA-approved cholinesterase inhibitors, tacrine should not be used, given the alternatives, its complex titration, and the associated risk of hepatic toxicity. The other three drugs seem similar in efficacy. They all appear to improve cognitive symptoms modestly in 15%–20% of patients and sometimes quite notably. In addition, they have functional benefits and may also delay the emergence of behavioral symptoms or reduce their severity. The evidence does not support their use as single agents to treat more severe neuropsychiatric or behavioral symptoms such as depression or delusions. Two exceptions may be apathy and visual hallucinations (see Chapter 8). The effect of these agents on the long-term progression of dementia has not been shown conclusively. Some studies suggest that they may reduce long-term cognitive or functional decline, but these studies are flawed due to high levels of dropout and the use of historical untreated comparison groups. One brain imaging study, part of a clinical trial, suggests that these drugs may have biologic effects on the size of the hippocampus or on the integrity of hippocampal neurons. In the absence of replication or a better understanding of the imaging measures involved, these data are not conclusive. At present, the efficacy of these agents is limited and in most patients may not extend much past 1–2 years after starting treatment. However, in our experience, some patients who respond well to them seem to have long-term benefits that warrant long-term treatment into more advanced dementia stages.

The mechanism of action of some cholinesterase medications has been shown in some cases to be broader than was once believed. Rivastigmine is also an inhibitor of butyrl cholinesterase, which may be more important in the degradation of ACh in later dementia. Galantamine is also an allosteric modulator of the nicotinic receptors. Both of these additional mechanisms of action may play a role in the pharmacology of these agents, but their clinical relevance has not been shown conclusively.

The practicality of the use of cholinesterase inhibitors in dementia is largely a matter of opinion since clinical trials that answer day-to-day clinical questions about their use have not been carried out. In this light, we offer our own recommendation, shown in Figure 10.2. As the figure shows, our preferred approach involves sequential use of these agents with careful monitoring for benefit. In general, we recommend them to all of our patients. This recommendation is based on a careful discussion of the pros and cons of their use with patients and involved family members. We make an effort not to raise expectations, and indicate that often it may become necessary to do a trial off a medication if there is no convincing evidence of a clinical response.

Based on our interpretation of the data to date, the risk–benefit ratio supports offering these agents for the treatment of mild to moderate AD. In addition, patients with DLB (Chapter 3) will likely benefit, as will patients with vascular dementia (Chapter 4), many of whom also have Alzheimer pathology. The use of these agents in more advanced dementia is less well supported by clinical trial data, but the benefits of their use probably outweigh the risks in patients with MMSE scores in the 5–10 range who are not very frail and have never been on them before.

In light of their comparability in efficacy for cognitive and functional symptoms, our first-, second-, and third-line choices among these agents are driven primarily by ease of use, dosing frequency, and side effect profile. Donepezil is used once a day and can be titrated to the maximal dose after 30 days of treatment, starting at 5 mg and increasing to 10 mg a month later. It also seems to have the best side effect profile from the point of view of gastrointestinal (GI) symptoms. Galantamine is used twice a day and requires a 3- to 4-month titration to the maximal effective dose. It is started at 4 mg twice daily, which is increased to 8 mg and then 12 mg twice daily over 3 months. In patients who tolerate it well, it can be increased to 16 mg twice daily if they fail to show a clear benefit on a lower dose. Galantamine has an intermediate side effect profile. Rivastigmine is started at 1.5 mg twice daily and increased to 3 mg and then 4.5 mg, the effective dose of 6 mg twice daily every month. In our experience, it is the least well tolerated of the three from the point of view of GI symptoms.

When patients are placed on a cholinesterase inhibitor, the clinical response should be rated by at least one and preferably several of the following: (1) a measure of cognition, such as the MMSE; (2) a measure of overall functioning, such as a clinical global impression (CGI) or an ADL scale; (3) a specific memory examination; and (4) the considered opinion of one or more caregivers who know the patient well. It is useful to discuss with caregivers a functional loss that occurred most recently (e.g., the patient no longer can set the table for dinner) and then see if treatment is followed by recovery of that function, which would be a strong indication of benefit. If no improvement is evident after 6 months, a trial period off the medication is indicated.

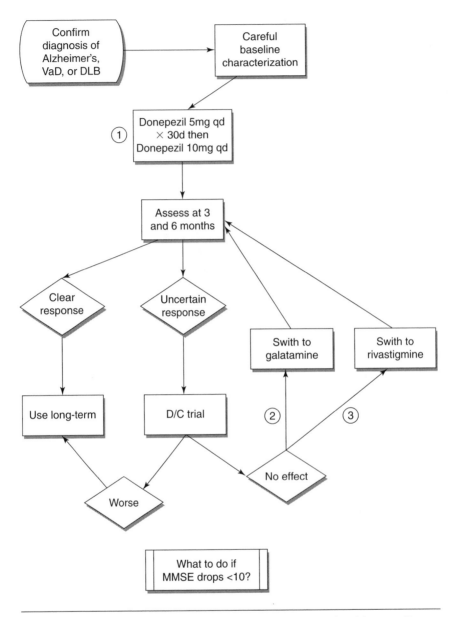

FIGURE 10.2 Use of cholinesterase inhibitors in patients with Alzheimer disease. D/C, discontinue; DLB, dementia with Lewy bodies; MMSE, Mini-Mental State Examination; VaD, vascular dementia.

Trials off carry the risk of accelerated decline and thus should be accompanied by careful monitoring by the caregiver at home and rapid return to using the medication if a rapid or even modest decline becomes evident. For many patients, use of these drugs induces a marginal improvement and then an apparent plateau or decline that is sustained for 6–12 months, which is an acceptable benefit. However, other patients have a clear response by all criteria. In one of our patients the MMSE increased by 7 points after treatment with donepezil. One of the advantages of trials off is that patients who do not benefit from one cholinesterase inhibitor will sometimes benefit from a different one. One of our most dramatic experiences, although surely a very rare patient, showed 3- to 7-point increases on the MMSE every time she went on one of four sequential cholinesterase inhibitors, even after showing MMSE declines while on an agent for many months. For safety reasons, mostly due to concerns about cardiac effects, the above cholinesterase inhibitors should not be used in combination with one another, or in combination with physostigmine or edrophonium (Tensilon), which are also cholinesterase inhibitors used to treat myasthenia gravis.

The most common side effects of cholinesterase inhibitors reflect increased central and peripheral cholinergic activity. The most common one is GI upset. All three drugs cause increased acid secretion in the stomach (because they increase ACh levels there). Nausea, vomiting, increased bowel motility, and diarrhea are also reported in many patients. In more advanced dementia, the GI symptoms often manifest as refusal to eat or weight loss, to which clinicians must be alert. Less commonly, they cause muscle cramps, bradycardia, or exacerbations of asthma.

TREATMENT OF NONCOGNITIVE NEUROPSYCHIATRIC SYMPTOMS

Autopsy studies suggest that damage to specific groups of brain cells and neurotransmitter systems is involved in the development of several disturbances in dementia. The best evidence relates decreased neuronal counts in the locus ceruleus to depression in AD, the primary source of brain norepinephrine, and the dorsal raphe nuclei, the primary source of brain serotonin. These areas may also be affected in clinical depression not associated with AD or other neurologic conditions. Antidepressant medications that act to increase norepinephrine or serotonin levels at these nuclei are theoretically likely to improve depressive symptomatology. Placebo-controlled trials have demonstrated that citalopram and sertraline, antidepressants that primarily affect the serotonin system, can reduce the depressive syndrome of AD. Another study found that amitriptyline, an antidepressant that primarily affects the norepinephrine system, is as effective as fluoxetine in treating depression associated with AD. This suggests that medications that augment either the serotonergic system or the noradrenergic system (or both) are likely to diminish depressive symptomatology. Three studies have shown that depression after stroke responds to nortriptyline, suggesting that depression occurring in vascular dementia is amenable to therapy.

In autopsy data, delusions and hallucinations in AD have been associated with relative preservation of the dopamine system in light of cholinergic system loss in the course of widespread damage to the brain. This suggests that an imbalance in the dopaminergic and cholinergic systems may be responsible for the development of these symptoms in some cases. It should be no surprise that delusions and hallucinations respond to medications that are thought to work by blocking brain receptors of dopamine. Drugs that block dopamine receptors have been shown to lessen psychotic symptoms (hallucinations and delusions) and physical aggression.

Despite these suggestive links between brain pathology and specific mood and behavioral symptoms, most of the treatment of noncognitive symptoms is based on clinical observation because the number of randomized, controlled treatment studies is small. Therefore, the decision about which medication to use is most often based on treatment success for the same symptom in another condition.

The remainder of this chapter will focus on these different classes of medications, indications for their use in treating the noncognitive symptoms of dementia, a discussion of how to use them, and an overview of their side effects and how to monitor them. Chapters 6, 8, and 9 discuss how to fit medication use into the overall plan of dementia care.

SPECIFIC MEDICATIONS

Antipsychotic medications

These were developed for the treatment of schizophrenia and other psychotic disorders. Antipsychotics are best thought of in two groups: the older typical or classical antipsychotics, such as haloperidol, thioridazine, or chlorpromazine, and the newer *atypical agents* such as olanzapine, risperidone, quetiapine, aripiprazole, ziprasidone, or clozapine. The typical agents all share the property of blocking dopamine receptors in the brain. For the most part, they are nonselective dopamine blockers, meaning that they block several subtypes of dopamine receptors. This may explain their side effects profiles since not all types of dopamine receptors are involved in the development of delusions or hallucinations. The atypical agents are more selective blockers of the D_2-dopamine receptors most closely associated with delusions and hallucinations and therefore tend to have fewer motors side effects. In addition, some of the atypicals have broader effects on the dopamine system (e.g., aripiprazole is a partial agonist of some dopamine receptors) whose clinical effect is uncertain. Atypicals are also antagonists of the serotonin 5-hydroxytriptamine-2 (5HT-2) receptors. The latter may explain some of their broader spectrum of clinical benefits in schizophrenia, against the *negative symptoms* of that condition, as well as their efficacy in mood disorders such as bipolar disorder.

Several lines of evidence suggest that antipsychotic agents are good treatments for delusions, hallucinations, or the agitation associated with AD, particularly if the delusions and hallucinations are leading to troublesome behaviors such as physical aggression. Several published, placebo-controlled, masked clinical trials demonstrate that, despite notable improvements in the placebo-treated groups, all atypicals have at least modest efficacy in treating these symptoms. However, it is not always possible to determine whether a patient with dementia, particularly in the later stages, is experiencing a delusion or a hallucination. Therefore, it is appropriate, at times, to consider using an antipsychotic agent for patients in later stages of dementia, who are aggressive, noisy, or intrusive, even if a specific delusion or hallucination cannot be elicited in the mental status examination or by the history.

The choice of antipsychotic medication is based primarily on the side effect profile since clinical trials suggest that all antipsychotic agents have comparable efficacy in treating delusions and hallucinations. However, at the time of this writing, no clinical trials have been published that compare the efficacy of different antipsychotics. The National Institute of Mental Health (NIMH) Clinical Antipsychotic Trial of Intervention Effectiveness (CATIE) study, initial results of which should be available in 2006, will provide such data on the comparative efficacy of atypical antipsychotics for psychosis or agitation in people with AD.

Clozapine, aripiprazole, and quetiapine deserve special mention since they are least likely to cause motor and extrapyramidal side effects and are thus especially useful in patients who suffer from PD or DLB. Typical antipsychotics and most other atypicals can severly worsen parkinsonism in these patients, and in fact can lead to very severe motor lock in DLB. The use of typicals in LBD patients has been associated with increased mortality, so they are relatively contraindicated for these patients. Therefore, quetiapine, aripiprazole, and clozapine are preferred for treating delusions and hallucinations in patients with these illnesses. While clozapine is not known to cause tardive dyskinesia, it is associated with a risk of bone marrow suppression in 2–4 per 1000 individuals. Therefore, regular, sometimes weekly, monitoring of white blood cell counts is necessary for several months and every-other-week monitoring thereafter. Therefore, quetiapine or aripiprazole are the first-line agents if an antipsychotic is indicated.

Antipsychotic medications differ in potency, that is, their effect per milligram, probably because these agents have different affinities (*stickiness*) for brain dopamine receptors. Higher-potency agents bind more tightly to dopamine receptors than lower-potency agents, resulting in the need for a smaller dosage.

The side effect profiles of antipsychotic medications also depend on their actions at multiple neurotransmitter receptors, including those that regulate movement, blood pressure, heart rate, and body temperature, as well as those that affect nausea and appetite. All antipsychotic medications can cause extrapyramidal side effects: parkinsonian features (tremor, stiffness, slowness, shuffling gait), dystonias (sudden, persistent contractions of muscles), and akathisia (a feeling of restlessness often manifesting as an inability to sit still). Most antipsychotics increase appetite and impair the ability to regulate body temperature. As a result, temperature extremes are especially dangerous. This class of medications also blocks ACh receptors in the brain and in the rest of the body, resulting in dry mouth, blurred vision, urinary retention, and constipation. Anticholinergic blockade is of particular concern in patients with dementia since it can worsen memory and other cognitive functions.

The blockade of ACh and histamine receptors causes sedation. This can be beneficial in patients with dementia who have a sleep disturbance, but because of their other side effects, antipsychotics should not be prescribed if sleep difficulty is the only problem. Blockade of norepinephrine receptors can lead to hypotension, particularly orthostatic hypotension. Orthostasis is of particular concern in patients with dementia who are debilitated since it can lead to falls and serious injuries.

Of note is that recent reanalyses of some of the clinical trials of atypical drugs in dementia have raised concerns about the cerebrovascular risks of atypical antipsychotics. This has led to FDA-issued warnings about this problem. The most recent data demonstrate an elevated mortality risk with *all* antipsychotics. Clinicians who choose to prescribe atypical antipsychotics for dementia patients should be aware of this small increased risk of cerebrovascular events and death from other causes. This risk may be especially increased in patients who already have evidence of brain vascular disease by history or on brain imaging. Thus, clinicians should carefully evaluate the risk/benefit ratio whenever considering the use of drugs in this class. Nevertheless, this risk remains low; therefore, we believe that clinicians can and should use atypical antipsychotics, with proper risk disclosure to patients and families, if a clinical indication for their use is present.

Less common side effects of atypical antipsychotics include skin rash, inflammation of the liver, and seizures (because these agents lower the seizure threshold). Rarely, patients develop a life-threatening complication called *neuroleptic malignant syndrome*, which is characterized by high fever, stiffness, and delirium.

Long-term use of drugs that block dopamine receptors can lead to the development of tardive dyskinesia (TD), a risk that is increased in older people. The risk of TD is much lower with the atypical antipsychotics compared to the typical agents. Tardive dyskinesia is characterized by involuntary movements most commonly affecting the face, cheeks, and tongue but also involving the limbs and trunk. Tardive dyskinesia is irreversible in 50% of individuals and can at times be quite disfiguring. It is often first noticed when the dose of the antipsychotic agent is lowered or discontinued. Therefore, the continued use of an antipsychotic agent should be based on a careful assessment of its benefits and risks. If TD develops, neuroleptics should be continued only if there is no alternative, if the benefits achieved are substantial, and if the risk of harm that would result from not taking the drug is significant. Such a decision should involve careful discussion with the patient and other decision makers who represent the patient.

Table 10.1 lists the common side effects of the different classes of antipsychotic agents. Higher-potency agents are more likely to cause extrapyramidal side effects and less likely to cause anticholinergic side effects. The reverse is true for lower-potency agents, but these have a higher propensity to induce hypotension. Atypical agents are listed separately because they have different receptor site blockage profiles. Before starting an antipsychotic, the clinician should assess the patient for symptoms of parkinsonism. The assessment should be repeated regularly, especially within the week of dose increases. When treating a patient with dementia with an antipsychotic agent (for indications with specific behavior problems, see Chapter 8), we typically choose quetiapine, risperidone, olanzapine, or aripiprazole. Typical agents are generally second line in this group of very frail patients because of their more serious side effect profiles.

The starting dose for quetiapine is either 12.5 or 25 mg at bedtime or a few hours before the symptoms are most prominent (e.g., noontime for late afternoon symptoms). The lower dose is preferred for more frail patients and for patients with PD or dementia with Lewy bodies. The dose can be increased rapidly as tolerated. The clinician should keep in mind that a total daily dose of quetiapine as high as 150–200 mg may be needed to fully treat delusions, hallucinations, or agitation in patients with dementia. Such doses can be well tolerated if the titration up is careful and the patients are closely monitored. Quetiapine is not available in an injectable, liquid, or rapid-action oral formulation.

Aripiprazole is started at 2.5 or 5 mg daily. Risperidone and olanzapine

Table 10.1. Antipsychotic Medications and Their Side Effects

Medication	Side Effects				
	Extra-pyramidal	Anti-cholinergic	Sedation	Hypo-tension	Tardive Dyskinesia
Typical Agents					
Haloperidol (Haldol)	++++	++	+	+	Yes
Fluphenazine (Prolixin)	++++	++	+	+	Yes
Thiothixine (Navane)	+++	+++	+	+	Yes
Perphenazine (Trilafon)	+++	+++	+	+	Yes
Atypical Agents					
Quetiapine (Seroquel)	0/+	+	++	0	Rare
Olanzapine (Zyprexa)	+	++	++	+	Rare
Risperidone (Risprerdal)	++	+	+	++	Rare
Aripiprazole (Abilify)	+	+	+	+	Rare
Clozapine (Clozaril)	0/+	++	++	++	Very rare

are good alternative first-line agents. Both are available in a liquid or rapid-action oral formulation (Zyprexa Zydis; Risperdal M tabs). Olanzapine is available in a short-acting injectable and risperidone in long-acting injectable formulations. The latter allow greater flexibility in dosing for very agitated or noncompliant patients. The starting dose of risperidone is 0.25–0.5 mg/day at bedtime, depending on the patient's degree of frailty. Risperidone doses of more than 2 mg/day rarely produce greater benefit than lower doses. The starting dose of olanzapine is 1.25–2.5 mg, depending on the patient's frailty, with increases of up to 7.5 mg/day being reasonable. Higher doses are not likely to be of help except in very rare patients. Clozapine may be started at 12.5 mg/day. Doses of over 100 mg/day are rarely needed or tolerated by most individuals.

The starting dose for haloperidol or perphenazine in dementia is 0.5 mg daily in early-stage disease and 0.25 mg daily in late-stage disease. We prefer to use one of these medications when patients are sleeping well, but are very driven or are moving a lot, since the motor effects may help slow them down (caution should be exercised to be sure that the movement does not represent akathisia, a symptom that would be worsened by one of these medications). Increases of 0.5 mg/day are well tolerated, with the best response occurring in the 2–4 mg/day range. Rarely are doses higher than 10 mg/day needed.

Antidepressant agents (Table 10.2)

The major indication for the use of antidepressants in patients with dementia is the treatment of affective mood disorders such as depression. There is evolving evidence that these agents are also effective treatments for delusions or hallucinations in patients who have mood symptoms and for agitation in the context of mood symptoms. Antidepressants, particularly SSRIs, have also been used in dementia to treat obsessive-compulsive symptomatology. Anecdotal case series and clinical experience also indicate that some antidepressants, especially bupropion and the SSRIs, can diminish behaviors indicative of executive dysfunction such as social inappropriateness, unprovoked aggression, disinhibition, intrusiveness, and hyperoral/stimulus-bound behaviors. The last are more likely to occur in late-stage dementia or in all stages of fronto-temporal dementia (FTD). Trazodone has been used with some success in treating anticipatory anxiety and preventing catastrophic reactions (see the Glossary). Finally, since trazodone is highly sedating and has relatively few other side effects, its is an excellent first-line agents for mild to moderate sleep disturbance in dementia patients in whom sleep hygiene interventions have failed.

The side effect profile also guides the choice of antidepressant. Table 10.2 lists the common side effects of the four classes of antidepressant. The first are the tricyclic antidepressants and include both tertiary and secondary amines. Second are the SSRIs. Third are other agents referred to as *atypical*. Fourth are monoamine oxidase (MAO) inhibitors, which require that the patient eat a diet low in tyramine.

The mechanism of action of antidepressants is believed to be the augmentation of norepinephrine, serotonin, and/or dopamine activity. However, many agents affect other receptors, including the ACh, alpha-adrenergic and beta-adrenergic receptors; these account for many of the effects on the cardiovascular system. The *serotonergic* side effects are due to overactivity of serotonin systems and include GI side effects (nausea, stomach upset, acid hypersecretion, and diarrhea), tremor, headaches, restlessness, and insomnia. Like other medications, antidepressants carry the potential for developing rashes, liver inflammation, falls, and bone marrow suppression. Tricyclics, and to a lesser extent SSRIs and other antidepressants, lower the seizure threshold and thus increase the risk of seizure. Buproprion has been associated with a higher risk of seizures.

A *serotonin syndrome* consisting of delirium, agitation, tachycardia, and hyperthermia (high temperature) occurs at high levels of serotonergic overactivity. Anticholinergic side effects are most prevalent with tricyclics and include blurred vision, dry mouth, memory loss, constipation, and urinary re-

TABLE 10.2. Antidepressant Medications and Their Side Effects

Medication	Sero-tonergic[1]	Anti-cholinergic[2]	Sedation	Orthostatic Hypotension	Cardiac Arrhythmia
Tricyclics					
Amitriptyline (Elavil)	++	++++	+++	+++	Yes
Imipramine (Tofranil)	++	++++	+++	+++	Yes
Notriptyline (Pamelor)	++	++	+	++	Yes
Desipramine (Norpramin)	++	++	+	++	Yes
SSRIs					
Fluoxetine (Prozac)	+++	0	0/+	0	Rare
Sertaline (Zoloft)	+++	0	0/+	0	Rare
Citalopram (Celexa)	+++	0	0	0	Rare
Escitalopram (Lexapro)	+++	0	0	0	Rare
Paroxetine (Paxil)	+++	+	+	0	Rare
Atypical Agents					
Venlafaxine (Effexor)	++	+	+	Increased blood pressure	Yes
Trazodone (Desyrel)	+	+	+++	0/+	Rare
Buproprion (Wellbutrin)	0/+	0	0	Increased blood pressure	Rare
Mirtazapine (Remeron)	++	++	+++	++	Rare
MAO Inhibitor					
Tranylcypromine (Parnate)	0	+++	++	+++	Rare

Side Effects

[1] Dizziness, headache, tremor, gastrointestinal upset.

[2] Blurred vision, dry mouth, constipation, urinary retention.

MAO, monoamine oxidase.

tention. Tricyclic antidepressants tend to be sedative, while SSRIs are more likely to be activating.

Tricyclics are more likely than other classes to have adverse effects on the cardiovascular system, particularly after an overdose or when levels are toxic. Arrhythmias are due to a slowing of electrical impulses conducted through the heart. The overdose risk is of particular concern with the use of antidepressants since patients who are prescribed them are at high risk for suicide due to their mood disorder. In addition, patients with dementia are at risk for accidental overdose. Because of their cardiotoxicity, tricyclics have a higher mortality after an overdose than other classes of antidepressants.

When an antidepressant is indicated, we most often begin with a low dose of an SSRI. A recent consensus panel of dementia experts suggested that in the dementia setting, sertraline or citalopram (or its enantiomer, escitalopram) are the recommended first-line agents because they have the best available efficacy data and fewest side effects. The starting dose of sertraline is 25–50 mg/day, and that of citalopram is 10–20 mg/day (10 mg escitalopram); lower doses should be use in more frail individuals. Alternative first-line agents include fluoxetine, 10 mg (the only SSRI available as a generic), and paroxetine, 10 mg. If there is no response, the dose can be doubled in 7–10 days. Fluoxetine is best increased at 1- to 2-week intervals due to its long half-life.

The Depression in Alzheimer's Disease Study (DIADS), a randomized clinical trial, has shown that 100–125 mg sertraline may be needed for maximal efficacy. This dose is twice that commonly prescribed in primary care to older patients. This finding leads us to increase the dosage to this level, if safe, before considering alternative drugs or treatments. If the patient's mood begins to improve, the dose should not be increased until the patient shows a plateau in improvement but has not returned to baseline. Usually, a treatment a response, if any, will be evident by 4 weeks. It is reasonable to switch treatment approaches if no benefit has been seen. However, it may take 2 months for the maximum benefit to be reached. Therefore, an antidepressant should be increased to the maximum dose and continued for 6–8 weeks before it is considered a treatment failure. Peak doses of these agents in dementia patients are: sertraline 200 mg/day; citalopram 40 mg/day; escitalopram, 20 mg/day; paroxetine, 50 mg/day; and fluoxetine, 60 mg/day.

Starting doses of second-line agents include venlafaxine, 25 mg bid (peak, 350 mg/day); bupropion, 75 mg/day (peak, 350 mg/day); nortriptyline, 10 mg at bedtime (increased to a blood level of 100–150 mg/dl); and mirtazapine, 7.5–15 mg at bedtime.

Trials of several different antidepressants may be needed before an effective agent is found. We rarely prescribe more than one antidepressant in patients with dementia. If tricyclics are to be used, an electrocardiogram should be checked prior to their prescription. If heart block or conduction delay is present or develops, tricyclics should be avoided or discontinued if possible.

Mood stabilizers

Mood stabilizers are a diverse group of agents that putatively share the ability to stabilize fluctuations in mood. They are effective treatments for mania or hypomania and appear to have efficacy for explosiveness, irritability, violence, noisiness, disinhibition and *frontal* behaviors, now referred to as the *executive dysfunction syndrome*. Several, such as divalproex sodium and carbamazepine, are also excellent anticonvulsants and are most useful in stabilizing mood or irritability in the context of a seizure disorder or brain injury from trauma or stroke.

Divalproex sodium (DVS)

Originally developed as an anticonvulsant, divalproex sodium (DVS) is an effective treatment for bipolar disorder and is considered by some to be a first-line agent for the treatment of mania. Its efficacy for mania generalizes to manic and hypomanic-like syndromes associated with dementia. Two randomized trials and several care series support its efficacy in treating explosive behaviors in nursing home patients with dementia, although the trials have significant methodologic weaknesses. Its side effects include sedation, nausea, gait instability, confusion, poor coordination, falls, and, with high doses, delirium and somnolence. It can cause liver inflammation, aplastic anemia, and other hematologic abnormalities. Divalproex sodium is less likely than carbamazepine to cause a rash. A blood level of 50–100 ng/dl is considered to be the therapeutic range. Typically, DVS is started at 125 mg po once a day in late dementia or twice a day in early disease. Liver tests should be performed weekly when the drug is started. If there is no benefit, the dose can be increased by 125 mg po daily every 2–7 days with blood level monitoring. If there is no improvement 2–3 weeks after the peak dose is reached, a different medication should be considered.

Carbamazepine

Originally developed as an anticonvulsant, carbamazepine is an effective antimanic agent that can stabilize mood and may reduce the recurrence of depression and mania in bipolar mood disorder. It may be particularly useful in patients who are *rapidly cycling*. In dementia, one randomized, placebo-controlled trial and anecdotal evidence suggest that it is efficacious in patients who are aggressive and agitated. Its benefit in treating explosiveness and irritability is less well established. Its main side effects are gait instability, skin rash, sedation, slurred speech, poor coordination, falls, and tremors. Other toxic symptoms include a drunken-like state and delirium. Carbamazepine can suppress the bone marrow, causing aplastic anemia and/or granulocytopenia. Careful monitoring of hematologic parameters is important in the early phases of carbamazepine treatment. Carbamazepine can also cause liver toxicity. This necessitates monitoring of liver tests early in treatment.

Before starting carbamazepine, a complete blood count should be obtained at a baseline. In elderly patients with dementia, carbamazepine is usually started at 100 mg orally once or twice a day. Gait should be closely monitored as the dose is increased by 100 mg/day at 2- to 7-day intervals until a response occurs, toxicity develops, or blood levels reach the 5–10 ng/dl range (at which therapeutic efficacy is most likely to occur). If there is no response 2–3 weeks after the peak dose is achieved, another agent should be considered.

Lithium carbonate

Lithium carbonate has been the mainstay treatment of mania and hypomania for 35 years and is used when manic-like symptoms appear in the context of dementia. Lithium may also have efficacy in the treatment of irritability and explosiveness in late-stage dementia. Lithium has antidepressant properties as well, particularly when added to a standard antidepressant that has been partially effective. At times it is used in combination with other agents such as antipsychotics, carbamazepine, or valproic acid. However, combined use with other drugs should be undertaken with extreme caution because of the risk of delirium.

Lithium is said to have a low therapeutic index. This means that the difference between a therapeutic dose and a toxic dose is small. Even at therapeutic levels, lithium often causes tremor, gait unsteadiness, sedation, and increased appetite. Lithium carbonate can cause diabetes insipidus, a disorder of the kidneys that results in an inability to concentrate urine. This leads to symptoms of large, frequent urination (polyuria) and drinking large amounts of liquid (polydipsia). Since lithium can suppress production of thyroid hormones and affect kidney functioning, careful monitoring of serum creatinine and thyroid hormone is important. Creatinine should be measured every 3–6 months in elderly patients taking lithium. Before starting lithium, serum creatinine and thyroid-stimulating hormone should be checked. In patients with dementia, lithium is started at 150 mg po daily. Five to seven days later, the serum lithium level is checked and the dose increased proportionately to the intended blood level (usually 0.2–0.5 ng/dl). This means that if the blood level is 0.2 ng/dl and the dose is doubled, the level is likely to reach 0.4 ng/dl after 6 weeks. Patients who cannot be given tablets or capsules of lithium carbonate can be given liquid lithium citrate.

Lithium should be increased cautiously because the therapeutic index is low. One advantage of lithium is the availability of blood levels that provide valuable input about whether individual doses are likely to work. An occasional elderly patient can tolerate and requires a blood level of 0.8 ng/dl, but patients with dementia frequently develop signs of toxicity when the blood level is greater than 0.5–0.6 ng/dl.

Beta blockers

Propranolol, atenolol, and other beta blockers have efficacy in treating explosive behaviors and akathisia. Propranolol has also been studied in patients with dementia in nursing homes. It can be cautiously prescribed for patients with dementia, particularly those in later disease stages, who exhibit driven behaviors, restlessness, explosiveness, and/or agitation and have not benefited from other therapies. Beta blockers are not effective treatments for mania or manic-like syndromes seen in dementia. The side effects of beta blockers include slowed heart rate, cardiac arrhythmia, low blood pressure with orthostatic changes, nausea, vomiting, rash, bronchospasm (particularly in patients with chronic lung disease), and delirium. Bone marrow suppression, liver irritation, and a lupus-like reaction have also been reported with beta blockers but are very rare.

Sedatives, anxiolytics, and other agents used for sleep

This is a diverse group of medications including chloral hydrate, zolpidem, buspirone, antihistamines (such as diphenhydramine and hydroxyzine), and benzodiazepines (such as lorazepam, oxazepam, diazepam, flurazepam, and clonazepam). These medications have been used for three general types of problems in patients with dementia: (1) sleep disturbance, particularly insomnia and sleep/wake cycle disorders, (2) agitation/aggression, and (3) and anxiety. While they appear to be most effective in dealing with sleep disorders, controlled studies of dementia-related sleep disorder have not been published. Their ability to treat agitation and anxiety in dementia (primarily anxiety as perceived by observers) is not well supported by the literature. Buspirone is reported in several case series to be effective in treating agitation and aggression, but the results of double-blind, placebo-controlled trials have not been reported.

Given the extensive risks associated with these agents, including addiction, and their high propensity for inducing pharmacologic tolerance, drugs in this category are not used as first-line agents for the treatment of agitation or anxiety. Their main use is in promoting sleep, stabilizing the sleep cycle, or providing sustained sedation for patients who would be unmanageable otherwise.

Side effects of chloral hydrate, zolpidem, and benzodiazepines fall into three general groups: worsening of the symptoms of dementia (such as amnesia, disorientation, and disinhibition), gait disorder and falls, and physical dependency. These three groups of agents have in common pharmacologic activity at the benzodiazepine receptor that promotes the actions of gamaaminobutyric acid (GABA), a major brain inhibitory neurotransmitter. This has a tranquilizing effect on the central nervous system with no appreciable effect on the respiratory or cardiovascular systems at pharmacologically active doses. In contrast, buspirone has a high affinity for one subtype of serotonin receptors and low affinity for a dopamine receptor but no affinity for benzodiazepine receptors. Its mechanism of action is unknown. It differs from the other agents discussed here by having no abuse or dependency potential.

Chloral hydrate

This agent, used in doses ranging from 500 to 2000 mg/day, is highly effective in producing sedation in patients with dementia but has fallen from favor because of its likelihood of causing daytime drowsiness and because safer agents are now available. It should be used to improve sleep or sedate patients in whom other agents cannot be used. The common side effects of chloral hydrate are sedation, blurred vision, falls, disorientation, delirium, and worsening cognition.

Antihistamines

There are many antihistamines, several of which are sold over the counter as sinus medicines or sleep aids (SleepAid, Sominex, Benadryl, and others). Diphenhydramine (Benadryl) and hydroxyzine (Vistaril, Atarax) are very occasionally prescribed for their anxiolytic and sedating properties in patients with dementia. Side effects include drowsiness, dry mouth, tremors, anticholinergic delirium, and, rarely, convulsions. Oversedation may increase the risk of falls. Given these side effects, we believe these medications should be avoided or used for only very short time periods. Diphenhydramine and hydroxyzine are started at 25 mg at bedtime and increased to 100 mg.

Benzodiazepines

For many years, this was one of the most widely prescribed classes of drugs in dementia patients because of its anxiolytic and tranquilizing effects. Individual agents are chosen on the basis of the rapidity of their onset of action and on their half-life or time until the blood level falls 50%. More rapid onset of action is beneficial for patients who have a sleep disorder. A long half-life is associated with lower abuse and dependency liability. In the short term, benzodiazepines can produce beneficial calming and sedation; in many patients with dementia, they can cause paradoxical reactions with disinhibition and a worsening of behavioral disorders. Their use for more than 4 months has not been adequately studied in any group of patients. This, coupled with the high likelihood of tolerance and dependence on these agents, makes their use in dementia risky. Adverse reactions commonly occurring at the beginning of treatment include sedation and unsteadiness. Disorientation, nausea, headaches, sleep disorder, and rash occur less frequently. Lorazepam and clonazepam are the most widely used of these agents in dementia. Their use has been encouraged by their exclusion from nursing home regulations affecting psychotherapeutic agents in the United States. Lorazepam (Ativan), 0.25–2 mg/day, is given in three or four divided doses when an intermediate half-life agent is needed, while clonazepam, 0.25–2 mg/day given once or twice a day, is preferred for its longer half-life.

Zolpidem (Ambien)

This is a nonbenzodiazepine hypnotic that also has activity at the GABA receptors. It appears to have less dependence liability than benzodiazepines. It is an effective hypnotic at doses of 5–10 mg before bedtime. Side effects include residual sedation the next day, headache, dizziness, and diarrhea.

Zalpelon (Sonata)

This is also a nonbenzodiazepine hypnotic with activity at the GABA receptors. It appears to have less dependence liability than benzodiazepines. It is an effective hypnotic at doses of 5–10 mg before bedtime. The starting dose in the elderly is 5 mg. Side effects include residual sedation the next day, headache, dizziness, nausea, and confusion.

Buspirone (Buspar)

This is an antianxiety agent whose mechanism of action is poorly understood. It has been shown to reduce the symptoms of general anxiety disorder in younger patients, and there is some evidence that it improves agitation and anxiety in patients with dementia. Its main side effects are dizziness, drowsiness, nervousness, and nausea. Diarrhea, numbness, headaches, weakness, and sweating have also been reported. The starting dose is 5 mg bid-tid. Total daily doses of 60 mg or higher appear to be safe.

Medications used to treat movement disorders seen in dementia

The most common movement disorders seen in dementia patients are parkinsonian features such as slowness, tremors, shuffling gait, and rigidity (which may be seen in AD, Lewy body dementia, and PD or as side effects of an antipsychotic agent). Dyskinesias (excess movements) such as chorea, athetosis, and myoclonus are also observed in the dementias. Parkinsonian features, caused by reductions of striatal dopamine levels or by imbalances of brain ACh/dopamine ratios, respond to agents that augment brain levels of dopamine or which reduce brain levels of ACh. Therefore, L-dopa (a precursor of dopamine), amantadine (a direct dopamine agonist), and bromocriptine (also a dopamine agonist) can be used for this purpose. Additionally, trihexyphenidyl and benzotropine are effective treatments of parkinsonian symptoms based on their anticholinergic activity.

L-dopa

This is a precursor of dopamine that acts by increasing brain levels of dopamine and parkinsonian symptoms. If administered alone, L-dopa is degraded in the stomach and has no activity in the central nervous system. Therefore, it is typically given in pills combining L-dopa and carbidopa, which blocks the peripheral breakdown of L-dopa, usually in a 10:1 ratio. L-Dopa is typically administered at a starting dose of 200 or 400 mg/day (of L-dopa) in divided doses, although doses as high as 250 mg six to eight times a day can be used. A sustained-release form of carbidopa/L-dopa containing 250 mg of L-dopa is also available because the half-life of L-dopa is short. Side effects of carbidopa/L-dopa include choreiform, dystonic, and other involuntary movements, delusions, hallucinations, and nausea. Less frequently, patients may develop palpitations, orthostatic hypotension, anorexia, vomiting, and dizziness. Gastrointestinal side effects and liver inflammation are much less common. L-Dopa can exacerbate delusions and hallucinations while reducing the movement disorder, especially in patients with dementia. This, in turn, might necessitate higher doses of an antipsychotic agent, which can further worsen the parkinsonism. Thus, patients with parkinsonism and dementia often do best when antipsychotics with less liability for parkinsonian effects, such as risperidone or clozapine, are used. For patients with PD, management can become quite complex because high doses are needed to treat the movement disorder but also induce side effects.

Amantadine

This agent was originally developed as a prophylaxis against influenza (the common flu). It has been found to directly activate postsynaptic dopamine brain receptors. It is an effective treatment for parkinsonian symptoms and produces augmentation of dopamine activity in general. Doses between 50 and 300 mg/day are typically required. Amantadine is cleared by the kidneys. Therefore, the dosage should be adjusted downward in patients with renal insufficiency. Its main long-term risks include worsening of renal insufficiency, delirium, delusions, hallucinations, and GI upset.

Bromocriptine

This is a dopamine receptor agonist that activates postsynaptic receptors. It is usually used to treat PD and other dopamine deficiency states. Typical starting doses are 0.5–2 mg/day with the most effective doses being in the 5.0–7.5 mg/day range, with 15 mg being the maximum recommended safe dosage. Adverse side effects afflict as many as 70% of patients who receive bromocryptine. Nausea affects up to 50% of patients, and headaches and dizziness affect 15%–20% of patients. Other side effects include fatigue, lightheadedness, abdominal cramps, nasal congestion, constipation, diarrhea, and drowsiness. Given its side effect profile, bromocryptine is best used after attempts to help the patient with L-dopa and amantadine have failed.

Tolcapone

This recently approved agent slows the breakdown of dopamine and thereby increases the amount of dopamine in the synapse. It has been found to augment the use of L-dopa in the treatment of PD.

Agents useful for executive dysfunction syndromes such as disinhibition, social inappropriateness, and others formerly known as frontal symptoms

Executive dysfunction is thought to be related to imbalance in the dopamine and serotonin systems in the frontal lobes and subcortical nuclei (see Lyketsos, Rosenblatt and Rabins, 2004). Two groups of executive dysfunction have been described. One is the *productive* groups, in which patients are disinhibited, stimulus-bound, intrusive, wandering, distractible, or engage in repetitive behavior such as hoarding, tapping, and vocalizing. The other group of symptoms are *nonproductive* and include apathy, social withdrawal, and amotivation. Medications that augment dopamine and serotonin neurotransmission may be useful for these symptoms, but no adequately designed study is available that establishes their efficacy, despite some promising early case series. Amantadine, L-dopa, bromocriptine, and bupropion all augment dopamine neurotransmission and are agents of first choice for patients with productive executive dysfunction syndromes. An extensive descriptive literature, mostly focused on patients with brain trauma including inattention, mild dementia, disinhibition, or explosiveness, documents benefit from these agents. Evidence, mostly from the brain trauma literature, suggests that stimulants such as methylphenidate (given their dopamine-augmenting properties) are useful treatments of these executive syndromes. The SSRIs (discussed under antidepressants) also have utility in the treatment of both productive and apathetic executive dysfunction symptoms.

Psychostimulants

Methylphenidate and other psychostimulants may also have efficacy in the treatment of apathy, social withdrawal, and nonproductive frontal syndromes. These agents are available both in short half-life and sustained-release forms. They are best started at low doses and increased incrementally when treating patients with dementia. Starting methylphenidate at 5 mg once a day and gradually increasing to as much as 40–50 mg/day can lead to benefit in dementia patients. The most common adverse effects are nervousness and insomnia, which can usually be controlled by reducing the dosage. Other reactions include hypersensitivity, anorexia, nausea, dizziness, palpitations, headache, dyskinesias, tachycardia, blood pressure changes (both increased and decreased), cardiac arrhythmias, weight loss, and abdominal pain. Delirium has also been reported. There is a risk of dependence (addiction) on these medications and of abuse by others.

OTHER BIOLOGIC THERAPIES

Brain surgery

Brain surgery is indicated in dementia patients to treat a condition believed to be the primary cause of dementia. The most common examples are surgery for the removal of a brain tumor, surgery to remove a subdural or other hematoma that is pressing on the brain tissue, or surgery to place a ventriculo-atrial shunt to better drain cerebrospinal fluid. Surgery may be necessary for reasons unrelated to the dementia and should be approached with caution. Finally, since carotid endarterectomy can reduce the risk of stroke in certain patient groups, this may be indicated in the treatment of certain cases of vascular dementia.

Bright light therapy

Patients who suffer from depression, both major and minor, and who have sleep disorders may benefit from treatments with bright lights. The main rationale for the use of bright lights for sleep disorder is that patients with dementia, particularly when institutionalized, do not have sufficient exposure to stimuli that maintain a stable 24-hour circadian rhythm. Instead, they tend to have longer circadian rhythms of 30–36 hours or to have erratic, nonentrained sleep/wake cycles. The use of bright lights in the morning or evening has been shown in several, but not all, controlled studies to stabilize circadian rhythms and improve both sleep and behavioral disorders in patients with dementia. The effect of bright lights on mood disorder in dementia is not well researched.

However, the provision of bright lights to dementia patients is complicated because effective treatment requires that patients' eyes be open and that they sit close to the lights for a sustained, regular period of time. Typically, patients are given bright light therapy sitting 3–4 feet away from a 10,000-lux commercially available *light box*. If the goal is to advance the sleep/wake cycle, that is, have patients go to bed later and wake up later, the lights are provided in the evening for 30–60 minutes, often between 5 and 6 P.M. If the goal is to delay the cycle, that is, have the patient go to bed earlier and wake up earlier, then treatments of 30–60 minutes are given in the morning before 10 A.M. Two weeks may be required for a response, and patients who respond will need to be maintained on bright light therapy for 4–6 weeks to sustain the benefit. No studies have determined whether bright lights should to be continued in the long term to stabilize the sleep disorders of dementia patients.

Electroconvulsive therapy

Electroconvulsive therapy (ECT) is the most effective and one of the safest treatments for severe depression. However, there is little research on its use as a treatment for depression in patients with dementia. Electroconvulsive therapy is particularly effective in patients with life-threatening depression, such as those who are acutely suicidal or have stopped eating. In a case series study of 31 patients with dementia and depression who received ECT, we found encouraging results. All patients had a progressive, degenerative dementia, usually vascular dementia or AD. They received an average of 9 ECT treatments, with one patient receiving a total of 23. Most individuals had a substantial reduction in depression, and 40% recovered fully. While 49% of the patients developed delirium at some time during the hospitalization, it had resolved in all individuals. The average patient gained 1.5 points on the MMSE. The risks of ECT include an adverse reaction to general anesthesia, skin bruises, prolonged seizures, fracture, temporary memory loss, delirium, and, very rarely, death. Given the adverse publicity ECT has received over the years if used in dementia patients, specialists should be involved and time should be allowed to discuss the pros and cons with patients and families.

11

Prevention, Early Detection, and Mild Cognitive Impairment

The prevention of disease and its sequelae is the ultimate aim of medicine and public health. For convenience, experts divide prevention into three levels: *primary* prevention, the absolute avoidance of the disorder; *secondary* prevention, the diminution of morbidity, for example, by early identification or prompt treatment; and *tertiary* prevention, the avoidance of morbidity that results from maximal ideal treatment. In some ways, the other chapters of this book are about tertiary prevention because they present what we believe are the best available options for care and because their provision will result in maximal function and minimum of morbidity. This chapter will focus on the little we currently know about the primary prevention of dementia, on future avenues for primary prevention, and on current evidence regarding secondary prevention.

At the beginning of the twentieth century, 20% of individuals in mental hospitals suffered from *neurosyphilis,* that is, infection and inflammation of the brain and central nervous system caused by direct invasion of it by the syphilis spirochete. Today neurosyphilis is a very rare condition. Its near elimination provides several lessons that are applicable to the prevention of other forms of dementia.

The number of cases of syphilis began declining around 1930 as methods and mechanisms were developed by public health specialists to identify persons who had had sexual contact with infected individuals. In the mid-1940s, penicillin became widely available and was found to be very effective against syphilis. This specific treatment led to further dramatic declines in the occurrence of syphilis infection in general, and neurosyphilis specifically, because involvement of the nervous system usually occurs months to years after the initial infection. Thus, the near elimination of the dementia and psychiatric disorder due to syphilitic brain infection resulted from both the availability of a specific biologic therapy (primary prevention of neurosyphilis) and the development of public health measures to detect and promptly treat those exposed (secondary prevention).

Similar success has occurred with the virtual elimination in many parts of the world of pellagra, a disease characterized by skin disease (dermatitis), GI symptoms (diarrhea), and dementia. Pioneering work by Goldgaber demonstrated that it was due to a dietary deficiency, and that it could be treated and prevented by supplementing the diet with B vitamins. Further study demonstrated that niacin and tryptophan deficiencies were responsible. The elimination of pellagra was accomplished by supplementing a universally used substance, flour, with niacin and other B vitamins. As a result, almost all individuals are protected from developing pellagra, even though the disease was caused by eating a diet deficient in B vitamins in only two groups of individuals: the poor and those subsisting on a restricted vegetarian diet.

An apparent recent success in dementia prevention is the near elimination of vCJD or *mad cow disease* within a decade of its discovery. As discussed in Chapter 3, this form of dementia is thought to have been introduced into cattle by the use of feed made from infected sheep and cattle. Even though there is still no effective treatment for vCJD , its incidence dropped dramatically once knowledge of how the agent causing the disease was spread led to a change in cattle feeds. This, coupled with a system of early identification of affected cows and the elimination of other animals that ate the same cattle feed, has led to a marked decline in the number of human and cattle cases. Thus, primary prevention in humans has resulted from primary and secondary prevention by eliminating the vectors or *carriers* that spread the infection to cows and humans.

A third example of currently available prevention is the possibility of decreasing the prevalence of the second most common cause of dementia, brain vascular disease. It is now well established that hypertension, atherosclerosis (*hardening of the arteries* due to the accumulation within arteries of cholesterol and inflammation-hardened material that can break off or weaken blood vessels and so cause stroke and decreased blood flow to the brain), hypercholesterolemia, and diabetes-caused blood vessel disease contribute to the development of vascular dementia (and perhaps AD). Evidence is just starting to accumulate that the treatment of hypertension (a form of secondary prevention of blood vessel disease) and the declining incidence of stroke can reduce the incidence of dementia, (primary prevention of dementia). To date, the studies demonstrating this have been relatively small and have primarily targeted other outcomes, such as the prevention of stroke or the preservation of memory, but evidence is accumulating that the treatment of high blood pressure, elevated cholesterol, arteriosclerosis, and diabetes by means of medication, diet, and physical activity decrease the likelihood that dementia will develop.

APPROACHES TO PREVENTION

The above paragraphs demonstrate the methods by which strategies to prevent dementia can be defined. First, as the causal biology of a specific illness is defied, scientists may identify methods to stop dementia from beginning (primary prevention). Even if the beginning of dementia cannot be stopped, early recognition of a biologic process could lead to strategies to prevent the progression from minor symptoms to full-blown disease.

Another strategy suggested by the examples described above is the identification of risk factors for developing a disease (e.g., exposure to syphilis, even though many individuals exposed to syphilis do not develop central nervous system disease). For example, many risk factors have been identified that increase the likelihood of developing AD. These include older age, having a family history of dementia, being female, head trauma, vascular disease, having the *e*4 allele of the Apolipoprotein E (APOE) E4 gene, and Down syndrome. Possible risk factors include lower education, early-life depression, low antioxidant intake, and lower physical and mental activity. Prevention may result from lessening the exposure to those risk factors that can be manipulated (head trauma, physical activity, diet) even *before* the biologic mechanisms by which these increase the risk of dementia are known. Such treatments may involve medications, but may also require an understanding of how to change the diet and activity levels of large numbers of people, approaches that have been able to decrease rates of smoking but not to reduce substance abuse, obesity, or other ills of modern life.

Study of the biology of many dementias may lead to the development of strategies for prevention even if the individual diseases have very different causes. For example, many of the degenerative dementias, including AD, DLB, and HD, appear to result from the accumulation of abnormal proteins in the brain. If scientists could develop methods to prevent the accumulation of these abnormal proteins, methods to enhance the body's innate mechanisms for removing such abnormal proteins, or methods to remove these proteins once they have formed, then the morbidity of the disease could be prevented even though the disease itself is not eliminated

WHO WILL BE TARGETED FOR PREVENTIVE INTERVENTIONS?

As is probably evident from the examples and the above discussion, the choice of a target for any preventive intervention depends on the biology of the dementia, the strength of the particular risk factor or agent being targeted, the monetary cost of the intervention, other potential benefits of the intervention, the toxicity or unwanted effects of the preventive intervention, and the risk status of the individuals being targeted.

Thus, interventions targeting vascular risk factors should have widespread application because many risk factors have been well established and because the benefits would likely include a lower incidence of stroke, myocardial infarction, and other complications of atherosclerosis in addition to the benefit of diminished risk for vascular dementia and possibly AD. Likewise, if physical and/or mental exercise interventions are proven to prevent AD, they may be widely recommended because they too may prevent vascular disease and depression and are of low risk in properly screened individuals. On the other hand, a preventive strategy that relies on a treatment with significant toxicity may be recommended only for those at genetic risk for developing the disease.

CHARACTERISTICS OF TESTS USED TO IDENTIFY THOSE TARGETED FOR PREVENTIVE INTERVENTIONS

An in-depth discussion of the characteristics of tests used to identify those at risk for developing a condition is beyond the scope of this book. However, the following paragraphs will introduce the reader to a few terms and concepts that will illuminate how decisions are made about the choice of screening tests.

Sensitivity refers to the likelihood that a test will properly identify those who *are* at risk for developing a condition. *Specificity* refers to the likelihood that a test will properly identify those who are *not* at risk for developing or having the disorder being screened for. Each of these is important in establishing the value of a test or screening procedure, since screening should identify both those who should and those who should not have the preventive intervention. Therefore, the ideal test should have high sensitivity and high specificity. Importantly, the sensitivity and specificity of a test do not depend on how prevalent a condition is in the population.

The phrase *positive predictive value* refers to how likely a positive test is to accurately indicate whether a person has the condition of interest. *Negative predictive value* refers to the likelihood that a negative test accurately indicates that a person does not have the condition of interest. In contrast to sensitivity and specificity, these measures *are* dependent on how prevalent a condition is in the population being treated. For example, HIV testing is not recommended for everyone because even though the test has good sensitivity and specificity, a positive test is equally likely to indicate that a randomly selected person has or has not been exposed to HIV. That is because being HIV positive is still uncommon, so that even if the test is accurate in 999/1000 instances, the 1 time out of 1000 it is inaccurate is about as frequent as the 1 time out of 1000 that a person will accurately be HIV positive.

This has already been shown to be an issue in testing for AD. Tests that rely on the presence of elevated beta-amyloid or tau protein levels in spinal fluid, blood, or urine are elevated often enough in those without AD that the test are not currently useful for population testing. However, in particular populations, for example those with one or two APOE *e*4 alleles or those who have been found to have memory impairment, a positive test may indicate accurately enough that a person is at risk for future AD.

THE EARLY DETECTION OF DEMENTIA

Research by us and others has found that only one-third of people who suffer from cognitive decline are recognized by their physicians as having dementia. While skeptics may argue that the lack of effective treatments and secondary prevention suggests that no harm results from this lack of recognition, we disagree. Early detection of dementia can have the following benefits at present. First, the occasional case of fully treatable and reversible dementia benefits from early detection because early detection minimizes the suffering and complications from the causative disorder. Also, some evidence suggests that potentially treatable causes of dementia, such as hypothyroidism and lack of vitamin B_{12}, can result in irreversible brain damage if present for long periods of time. Secondly, early detection can help the patient make plans, ensure that documents such as a will and an advance directive are written, and provide an impetus for the individual to discuss desires for future care with the appropriate individuals. A third justification for early detection is protection against being taken advantage of in the early stages of dementia by unscrupulous individuals and organizations. A fourth support for early identification is the information and explanation that family and other loved ones can receive and the improvement in quality of life that the patient and loved ones can gain from being properly informed.

The development of methods for early detection will also be important for research and future treatment. From a research perspective, secondary prevention will probably be most effective if it is initiated as early as possible, that is, at the very beginning of symptoms. Thus, the development of methods for identifying cognitive decline very early will allow for research to determine if dementia can be prevented and cognitive changes reversed. Also, most researchers and clinicians believe that the earlier a treatment can be initiated, the greater the likelihood of avoiding permanent, irreversible brain damage. For these reasons, among others, researchers have focused on early detection of what is thought to be the very earliest evidence of dementia, conditions known as *mild cognitive impairment* (MCI) or *cognitive impairment, not dementia* (CIND).

BETWEEN NORMAL AGING AND DEMENTIA: MILD COGNITIVE IMPAIRMENT, COGNITIVE IMPAIRMENT, NOT DEMENTIA, AND PREDEMENTIA

The observation that some older individuals become mildly forgetful as they age dates back to the earliest medical writings. In the modern era, the first epidemiologic study of dementia, carried out in the northern English city of Newcastle-Upon-Tyne, identified a group of individuals who did not fit clearly into the cognitively normal group or the dementia group. A follow-up study of these individuals revealed that more than one-third progressed to dementia over a 5- to 7-year period.

In the 1970s, the Canadian psychiatrist V. A. Kral described a group of patients suffering from what he called *benign senescent forgetfulness*. These patients complained of memory decline and had subtle changes on memory testing that he believed were compatible with normal aging. However, when he followed them long-term, he found that a significant proportion (~90%) had developed dementia, leading him to conclude that the condition was not so benign after all. In the 1980s, the neurologist Ronald Peterson began studying a group of individuals who were thought by their physicians to have memory difficulties but who did not meet criteria for dementia. In an elegant series of papers over the subsequent two decades, he reported that about 12% of these individuals developed dementia each year. Thus, he concluded that these individuals, whom he categorized as suffering from MCI, had a condition that was a precursor or an early manifestation of dementia.

At about the same time, a population-based survey called the Canadian Study of Aging labeled a similar group as having CIND. While those in Peterson's MCI group were identified as having only memory impairment, the CIND group was defined as having a decline in any area of cognition but not meeting criteria for dementia.

At present, most researchers and clinicians agree that there is a group of patients who have suffered some decline in cognition but who do not meet criteria for dementia. There is no consensus on what criteria should be used to identify such individuals. In addition, there is no consensus on whether these individuals suffer from the earliest form of dementia or have a syndrome that is a risk factor for developing dementia. This chapter will review the current views and controversies on these topics, and identify those issues on which there is widespread agreement and those on which there is significant disagreement.

Are There Several Types of Mild Cognitive Impairment/Cognitively Impaired/Not Dementia?

The most common presentation of cognitive decline that does not meet criteria for dementia (or delirium) is decline only in memory. It is this group that has been studied the most and to which we will refer as having MCI, because the criteria proposed for this syndrome include decline in memory without other cognitive impairments. This has also been refered to as amnestic MCI.

Another presentation of cognitive decline not meeting criteria for dementia, almost as common as amnestic MCI in our research, characterizes individuals with cognitive impairments in nonmemory realms such as executive function, visuospatial function, and language. Some individuals in this group have mild declines in multiple areas of cognitive function, including memory, but do not meet criteria for dementia because the declines are mild.

Evaluation

Patients complaining of memory loss or of decline in function should be examined thoroughly, as discussed in Chapter 2. Neuropsychological testing is especially helpful, as it provides a thorough assessment of many areas of cognitive function, because it is sensitive to detecting mild impairments, and because many tests have normative data that allow for age and education adjustments. Even if the test results are equivocal, a thorough neuropsychological testing battery provides a baseline that can be compared to subsequent testing. We often obtain repeat testing in 9–12 months if the diagnosis is unclear.

One of the challenges in diagnosing CIND or MCI is the distinction between the usual or normal changes that occur with aging (primarily in free recall and speed of performance) and the early symptoms of dementia. The presence of a functional impairment that is linked to the cognitive change is one indication that a pathologic process is likely to be developing, but research has not yet identified criteria that can be used with confidence in individual cases to predict who will develop dementia within a relatively short period of time. Not surprisingly, the more severe the MCI or CIND, the more likely that the symptoms are early indicators of dementia.

TREATMENT

As of late 2004, no pharmacologic or nonpharmacologic treatment had been demonstrated for MCI. Several trials of cholinesterase inhibitors have not shown efficacy on the primary outcome, although reanalyses have found suggestions of mild short-term benefit. We believe the lack of benefit on the primary outcome that was chosen at the initiation of the study is what should be emphasized. While there is no evidence that treatment of hypertension, hypercholesterolemia, or diabetes may stave off progression of MCI or CIND to dementia, the benefits of reduced vascular disease that such treatment brings about support controlling these risk factors as much as is safe and possible. Research on normal aging individuals has shown that lessening anxiety about usual aging changes can benefit memory performance. No such data have been reported for MCI or CIND, but acknowledging the frustration that accompanies declining memory and encouraging the person with MCI to remain active in areas that are enjoyed has face validity.

WHAT SHOULD INDIVIDUALS AT RISK BE ADVISED NOW IF THEY WANT TO DECREASE THEIR RISK FOR ALZHEIMER DISEASE OR OTHER DEMENTIAS?

We are often asked by the children, brothers, or sisters of individuals with AD or vascular dementia what we would recommend for prevention. At present, we know of no preventive interventions that can be supported by appropriately designed prospective prevention trials. Nevertheless, we do believe that the evidence linking vascular risk factors to AD is strong enough, and that they have been shown to lower the risk for stroke, myocardial infarction, and death, that any added benefit for possibly lowering the risk for developing AD supports their adoption by all adults. Likewise, we believe the benefits from exercise and social/mental activity are so significant that all adults should participate actively in both if approved by their physician. We suggest that this is especially true of those with symptoms of MCI/CIND, even though data are not available to support their widespread adoption. However, we recognize that individuals who have never been physically active or who have not enjoyed attending group activities will have a difficult time beginning such activities. Therefore, we encourage people to do so, but do not make a strong recommendation because there is no good scientific study demonstrating cognitive benefits.

12

TERMINAL CARE

Most dementia syndromes are progressive and lead to an end stage of severe disability. In much of this book, we emphasize the differences among the dementing illnesses and link those differences to specific treatment approaches. However, the end stage of most dementias is a great equalizer. The problems become similar and the approaches similar. While some differences among individuals remain and different diseases have some distinct abnormalities, this chapter will deal with general approaches, because these distinctions have less clinical import. The chapter will describe the features of end-stage dementia, discuss the care issues commonly encountered, and describe ways to assist family members in making decisions about the end stage.

THE TERMINAL PHASE OF DEMENTIA

In advanced dementia, all realms of cognition are severely impaired. Memory for recent and remote events is almost absent. Language production and comprehension are markedly compromised, and speech ranges from an ability to say a few words or syllables to babbling or muteness. Because of severe apraxias, most patients have a very unsteady gait and are unable to walk, cannot feed themselves, and have impaired eating, chewing, and swallowing. Agnosia progresses to the point that patients recognize little of the world around them and few of the people around them. Patients may not look at others even when spoken to. Death is commonly attributable to complicating infections such as pneumonia, but malnutrition is a common contributor.

Two studies provide information on predictors of death. The Predictors Study followed a group of outpatients for 5 years and found that those with psychosis and extrapyramidal symptoms were more likely to die. A study by Volicer and colleagues (1993) developed a formula to predict life expectancy of 6 months or less in patients who develop fever. Older age, greater severity of dementia, and palliative care in a hospital within 6 months predicted mortality within 6 months. Volicer et al. recommend that this formula be used to certify patients for the Medicare Hospice Benefit. The National Hospice Association has also developed guidelines to predict which patients with dementia are likely to die in the next 6 months. It is based on Reisberg's Functional Assessment Staging of Alzheimer's disease (FAST) staging and is presented in Table 12.1. Risk factors for death include being nonambulatory, immobile, unable to dress or bathe, having frequent urinary and fecal incontinence, and being unable to communicate more than six words.

In a 1994 study, Collins and Ogle determined where patients died and the types of service provided prior to death. Forty-two percent of patients died at home, 32% died in nursing homes, and 26% died in hospitals. The home patients had few or no home health services 90 days prior to death. On the other hand, studies from Alzheimer Disease Research Centers find that 90% of those in the study enter a nursing home before death.

Wishes of patients and families in terminal phases

Currently, few elderly individuals have advance directives of sufficient detail to guide decision making in the terminal stage of dementia. Additionally, defining for an individual what a good quality of life constitutes in someone who is severely demented is problematic. Few individuals can realistically look ahead to evaluate what kind of interventions they would want in a particular situation at the end of life. It is true that it is hard for many to imagine that someone even severely impaired can be healthy and happy. Since few elderly persons have very detailed advanced directives, decisions about their care inevitably fall to others—surrogates—almost always a family member. Given the difficulties inherit in anticipating every possible situation that will need a health care decision, it is preferable to have the patient designate a durable power of attorney for health care early on. Ideally, that person would have an intimate knowledge of what the values of the individual were and a sense of how the individual would want his or her care organized.

In a study of caregivers receiving care at the Johns Hopkins Alzheimer Disease Research Center, the majority of family members were unaware that choices about the method of care, such as diagnostic tests, transfer to the hospital, and feeding tubes, were theirs to make in the terminal phase. Many had little confidence that professionals would allow or enable them to be part

TABLE 12.1. Guidelines for Determining Mortality in the Next 6 Months

I. Functional assessment staging
  A. The patient should be at or beyond stage 7 of the functional assessment
    staging scale (Table 1.5)
  B. The patient should show all of the following characteristics:
    1. Unable to ambulate without assistance
    2. Unable to dress without assistance
    3. Unable to bathe
    4. Urinary and fecal incontinence
    5. Unable to speak or communicate meaningfully

II. Presence of medical complications
  A. Presence of co-morbid condition to warrant sufficiently severe treatment,
    whether or not treatment was given
  B. Co-morbid conditions commonly associated with dementia
    1. Aspiration pneumonia
    2. Pyelonephritis or upper urinary tract infection
    3. Septicemia
    4. Decubitus ulcers, multiple, stage 3–4
    5. Recurrent fever after antibiotics
  C. Difficulty swallowing food or refusal to eat
    1. Patients who are tube fed must have a documented impaired nutritional
    status

Source: National Hospice Association.

of the discussion. Even in the few families who had thought ahead and made decisions about methods of care, those decisions were rarely documented in a letter to an attending physician for home-dwelling patients or in the medical records of nursing home residents. Most families assumed that "the doctor knows what we want," and yet, physicians change in nursing homes and those who will implement decisions, the nursing staff, have very high turnover in long-term care. In many nursing homes, discussions about end-of-life care take place between the social worker and the family, not the direct health care providers.

The Gerontological Society of American surveyed 2300 professionals and family members and posed the question "What is appropriate health care for end-stage dementia?" Seventy percent of those surveyed favored the least aggressive level of care. Those family members who had had a discussion about terminal care were more likely to choose the least aggressive level. Older family members were also more likely to choose the least aggressive care. Ninety percent of individuals surveyed felt that hospice care was appropriate for end-stage dementia.

Hospice services have been used more for patients with dementia in the past few years, and 5%–10% of patients in hospices in the United States have a primary diagnosis of dementia. In one study, more for-profit hospices cared for patients with dementia than not-for-profit centers, but difficulty in predicting survival in dementia remains a major barrier to the use of hospice care.

The best way to help a family make decisions about end-of-life care in dementia is to provide information about the options and their likely consequences. Questions should be encouraged, and the discussion may need to be repeated several times. Ideally, decisions can be made in an unhurried fashion so that the emotional implications of the choices can be reviewed when appropriate.

BENEFITS AND BURDENS OF MEDICAL INTERVENTION IN TERMINAL PHASES

The medical benefits of cardiopulmonary resuscitation (CPR) and permanent gastrostomy feeding are unclear. Less than 2% of nursing home residents who receive CPR care are successfully resuscitated. Even when a cardiac arrest is witnessed and skilled personnel conduct the resuscitation, the success rate is no higher. Virtually no one with end-stage dementia who is resuscitated in a hospital survives to leave the hospital.

There is no evidence that tube feeding decreases the incidence of infections or aspiration of food and fluid into the lung. In one study that followed 36 nursing home residents for 18 months, no patient's functional status improved after insertion of the percutaneous endoscopic gastrostomy tube. Complications occurred in approximately 35% of the patients. These included hospital admissions and emergency room visits for problems such as tube obstruction (46%), tube migration (17%), leakage (13%), local wound infections (4.3%), bowel obstruction (4.3%), and GI bleeding or gastritis (4.3%).

Another common problem in end-stage dementia is elevation of temperature. In efforts to determine the utility of diagnostic tests and antibiotic therapy in end-stage febrile demented patients, Ludislav Volicer and colleagues (1993) assessed fever episodes in 75 patients with AD residing in a Veterans Administration nursing home. Seventy-five patients developed fever episodes. All underwent a diagnostic workup including blood cultures, suctioning of sputum samples, and urinary culture.

In 30% of the individuals, the cause of the fever was not detected. The use of antibiotics and diagnostic testing did not affect survival. Likewise, when compared to a group of patients who were treated symptomatically with oxygen, pulmonary toileting, hospice nursing, and antipyretics, patients undergoing testing and antibiotic treatment did not survive longer.

The transfer of patients with end-stage dementia to an acute hospital for the treatment of pneumonia and sepsis also poses many challenges. They must be transferred by ambulance and are put under the care of acute hospital staff who are often not skilled in caring for patients with severe cognitive impairment. They often must be restrained in bed to prevent them from falling out of bed or pulling out intravenous lines (IV's) and frequently must be sedated and restrained for diagnostic tests. They are also at high risk of developing a hospital-acquired infection because of their debilitated state.

Nevertheless, the decision to limit diagnostic testing and antibiotic therapy is a difficult one for many individuals. We discuss some of the ethical and moral aspects of decision making in the next chapter.

GOOD CARE UNTIL THE END

A focus on meticulous personal care must not be abandoned even in those who are profoundly demented. In addition to the medical interventions agreed to by the patient, family, or surrogate, the priorities of care at the end of life in dementia include careful attention to feeding, skin care, elimination, oral hygiene, and grooming. These will each be discussed. A discussion of other terminal phase issues follows.

Feeding problems

The issue of feeding is so inherently embedded in the role of caregiving that it commonly presents difficulties to nurses and family caregivers alike. Ethical issues raised by feeding are discussed in Chapter 13. Feeding problems commonly encountered in the patient with end-stage dementia include loss of appetite, not opening the mouth, sleeping through meals, "cheeking" food, being unable to swallow safely, and choking.

Measures that promote feeding and decrease the risk of choking include:

- Giving lukewarm liquids
- Keeping the head of the patient's bed at a 45-degree angle
- Using relatively thick liquids
- Using a straw with patients who can still suck
- Feeding patients slowly, one sip at a time, with liquid nutrients once they cannot swallow solids or pureed foods, or using a straw with patients who can still suck

Stroking the throat or changing from a solid to liquids in midmeal can sometimes help clear the oral cavity.

Skin care

Meticulous attention to skin care is essential, particularly if pressure ulcers (decubitus ulcers or decubiti) are to be prevented. The mainstays of good skin care include:

- Protecting bony prominences.
- Regularly inspecting the skin and documenting when redness appears.
- Turning and repositioning regularly. Moving every 2 hours is commonly recommended.
- Massaging at risk areas.

Massaging helps improve the circulation and provides a way of interacting with the patient. It also provides relaxation and pleasure for the patient. Common places and pressure points that should be inspected routinely for breakdown include the toes, heels, ankles, knees, buttocks, lower back, shoulder blades, breasts, ears, and elbows.

Unfortunately, skin breakdown can occur even with the increased vigilance, attention to nutrition, and steps listed above. The risk is lowered by avoiding the extremes of moisture and dryness and by taking steps to avoid skin tears. Shearing of skin occurs when the skin is pulled in the opposite direction to the weight of the bone—for example, when patients are pulled up in bed while their skin adheres to the sheet. Therefore, it is important to teach caregivers, professionals, and family members to use draw sheets and to avoid pulling patients or turning them if the sheets are moist.

Bowel care

Caregivers must meticulously record voiding and bowel movements. If no bowel movement occurs after 3–4 days, milk of magnesia should be followed by oral medications that provide bowel stimulation and, if that is unsuccessful, suppositories. No patient should repeatedly go more than 4 days without a bowel movement and then be given enemas, unless all other steps fail. If suppositories are needed, they should be given before breakfast. Constipation can be minimized by providing a diet that includes adequate fiber and at least 2 liters of liquids per day.

Several new incontinence products contain gel inserts that retain large amounts of fluid. These reduce the frequency with which diapers and bed sheets need to be changed. Some incontinence products have color-coded strips that change color when moist; this helps caregivers recognize when a change is necessary and lessens the need to disturb the patient. Frequent checks and changes of diapers at appropriate intervals can minimize the development of rashes and secondary infections.

Oral health

Oral health is one of the most challenging aspects of nursing care in terminal phases. Problems include xerostomia or dry mouth, tooth loss, dental caries (cavities), periodontal disease, and oral cancers.

Oral hygiene should include tooth brushing at least once a day after the largest meal. The mouth should be inspected after each meal and cleared of dried mucus and food using a gauze-wrapped tongue blade (to prevent aspiration) that has been moistened with water or a saliva substitute. The tongue should be brushed regularly since it can collect bits of food and infected material. When dry mouth is present, artificial saliva may be used. It can provide comfort and prevent dried contents from being aspirated. Dental caries and tooth abscess cause pain and are common reason for patients to refuse to eat and lose weight. Therefore, teeth that are decayed should be considered for removal.

Mouth care in uncooperative demented patients is especially challenging. Caregivers should never stick their fingers between a patient's teeth. They should get help from others and ask them to hold the patient's head and hands. It is important to be persistent in providing mouth care since it is extremely important to the health of the patient. Sometimes pressing between the cheeks and the jaw with the thumb will open the mouth. Four to five tongue blades wrapped with gauze and adhesive tape should be used if it is necessary to keep the mouth open while providing care. Sedation with a short-acting benzodiazepine such as lorazepam is sometimes needed before dental care can be provided.

Maintaining dignity

Measures that maintain patients' dignity benefit them and ensure a pleasant environment for family and staff. Patients who wear glasses and hearing aids should be encouraged to use them, although this cannot always be accomplished. Hair should be groomed neatly in a style to which the patient was accustomed. Good mouth care diminishes foul odors and unattractiveness. Patients should be kept in their own clothes rather than in hospital gowns. Women who wear dresses can be dressed by cutting the dress up the back and putting it on the patient. This avoids turning or moving the patient but keeps up her appearance.

Patients should be spoken to and called by their name even if they cannot speak and do not look at the examiner. Many individuals respond to touch in a positive fashion even when they do not communicate in any other way.

Roper argues that for each symptom there is a logical treatment that can alleviate it. For thirst, mouth swabs can prevent dryness and ice chips or oral intake can keep the mouth moist. Dry, inelastic skin can be eased with soft mattresses, careful lifting and turning, and the elimination of soaps that will dry the skin further. Elevated temperature can be addressed with alcohol swabs, cool baths, a fan, light clothing, and bedcovers. Apprehension and restlessness can be addressed with frequent stroking and antianxiety medications.

Seizures

Ten percent of late-stage patients develop seizures. These can often be controlled with antiseizure medications, but an occasional patient cannot tolerate the doses needed to control the seizures. If such patients are not at risk for harm from hitting against bed rails or falling, anticonvulsants may not be necessary. Bed rails can be padded to protect the patient.

Oxygen can be given if respiratory distress is present, but this is rare. The use of oxygen in the terminally ill is of unproven benefit, but patient comfort should guide the decision to provide it.

Is dehydration painful?

Clinicians are frequently asked if the lack of fluid intake that commonly accompanies the dying process in end-stage dementia is uncomfortable. This is a reasonable question since most people experience thirst as uncomfortable. However, the evidence suggesting that dehydration in terminal dementia is uncomfortable or painful is limited.

Thus, it is not clear that starting IV rehydration actually improves patient comfort. The issues of feeding and hydration in terminal dementia are frought with many ethical dilemmas, some of which are discussed in Chapter 13. The benefits and burdens of any treatment should be discussed thoroughly with whomever is making treatment decisions before therapy is initiated. Some have suggested that dehydration has advantages for terminal patients because reduced urine output lessens incontinence and because diminished GI and pulmonary secretions lessen coughing, choking, vomiting, and a drowning sensation. The electrolyte imbalances, acidosis, uremia, hypercalcemia, and hypervolemia that accompany dehydration can also lead to analgesia and lethargy, and this further complicates the decision-making process involved in deciding whether to start an IV.

Use of restraints and causing emotional upheaval

Terminal dementia patients are almost always calm prior to their death, especially if the environment is calm, familiar, and warm. Restraints are almost never needed and should be used only if bed rails are not adequate to prevent harm. If patients are in pain, anxious, experiencing air hunger in spite of oxygen or uncomfortable, opioid analgesics (orally, intramuscularly, per rectum, or intravenously) should be used to relieve suffering. The short-acting benzodiazepine lorazepam may be used to reduce fear and anxiety. In the rare occurrence of delusions or hallucinations that are upsetting a patient or causing danger, antipsychotics should be used. If medication administration is causing problems or medications are providing no benefit, they can be discontinued.

Assisting Families in End-Stage Dementia

All family members who are interested, even those who have not seen the patient for quite some time, should be informed that the patient is likely to die soon. Questions should be answered as honestly as possible but ignorance admitted to when the answer is unknown.

Family members should be shown how to carry out comfort measures such as moistening the patient's lips with a cool cloth and using lotion to massage the extremities. They should be encouraged to continue talking to their dying relative and to maintain their connection with the patient as long as possible.

Hospice Care in Terminal Dementia

There are more than 2000 hospice programs that serve communities throughout the United States. Cancer was the original focus of hospice care, but it has been extended to other end-stage illnesses, including renal disease, AIDS, ALS, heart disease, lung disease, and AD. The National Hospice Organization has published guidelines for determining short-term survival in patients with AD that are used nationally (Table 12.1). The focus of hospice care is on palliative care, that is, comfort and quality of life. Hospice care can be provided in the patient's home, in a hospice, or in a nursing home.

Upon the Death of the Patient

The process of caring for someone with dementia has been described as "the funeral that never ends." Some caregivers will state that their loved ones were "gone" many years prior to their physical death. The profound changes dementia causes in the patient and the long nature of the illness can result in an awkward experience at the end.

A variety of reactions by family members may be observed; two scenarios are common. In the first instance, the caregiver is intellectually prepared for the death of the patient but experiences intense sadness at the actual event. Persons in this situation often express surprise and occasional embarrassment at their "lack of control" over their feelings. It is useful to inform them that intellectual and emotional reactions are different and that upset is an integral part of the grieving process.

In the second scenario, the funeral process becomes awkward when the caregiver feels relief that the death has finally occurred. Often, persons who have not been directly involved in caregiving will attend funeral or memorial services. They may feel shocked and intensely saddened, and may be puzzled or even critical of the primary caregiver who does not express such feelings. Even within a family, the reaction to the death may be quite different for different members. Providing the explanation that all persons do not have to be at the same place in grieving can be reassuring to such families.

As in other chronic illnesses, it can be difficult to recall how life was with patients when they were well. In time, that is possible for most and is a sign of recovery. Our practice is to meet with surviving family members several months after the death when possible and if they agree. This meeting is often initially upsetting, as it is the first visit to the office without the patient. The meeting provides an opportunity to review the patient's life before the illness and to provide praise for a long ordeal of caregiving. Many families report that such meetings release them from the mourning process and allow them to continue their lives.

THE ISSUE OF AUTOPSY

In our experience, the issue of autopsy confirmation of the diagnosis of AD arises commonly. As reviewed earlier, when the diagnostic procedures we recommend are followed, the diagnosis of AD is confirmed at autopsy over 90% of the time. Thus, the autopsy is not necessary in most cases to make a diagnosis. However, autopsy confirmation is reassuring to some that nothing treatable was missed. In families where several persons have had AD, the need to positively confirm the diagnosis may be important because of concerns about risk and possible prevention in surviving family members. When the autopsy is conducted as part of a research study, an added benefit is possible because the information gained from the autopsy adds to the body of knowledge about dementing illnesses and can thus help future generations. For many, this is a source of pride that something positive was gained from an unfortunate illness.

13

ETHICAL AND LEGAL ISSUES

Chronic illnesses like dementia raise many ethical, moral, and legal issues. Discussions of ethical issues are often frustrating because they do not end with an expert telling clinicians the "right" thing to do. Nevertheless, an open discussion of ethical concerns is important because it alerts practitioners to an important aspect of what they do and identifies issues that clinicians may be unaware of. Discussion sometimes leads to consensus on the appropriate action, and at other times clarifies the available options. This chapter will first discuss six ethical issues that arise in dementia care and then use these examples to develop several principles that guide our practice. It is followed by a discussion of the most common legal issues that arise in the care of dementia patients.

ETHICAL ISSUES

The person with memory problems who doesn't want to be evaluated

It is common for individuals with memory impairment to be unaware that they have a problem. When memory problems are brought to their attention, some are happy to seek medical attention but others refuse an evaluation. What can a family member or professional do when evaluation is refused? Several issues are clear. It is impossible to force individuals to seek medical care if they do not want it unless the situation is acutely life-threatening. As a culture, we have established, and the courts have confirmed, the right of a competent individual to refuse treatment. The difficult issue that arises in individuals with memory loss is whether they actually have the capacity to make an informed choice to refuse evaluation and treatment.

It is appropriate and ethical for family members, friends, physicians, and others to encourage and even urge a person with memory problems to have a complete assessment. At times, individuals will agree to be evaluated if a family member or close friend accompanies them to the doctor. For the vast majority of people, frequent encouragement, even nagging, will eventually lead to their seeing a physician. However, if a person continues to refuse a medical assessment, there is little that can be done to force an evaluation unless a clearly dangerous situation occurs. In some communities a Geriatric Evaluation Service can force an evaluation, but usually only when a clear danger is present.

When a person who is reluctant or unable to acknowledge a memory problem has a doctor's appointment, the family should consider calling ahead to alert the physician that a problem exists. This will ensure that the proper medical assessment is done. It will also alert the physician that there are important social or practical questions, such as living alone and driving, that need to be addressed.

Principles

Unless there is clear evidence of danger, a person should not and cannot be forced to undergo an evaluation for memory disorder. Persistent encouragement can often lead the reluctant individual to agree to an evaluation.

The person who lives alone

Most dementing illnesses ultimately rob people of their independence. When questions arise about a person's ability to live alone, a professional evaluation of the many abilities needed to be independent should be sought. Among the questions to be reviewed are: Can the person find her way around the neighborhood or does she get lost even occasionally? Is he able to prepare proper meals? Can she recognize an emergency situation, and does she know how to get help (using the telephone, dial 911)? Is there someone available to keep an eye on him?

Competent adults have the right to choose where they want to live. Most of us would interfere with this right only in extreme circumstances. In the majority of instances, the person with dementia can eventually be convinced that the move to a safer environment is necessary. However, when there is a significant likelihood that harm would come to the person or to someone else by wandering, malnutrition, fire, or failure to take medication, we should intervene to protect the person. If the person cannot be convinced and clear danger is present, then a legal solution should be sought.

It is often possible to find intermediate solutions to a dilemma such as this. For example, even when people are unable to live alone, their impairments may not necessitate placement in a nursing home. Options include hiring a home companion, having the person attend a day-care center while family members are at work, or moving to a small group home. These examples illustrate that many ethical dilemmas can be solved by finding a middle ground between two extremes. In this situation, individuals may not fully have the ability to determine their living situation, but they can be helped by being given a set of options and encouraged to choose among them.

Principles

Attempts should be made to maximize choice, even in an impaired individual. Offering a range of options can sometimes preserve a person's right to choose, but from a limited menu of choices.

Should anyone with dementia be allowed to drive?

Driving presents difficult clinical and ethical dilemmas. For many individuals and their spouses, driving is necessary to retain an active life and independence—important goals in the treatment of dementia.

However, driving is a complex skill that depends on many physical and cognitive skills. It is impossible to identify exactly when in the course of dementia the ability to drive safely is lost, but all progressive dementing diseases ultimately impair the skills needed to drive.

Some clinicians have concluded that any person with a diagnosis of dementia should stop driving because we cannot know when driving ability is lost and because impaired driving places others at risk. Others argue that there must be evidence of danger such as poor performance on neuropsychological tests that measure reaction time, judgment, or perception skills; a history of automobile accidents; or a failed driving test before a person should be forced to stop driving. Those holding this latter opinion note that driving can often be the only means of getting food from the grocery store, visiting others, and staying active. Preventing some individuals from driving may also adversely affect a spouse who is unable to drive.

There is universal agreement, though, that a person's privilege to drive should be revoked once there is clear evidence of impairment in the skills required for driving. It is only in the group of patients who have yet to show impairments that ethical dilemmas arise and significant disagreements exist.

Because impaired driving places others at risk of harm and because driving is a privilege, not a right, the standards for depriving a person of the privilege to drive are less strict than those for the two previous examples, refusing an evaluation and wanting to live alone. We recommend that all individuals who have received a diagnosis of dementia stop driving and be carefully evaluated prior to resuming driving. We base this conclusion on recent evidence that patients with even mild dementia have impaired driving ability and on the inability to know when the ability to drive first becomes impaired.

The recommendation to stop driving is easy to make if the person with dementia has someone else available who can drive. Even when the ability to drive seems intact, many patients stop driving on their own or on their family's or physician's recommendation. Difficulties arise when individuals persist in wanting to drive or if their families feel that their driving is a necessity ("It's the only way we can get groceries"). When these issues arise, we refer the patient to a driving school and sometimes also for neuropsychological testing. If the driving school or testing results suggest that there is danger, then a strong recommendation to stop driving is made. If legally permissible, the appropriate authorities should be notified. If the driving test and neuropsychological tests reveal no evidence of impairment that would interfere with driving, we inform the patient and family that we still believe some danger exists, that driving problems are likely to develop in the future, and that the person should no longer drive.

The laws regarding notification of the motor vehicle bureau that a person's driving ability is impaired varies greatly across the United States. In some states, physicians are required to report all persons with a diagnosis of dementia or AD to the motor vehicle authority. In other states, notification is not permitted because of confidentiality statutes. We believe this question should be settled legislatively since this is one way for society to express a collective opinion on a difficult issue over which clinicians disagree.

Principle

When danger to others exists, we are justified in depriving persons of something they want. However, since there is no consensus on when the driving privilege should be revoked and since driving is a legally granted privilege, the authorities who legislate and regulate this privilege should address the issue.

Should medications and restraints be used to control behavior and protect patients from harm?

One of the most distressing aspects of a visit to a nursing home is the sight of individuals secured in chairs or appearing to be drugged. As discussed in Chapters 8 and 9, patients with dementia commonly suffer from functional impairments or behaviors that are distressing to them and place the patient or others at risk of harm. A duty to protect the ill person from harm and distress is well established, but clinical practice also mandates that patients be treated in the least restrictive manner. The conflicting goals of protection from harm (and thereby limitation of freedom) versus maximization of independence underlie several of the issues discussed in this chapter. The ideal solution usually involves finding a midpoint that allows as much freedom as seems safe *and* provides the least amount of restriction that will minimize danger and distress.

If a behavior in question presents no danger to the patient or others and no significant distress to the patient, then it should probably be allowed to continue (see Chapter 8 for examples). If a psychiatric disorder (in addition to dementia) is the cause of the behavior problem and the patient is likely to benefit directly from treatment, then therapy should be given strong consideration. When neither danger nor benefit is clear, the potential benefit to the ill person must be weighed against the potential for harm. In general, this means trying the least restrictive nonpharmacologic, nonrestraint approaches first (Chapters 8 and 9) and using medication when a specific indication for it is present. Physical restraints should be considered only for *specific indications* that are identified in the medical record when danger to self or others is present or significant emotional distress is likely in the ill person *and* if other alternatives have either been tried and have failed or if the danger is so acute that a less restrictive alternative is unlikely to prevent harm. In general, invasive therapies such as physical restraint should be continued only as long as the behavior or physical problem remains a danger and the treatment is documented to be helpful or protective of safety.

Principle

The least restrictive, safest, and most effective treatment should be chosen for each problem. Balancing these goals can be challenging. Not labeling an issue a problem is appropriate if neither the patient nor others experience harm or distress. Treatment is appropriate when distress or harm is possible or likely.

Is it ever proper to lie to a person with dementia?

A very distressing behavior associated with dementia is the constant repetition of a question or an incorrect statement. Some patients repeatedly ask to go home, ask where their parents are, or claim that a specific individual is harming them. Among the options open to managing this behavior are *distraction* (getting the person to think or talk about something else), *dealing with the underlying feelings* rather than the statement itself ("You sound lonely today"; "It sound like you miss your mother"; "Are you feeling lost?"), and *ignoring* the statement.

None of these approaches directly addresses the patient's concern. Rather, they redefine it, assume that there is some other concern that is actually being expressed, or ignore it. Directly addressing the issue (e.g., "Your mother is dead") is often harmful and rarely benefits the ill person.

Why are we comfortable using distraction or addressing the underlying feelings? Undoubtedly, part of the reason is that these approaches work. More importantly, though, these strategies enable us to interact meaningfully with demented individuals *and* diminish their upset. We prefer these approaches to blunt truth-telling (such as "Your mother's dead." or "You're going to live here the rest of your life") because they are less upsetting to ill individuals, allow us to communicate with them in a positive fashion, and benefit them by encouraging them to express their emotions.

Furthermore, blunt truth-telling does not benefit many people with dementia because they are often unable to remember or appreciate the truth. Since helping rather than hurting patients is our primary goal, it follows that distraction, discussing facing one's feelings, and ignoring can simultaneously benefit patients and avoid harming them.

Distraction and focusing on feelings are not lies, but they are not telling the full truth either. Unfortunately, there are times when these approaches do not work. When they fail, the ill person often becomes more upset, restless, angry, or even physically combative. Many practitioners report that they will say "Your mother will be here soon, don't worry" when she has been deceased for a number of years or "You're just staying here for a little while until your health gets better" when the person has permanently moved to a child's home or a nursing home. We believe this is lying and that this approach raises several awkward questions: Is this lying justifiable? Is lying ever justifiable? We believe the answer is "yes" and that this is one of the very few circumstances when it is.

Upset and distress are unavoidable aspects of living. As human beings, we have many means of adapting to loss and disappointment. Unfortunately, some persons with dementia are robbed of these adaptive mechanisms. They cannot remember new information, so the grieving process that human beings rely on to adapt to loss cannot evolve as it usually does. Some individuals with dementia cannot express themselves verbally and so cannot share with others their distress and concerns, another important mechanism to help them adapt. Adding to these problems is that many patients have a diminished capacity to learn from experience.

Dementing illnesses predispose people to emotional outbursts. Some individuals with dementia remain distressed and agitated despite reassurance, distraction, and emotional support, even if it is likely that such interventions would have been helpful to them before the onset of the dementia. In this situation the *inappropriate* response is the one that further distresses the patient. The *appropriate* response is the one that relieves distress. To our great discomfort, this sometimes involves lying.

We share the belief that lying is wrong. We believe lying can be justified only as a last resort and only when it is the sole means of relieving the distress of a person with dementia. One justification for lying in this circumstance is that, for the patient, the truth cannot be true. A statement that is true for us ("You live here now," "It sounds like you're frightened," "How do you think we should fix the place up?," "Your mother passed away several years ago") may *not* be true for people with dementia because the illness prevents them from knowing it. For them, their mother is still living and this is not where they live. For them, reality is different from what is true for us. Said another way, the lie or partial truth that we tell is an untruth *for us*, not for the patient. Since the purpose of our intervention is to relieve patients' distress, not to convince them of *our* reality, an untruth is often more beneficial than the truth. Ideally, all other approaches, including telling the truth once or twice and assessing if it benefits or harms the person, should be tried first.

Principle

Acting to reduce distress and to preserve a patient's dignity are important principles of dementia care. In most circumstances lying is unacceptable, but if it is the only way to relieve distress in a person who cannot benefit from the truth, then it is justifiable.

Who should make health decisions for a person who is severely incapacitated?

In the United States, most people believe that an individual's wishes expressed prior to becoming incapacitated should be followed if possible. Even with the availability of legal documents such as the durable power of attorney for health (discussed later in this chapter), it is difficult for people to predict and discuss ahead of time all the major decision points that reflect their views. Ideally, each of us will have discussed our broad desires with someone we trust and legally empowered them to express these wishes through an advanced directive. Often, however, neither of these has taken place. Who should make decisions for the incapacitated person?

Precedent and law empower the family to make substituted judgments in some states. In others, the trend is for legal representatives to be appointed. Which is more desirable? We believe the family should make substituted judgments unless there is reason to suspect that they are not acting on behalf of and in the best interest of the ill person. Our reliance on the family reflects our clinical experience that most families have their loved one's best interests at heart and have struggled to dignify and support the ill person. Most family members undoubtedly consider their own physical, financial, and emotional needs when making substitute judgments. However, family members rarely consider their own needs to the detriment of the patient's. When this does occur, a legal solution, such as a court-appointed guardianship, should be sought.

Occasionally, disagreements arise among family members or between the family and the health care provider. These can usually be resolved by helping family members and the treatment team work together to reach a consensus. When disagreements exist, the first step is to review the medical facts of the situation. The clinician should determine what is known about the specific problem under discussion, identify the options that are available, and discuss the likely outcomes of each approach. It may take several meetings to cover all the issues that need to be reviewed since most people are unaccustomed to discussing complex medical issues and because these discussions often occur in upsetting circumstances.

In the rare instance that family members cannot reach agreement, it is appropriate to seek help from others. If the family has not consulted clergy and they share a common religious background, this should be suggested. Social workers and medical consultants (both nurses and physicians) can be helpful. All hospitals and some nursing homes have ethics consultants who may be of help. Rarely, the family will need to see a new physician or nursing home because the current practitioner or institution cannot meet their needs. In extremely rare circumstances, legal adjudication must be sought.

Principle

Incompetent individuals should be *protected*. When they no longer have the capacity to decide for themselves, someone should make decisions for them. Ideally, this should be someone who knows their lifelong values and who will make decisions in their best interests. Family members are in the best position to stand in for the ill person because they can best represent the ill person's long-held beliefs and consider the person's best interests. Legal adjudication is necessary when disagreements cannot be resolved by time and discussion or when the ill person's best interests are not being considered by those making decisions.

Refusal to eat

Patients with dementia typically lose a few pounds per year as the disease progresses. In a minority of individuals, weight loss becomes a significant health concern and, for some, life-threatening. A small percentage of individuals with dementia actively resist eating. They push away the spoon or food when people attempt to feed them. Whenever food refusal or weight loss develops, it is necessary to determine whether an identifiable cause of the eating difficulty is present and whether the problem can be treated (see Chapter 9).

Dilemmas arise when no treatable cause for poor food intake is identified or when the ability to swallow appears to be permanently impaired due to the disease. If weight loss continues, severe debilitation and death become likely. What options are available? Attempts to feed the patient by mouth should continue as long as they are safe. This preserves eating as a natural function and provides a way of giving individualized care, attention, and love to an impaired person.

Most individuals with dementia who have life-threatening eating problems are severely demented. As a result, others must make decisions about artificial feeding. If the person's previously stated wishes can be reasonably accommodated, they should be given a prominent place in the decision-making process. How strongly they should influence the person who has authority to make the final decision is often a difficult question since the details of specific situations are almost never known ahead of time. Some would argue that a prior expressed wish must always be followed. We believe the circumstances of each decision require careful thought and that no absolute rule can be stated.

So-called *artificial feeding* is defined as feeding by blood vessel, usually by vein (intravenously) and rarely by artery or by a tube that is inserted either through the nose (nasogastric tube) or through the abdominal wall directly into the stomach (gastrostomy tube). A discussion of these options should be started as soon as it becomes evident that a patient is losing weight more rapidly than expected and no treatable cause is found. Ideally, this discussion should begin months before any decision must be made to allow the family or decision maker time to decide what actions they would like to take to address the problem and avoids the need to make a sudden decision. Most medical ethicists and courts agree that the placement of a nasogastric or gastrostomy tube is a specific medical intervention, not a normal aspect of feeding. We agree and believe that the choice *not* to use a feeding tube should be explicitly offered.

Is the placement of a feeding tube *desirable?* There is no single answer to this question (see Chapter 11). Feeding through tubes can provide balanced nutrition, thereby improving the body's function and prolonging life. On the other hand, feeding through a tube deprives a person of the pleasure and dignity of eating naturally and can lead to aspiration of food into the lungs. Being fed through a tube also deprives a person of the communal/sharing aspects of eating.

We also believe that a feeding tube can be removed at any time, just as any medical treatment can be stopped. Some individuals would disagree and contend that, since the individual is being starved, removal of a tube is always ethically inappropriate. Our opinion that feeding via a tube is a medical treatment is supported by the recognition that there are significant side effects of artificial feeding.

Because most patients who are unable or seem to refuse to eat are severely demented, they are almost never able to participate in a clear, consistent, and reasoned discussion about death, suicide, or refusing to eat. We believe it very unlikely that most individuals in this circumstance are *choosing* not to eat. Their severe cognitive impairment prevents them from appreciating the complexities of their circumstances. It seems particularly inappropriate to *assume* that food refusal results from a person's realization of the severity of his or her condition without telling us. We believe it is inappropriate to *guess* that not eating is a choice of the ill person without being told this directly and repeatedly by that person. Because depression is difficult to diagnose in patients with dementia, is potentially treatable, and is a cause of life-threatening food refusal, treatment for depression should be attempted if the possibility exists that it underlies food refusal.

If families are considering not placing a feeding tube in a person who resides in a nursing home, we urge them to discuss this directly with the staff and administration. Some nursing homes are unwilling to "let a person starve to death," but an increasing number see the placement of a tube in the patient as invasive and as an option that the patient or family can choose or reject. If it is chosen, a decision to remove the tube can be made in the future. Experience tells us, however, that the decision to remove a tube is very difficult emotionally.

One question that sometimes arises is whether inadequate food and fluid intake causes pain to the patient. This is impossible to answer with complete confidence. However, based on the reports of individuals who recover from severe dehydration and who report that they were not uncomfortable, we believe it very unlikely that this is a painful or uncomfortable state. Furthermore, patients who do not eat appear to be comfortable and do not complain of hunger. Thus, when caregivers ask about discomfort, we discuss our conclusion that it is unlikely.

The question of what to do for individuals with no available family, no legal guardian, and no well-documented evidence of prior desires is less difficult. While some argue that a third party, for example a court-appointed guardian or ombudsman, should make a decision based on an educated guess or a quality-of-life assessment of what this person might have wanted, we believe this is inappropriate. Since the sanctity of human life requires that professionals act to preserve life unless a fully competent person chooses otherwise, we believe that the lack of a person who is aware of the prior wishes of the ill person or the family's own wishes should lead professionals and society to act to support life.

Principle

There is no single right answer to the questions surrounding feeding tube placement. The patient's prior wishes have primary weight and should guide treatment. The professional should provide information and emotional support, raise questions, encourage discussion, and allow time for a decision to develop. Not feeding is an emotionally difficult option, but it can be ethically appropriate.

LEGAL ISSUES

Determining capacity or competency

In the United States, adults have the legal right to make all decisions for themselves and their children. *Competency,* the ability to make decisions, is automatically established when a person reaches the age of adulthood. It should be kept in mind, though, that *competency* and *incompetency* are legal concepts. A determination of incompetency must be made by a judge and indicates that the judge has found that the person lacks the ability to make responsible decisions.

The term *capacity* is a clinical concept that refers to the abilities a person needs to make decisions. Intact capacity requires three elements: (1) the ability to *comprehend* the issues at hand; (2) the ability to *choose freely,* that is, without the undue influence of others and without the determinative role of a mental illness; and (3) the ability to *communicate* the choice. A determination of incapacity implies impairments in at least one of these elements *plus* a diagnosable condition that is causing these impairments.

In the past, capacity was considered to be either present or absent. It is now recognized that a capacity can be partially present, and, in fact, many of those with impaired decision-making capacity have the capacity to make some decisions but not others. Indeed, only the most severely cognitively impaired lack the capacity to express some wishes and choices. For example, patients who cannot live independently or prepare meals can express a preference for clothing, choose if they would like to go on a trip, or ask for a specific food. Even individuals with severe dementia may have the capacity to express meaningful wishes about food or activity preferences.

The most important thing to keep in mind is that different *levels* of capacity are required in different circumstances. As a result, the clinician assessing capacity must examine both the person's abilities to comprehend and decide *and* the potential outcomes of a decision. If serious harm is likely, a greater burden is placed on the patient to demonstrate capacity. When harm is unlikely or nonexistent, there is little reason to invoke incompetency.

The inability to precisely define terms like *capacity* and *competency* is a source of frustration for some clinicians. However, medical decision making often requires balancing competing risks and benefits, and this is the central challenge in assessing the capacity to decide. Further complicating the issue, though, is the fact that decision-making capacity usually changes over time in dementia because most dementing illnesses cause progressive cognitive decline. It should be kept in mind that some medical conditions that impair decision-making capacity (e.g., delirium) are reversible. Thus, a person who suffers from a permanent dementia may undergo a sudden decline in capacity due to a urinary tract infection and then regain capacity after treatment.

This potential variability in capacity has several implications. First, if there is some potential for improvement in the patient's condition and a decision about capacity to choose does not need to be made immediately, it is better to delay a decision about decision-making capacity as long as possible. Even when an immediate decision must be made, repeat examinations over several hours may reveal periods of lucidity and retained decision-making capacity. Because the maximization of individual decision making is a widely held value in the United States, clinicians should seek as much information about the patient's desires as possible. This is not true in all cultural groups, however, since some groups emphasize group values over individual values. This emphasizes the point that the concepts of capacity and competency have strong components of cultural shaping. It is likely, therefore, that the definition of concepts such as competency and capacity will change over time and will vary among different cultures and legal jurisdictions.

As noted above, there are three central elements of a capacity assessment: *comprehension, choosing freely,* and *communicating* the choice. At a minimum, intact comprehension requires evidence that the person has identified the issue or issues that are being considered. A determination of intact comprehension can be made with greater confidence if the person is able to discuss the major options or issues and their potential outcomes or risks and benefits. *Choice* requires evidence that individuals know that a choice is being make and express a choice. Ideally, they will be able to give reasons for their choices, both pro and con. *Communication* requires that the person express the choice without influence and with some consistency.

The following paragraphs list seven issues the clinician can review when assessing if a person with dementia has intact decision-making capacity. They are also listed in Table 13.1. In the end, the clinician must make a clinical judgment based on the available information. Question 1 assesses whether the person comprehends the issue at hand. Questions 2–5 assess whether the person is making a choice. Questions 4, 5, and 6 are not required, but strengthen the evidence that a choice is being made. Question 7 addresses lack of duress and choice. If the person is able to meet all seven criteria, their capacity is intact. If they meet some but not all of the criteria, they may have partial capacity that is adequate for some decisions. When the capacity to decide is partially intact, the assessment of whether a person has the capacity to make a particular decision depends on the potential risks and benefits of that decision.

1. *Identify the issue at hand.* As a starting point, the patient should be able to state what the issue is. A capable person will be able to verbally repeat and summarize the question. Individuals who are unable to verbally communicate may be able to do so in writing. Persons with severe language disorders can be given four or five options; if they consistently choose the issue at hand, then this criterion would be satisfied.

   This criterion is aimed at ensuring that all parties are discussing the same issue. It does not assess whether the person understands the issue. Several of the subsequent criteria do assess the capacity to understand. Examples of meeting this criterion would be statements such as "The doctor says I need an operation" or "The social worker doesn't think I can live by myself."

2. *Can the person list the major options?* The ability to describe the major options or possible decisions demonstrates that the person appreciates that a choice among options must be made.

3. *Can the person state the most likely outcome or outcomes of each major option?* The ability to describe the potential outcomes of each option further demonstrates an understanding of the issue being discussed. The level of sophistication of this discussion will vary widely, depending on the patient's innate ability and willingness to cooperate. Statements such as "The doctor says I'll probably die if I don't get this operation" or "I know I could freeze to death if I sleep here" demonstrate knowledge of the potential outcome and support the conclusion that the patient has the capacity to comprehend the question.

4. *Does the person state a choice from among the options?* A key element of capacity determination is assessing whether the individual has

Table 13.1. Seven Elements in Deciding Capacity in
Dementia Patients

Can the dementia patient:

1. Identify the issue at hand?
2. State the major options to address the issue?
3. Know the most likely outcome(s) of each option?
4. State a choice from among the options?
5. Provide a reason that justifies the choice?
6. Show consistency over time?
7. Choose without coercion?

the capacity to make decisions. The demonstration that a choice has been made is central to this determination. Affirmative responses to the first three questions address the patient's ability to *consider* the specific question being discussed. This criterion establishes whether the person is expressing a specific *choice*.

5. *Does the person give a reason that justifies the choice?* This is positive evidence that a decision is being made. However, the inability or refusal to give a reason cannot be used as the sole basis for deciding that a person lacks capacity. Statements such as "Because that's what I want" offers no evidence. However, requiring that individuals give rational reasons for their decision imposes too strict a standard and would limit a person's ability to make an unusual or uncommon decision. On the other hand, a person's willingness to state reasons should be considered positive evidence that the decision-making capacity is intact.

6. *Is the person consistent over time?* While people must have the ability to change their opinions, the person who consistently repeats the same decision is offering evidence that a choice has been made. Indecision or changing a decision is not abnormal, but when the capacity of a person to make decisions is in question and the person is constantly changing, it is appropriate to question his or her decision-making capacity. The ability to give reasons for changing a decision should increase the clinician's confidence that the individual has made another choice. However, refusal to give reasons for a change or apparent inability to do so cannot, in itself, be used as evidence that a person lacks capacity.

7. *Is there evidence that the person's choice is being made free from co-*

ercion? Clinicians should attempt to elicit the person's choices in a setting in which outside influences on the decision-making process are minimized. Because it is clear that the way information is presented can influence the decision, the clinician should also attempt to ensure that the issue and choices are presented in as neutral a fashion as possible. Patients who give reasons derived from misperceptions that cannot be corrected, delusional ideas, or repeated misunderstanding and misstatements of facts are not able to choose freely and likely lack capacity.

If a given patient does not have the capacity to decide, then the clinician must identify a psychiatric or medical disorder that explains the incapacity. The reason courts empower clinicians to give expert testimony about capacity is that clinicians are trained to identify medical and psychiatric conditions that have caused the incapacity. Dementia, mental retardation, delusional depression, and schizophrenia are *potential* causes of impaired capacity. The mere presence of any one of these disorders, however, is not adequate evidence that a person is incapable of making decisions. Medical testimony that links the impairments in understanding, reasoning, and choosing to the conclusion that the person lacks the capacity to make decisions is a necessary aspect of the justification for concluding that a person lacks the capacity to make decisions.

Testamentary capacity

Testamentary capacity is the ability to write a will. In most jurisdictions, three abilities are necessary for intact testamentary capacity: (1) knowledge of assets, (2) knowledge of how assets are usually distributed, and (3) an explicit statement of how (and perhaps why) the person is choosing to distribute assets.

As can be seen, these are much more specific criteria than those listed previously for the capacity to decide other issues. One reason is that will writing is a very specific ability. Another is that will-making has a long tradition of importance, so case law has developed. Finally, leaving possessions to one's heirs has important links to family values and a strong tradition in many cultures. Therefore, courts are loath to overturn a person's wishes as expressed in a will, and the criteria for overturning a will are very strict. Thus, a person can be impaired in many areas of function and yet be fully able to prepare or change a will. Since a will can be contested, we suggest a specific assessment of the three issues listed in the prior paragraph if a person with dementia wishes to draw up or change a will.

Durable powers of attorney

Power of attorney is a legal term that refers to the delegation of legal powers. It usually delegates to another person (referred to as the *attorney*) the ability (*power*) to sign papers or carry out other legal processes. Because it is a delegation of a legal right, a person must be competent to delegate power of attorney *and* that person must remain competent for the power of attorney to be enforced. Intact capacity to decide is required because the individual retains the right to remove or discontinue the power of attorney at any time, and this ability would not be present if a court found the person incompetent.

Because the diseases that cause dementia often interfere with a person's capacity and often lead to incompetency, many states have passed laws that allow for the establishment of a *durable power of attorney.* This document appoints a personal representative (attorney) in the event that a person becomes incompetent. It is usually worded so that it comes into force only when incompetency develops, but it can be written as part of a standard power of attorney document. Thus, it can begin while a person is still competent and then continue if the capacity to make health or financial decisions is lost.

In some jurisdictions, the durable power of attorney is divided into several types. A common distinction is made between a durable power of attorney for health matters and for financial matters. Health matters relate to agreeing to medical care, signing for operations, and making life-and-death decisions. Financial matters usually relate to buying and selling of property and other monetary issues.

We recommend that all dementia patients set up a durable power of attorney that meets the laws in their state. This should be done as early as possible to prevent any questions about a patient's capacity to appoint an attorney. It allows patients to decide ahead of time who will manage their affairs and also avoids the necessity of having a judge assign a guardian.

Advance directives

In the past decade, many jurisdictions in the United States have set up legal documents by which individuals can direct others to make future health decisions for them if they become unable to do so themselves. The first such document was the *living will.* It describes peoples' wishes *if* they become terminally ill. In fact, decisions about terminal care are a small part of health care decisions, so the living will applies to only a small subset of health decisions, albeit an important one. A more recently developed document, called an *advance directive,* has been established in almost all states that allows competent individuals to designate who should make health decisions for them if they become incapacitated. It also allows persons to state specifically what they would like done in specific circumstances—for example, if questions about the use of feeding tubes, ventilators, and aggressive treatments at the end of life arise.

We see little use for the living will, as it is too narrow and inflexible and covers decision making only in terminal phases of an illness, a stressful but usually very brief period of time. On the other hand, we believe the advance directive is an important and useful document and encourage all of our patients who have capacity to draw one up to do so and to list general values. For patients who have one or more individuals whom they trust and with whom they can have a *conversation* about their specific values and wishes, we recommend that they appoint these individuals as their durable power of attorney and *not* list specific wishes. We make this recommendation because the details of most medical decisions are an important aspect of the decision-making process and cannot be known ahead of time. Having a trusted person or group of people making the decision that best reflects the values and wishes of a person offers the best method of respecting an incapacitated person's values. On the other hand, if someone who can represent a person's values is not available, we recommend that specific values be described in the document.

GENERAL CONCLUSIONS AND PRINCIPLES

Several principles can be derived from the above discussions. Attempts should be made to maximize the independence and self-determination of persons with dementia. While dementia often limits individuals' judgment and decision-making capacity, many persons with dementia have retained the capacity to decide some or all issues that control their health care. Attempts should be made to preserve whatever ability is retained.

Some dilemmas can be avoided by preventive ethics. Early discussion can avoid the need for rushed, last-minute discussions. All individuals should be encouraged to discuss with others their preferences regarding life support, surgery, and other significant interventions while they have the capacity to do so. We recommend strongly that all of our patients appoint a *durable power of attorney for health matters* who will be legally empowered to make decisions for them if they become disabled. Ideally, this will be done long before health problems develop.

A diagnosis of dementia in no way limits the person's access to adequate medical, social, and psychological care. Most mildly impaired individuals have the capacity to discuss, decide, and express their wishes. The presence of severe deficits should be taken as an indication that care must be carefully supervised and supported since the person is not able to defend himself.

A person chosen by the sick individual before she becomes incapacitated best supplies substituted judgment. Often this will be a family member but not always. A legal opinion should be sought only when the durable power of attorney has been designated when no family is available, when there is significant disagreement among family members, or when the family's or surrogate's self-interests appear to be affecting their choice of what is in the patient's best interest.

Most ethical dilemmas are solved by discussion. The clarification of medical, social, and financial issues, the expression of feelings and an exploration, of practical solutions almost always lead the interested parties to agree on an ethically acceptable course of action. *Consensus building* is an effective and attainable method of resolution. After the medical facts have been discussed, the potential options and their consequences should be reviewed. Choices can often be narrowed in this way and the discussion focused on specific questions and information.

Grief, anger, and guilt should be raised as issues if present. Airing these feelings openly can help clarify sources of disagreement. Such feelings are powerful shapers of the decision-making process. Their expression and clarification can allow the decision making to proceed.

14

CLINICAL GENETICS AND DEMENTIA

In almost all human diseases, there is an interaction between nature and nurture. For some diseases, such as HD, inheritance determines whether the disease will occur, while the environment may influence its age of onset, clinical presentation, and severity. Other diseases, for example head trauma or toxin exposure, are caused by environmental factors but are modified in clinical expression by genetic factors. In AD, multiple genes are involved, some of which cause the disease and others of which modify (increasing or decreasing) the likelihood of its occurring.

While our understanding of the clinical genetics of the dementias is in its infancy, clinicians caring for patients with dementia should have a basic understanding of genetics. Knowledge of genetic contributions to the cause and expression of dementia is likely to influence treatment in the future. In addition, understanding the pattern of inheritance will provide information on which genetic counseling should be based and provide guidance about when to refer to a genetic counselor. This is the process through which relatives, particularly offspring, of those afflicted with dementia can understand their own risk for the disease as well as the risk of their offspring.

This chapter will first outline basic genetic principles. Subsequently, genetic testing and genetic counseling as a whole will be discussed to set the context for the genetic counseling of persons related to patients with dementia. In particular, we will discuss presymptomatic testing, genetic counseling, and estimating risk. Finally, we will briefly apply knowledge gained from genetics to the care of patients with three diseases: AD, HD, and vascular dementia.

A GENETICS PRIMER

Chromosomes are complex molecules made up of deoxyribonucleic acid (DNA) that involve a variety of other proteins. They are carried in the nucleus of cells and have a very dense central point (centromere), from which a long arm (q arm) and a short arm (p arm) emanate. Each human cell carries a total of 46 chromosomes, all of which are arranged in pairs. Chromosomes 1–22 are referred to as the *autosomal* chromosomes. There are two copies of each. Humans also carry two sex chromosomes: women have two copies of the X chromosome, and men one copy of the X and one copy of the Y.

Genes are made up of long strings of DNA contained on chromosomes. Each human has about 100,000 genes. (The actual number has yet to be determined.) Each gene codes for a distinct protein. Proteins are the basic structural and functional foundation of the body. Since there are two copies of each chromosome, there are two copies of every gene, each of which is referred to as an *allele*. Because a copy of each gene comes from each parent, the two alleles are not always identical. This allows for redundancy, so that if we carry one aberrant gene, a second normal gene coding for the same protein may allow us to function as humans. The variation in amino acid sequence of a gene is called a *polymorphism*.

During reproduction each parent produces either sperm or ova, which contain half of their own genetic material. Thus, a father contributes to his sperm one copy of chromosome 1, one copy of chromosome 2, and so on. Half of his sperm contain a Y chromosome and the other half contain an X chromosome. The assortment of different chromosomes (and therefore genes) in individual sperm cells is random, allowing for a tremendous amount of variation. Similarly, the mother places in her ovum (egg) through the process known as *meiosis* one-half of her genetic material. When the sperm fertilizes the egg, the new human organism has a full complement of chromosomes (half from each parent). Because of this process of reproduction, individual genes are inherited as separate particles, independent of one another. Parental characteristics do not blend in offspring but rather are present in offspring as an aggregate of individual parts.

Genes vary in function, so it follows that specific diseases are associated with particular genes. Aberrations in some genes do not allow viability of the fetus and account for the relatively high rate of undetected spontaneous miscarriages. In some instances, it is possible to live a normal life with only one functioning gene. Under a biologic stress, however, having only one functioning gene may result in transient symptoms of a disease that resolve when the stress resolves. Aberrant genes may code for aberrant proteins that cause malregulation of other genes, leading to the expression of a disease in all those who carry it.

Several distinct inheritance patterns of disease have been described. In the *autosomal* patterns, a diseased gene is carried on 1 of the 22 non-sex chromosomes and is the cause of disease. If a single copy of the aberrant gene is sufficient to produce the disease, this is referred to as the *autosomal dominant* situation. A disease inherited as an autosomal dominant occurs in every successive generation and afflicts, on average, one-half of the offspring. Huntington disease is an example of this. Looking carefully at the pedigree (a genetic diagram) of an individual with dementia can help us appreciate whether the disease is being transmitted as an autosomal dominant.

In *autosomal recessive* inheritance, two copies of an aberrant gene are necessary to express the disease. In this way, the gene may be carried down several generations and remain silent because the offspring do not mate with individuals who also carry the aberrant gene. This is referred to as a *carried* state. Occasionally, there will be a chance pairing between two carriers of the gene, which results in the development of the disease in approximately one-fourth of their offspring—that is, in those who inherit two aberrant genes, one from each of their two healthy parents. Cystic fibrosis is an example of autosomal recessive inheritance.

The third general pattern of inheritance is referred to as *sex-linked*. If the abnormal gene is carried on an X chromosome, it behaves like a recessive. In women, who carry only one affected X chromosome, the disease will not be expressed because the gene on the other X chromosome is normal. However, in men, who have only one X chromosome, the disease will act as a dominant and will occur in every man who inherits the aberrant X chromosome. As a result, sex-linked diseases occur almost exclusively in men of a particular family and skip generations if there are no male offspring. Hemophilia is an example of X-linked inheritance. The final general category of inherited diseases is known as *multifactorial*. In this paradigm, several genes must be aberrant at the same time for a disease to develop. Inheritance is neither dominant nor recessive, and several generations may be skipped before it is expressed. Most of the common dementias have multifactorial inheritance.

A variety of genetic tests is available, and more are being developed. The simplest is a direct examination of the chromosome and is referred to as *karyotyping*. It involves drawing blood and examining peripheral white blood cells (lymphocytes) after chemical fixation of the cell in the nuclei. Under the microscope or by photographic enlargement, the general appearance of the chromosomes can be examined and gross aberrations such as large pieces of missing or duplicated chromosomes can be identified. Trisomy 21 (Down syndrome) is diagnosed in this fashion. Currently, most of the chromosomal conditions are diagnosed by karyotyping.

Other tests look specifically at the DNA by drawing blood or taking dead cell samples by gently scraping the mouth cavity or taking a piece of hair.

The simplest tests are the restriction fragment length polymorphism (RFLP) studies. It has been known for some time that if certain enzymes are added to DNA solutions, they cut the DNA at predetermined sites. DNA in the form of "DNA soup" can then be studied to look at the fragments left after cuts with different restriction enzymes. This process allows the creation of large libraries of what happens to normal DNA after it is cut with specific restriction enzymes. It then becomes possible to predict the lengths that different parts of DNA will be cut into when it is normal and cut with specific enzymes. Taking DNA from persons with different diseases and applying different restriction enzymes can lead to finding DNA of different lengths (and therefore different molecular composition) because of differences in sequence. Systematic comparisons of different lengths allow scientists to determine which segments of DNA may be involved in particular diseases. More elaborate tests then allow us to look at specific segments and regions of DNA and eventually allow the identification of specific genes involved in different diseases. Given the ability to directly examine DNA sequences, RFLP studies are losing their clinical utility.

Now that the human genome has been fully sequenced, it is possible to test for the presence or absence of aberrant genes for thousands of human diseases. In the future, it will be possible to test individuals for the presence or absence of individual aberrant genes in their genetic makeup even in the absence of disease. This will be done simply by drawing blood from the individual involved. Already this is possible with HD where the gene for the condition has been identified on the short arm of chromosome 4. Individuals at risk for this disease can now be tested and told with 100% certainty whether they will develop the disease. What they cannot be told is when it will develop or exactly what the symptoms will be.

These advances in genetic diagnosis have led us into a new era. They raise many problems as well as many possibilities. The experience at Johns Hopkins with presymptomatic testing for HD has been that the majority of individuals at risk for the disease are not interested in finding out whether they carry the diseased gene. With the proper approach, genetic counseling of those who *are* interested evolves smoothly. Genetic counseling and presymptomatic testing related to dementia are likely to become widespread in the years to come.

GENETIC COUNSELING AND PRESYMPTOMATIC TESTING IN DEMENTIA

Genetic counseling communicates information about the genetic aspects of dementia and provides support to relatives of persons with dementia. Genetic counselors are health care professionals who are trained in the technical and clinical aspects of a genetic disease, including dementia. The purpose of genetic counseling is twofold. The first is to provide general information about the heritability of particular dementia-causing conditions. This basically involves the communication of knowledge that has been acquired through research. Second, genetic counseling is intended to provide specific advice to relatives, typically children, of persons with dementia regarding their own risk of developing dementia.

Several steps are involved in genetic counseling: obtaining a complete history and pedigree, conducting an examination of the affected individual, ordering appropriate laboratory investigations, and counseling. As applied to dementia, genetic counseling involves the determination of a phenotype of the patient with dementia using the evaluation practices described in Chapter 2. When possible, the specific etiology of the dementia should be identified, that is, AD, vascular dementia, HD and so on. Pathologic diagnosis of the cause of dementia is important, although not always available. Finally, genotyping of the affected individual with respect to abnormal genes is conducted.

Perhaps the most important aspect of genetic counseling involves a careful understanding of the individuals who are seeking it. Their motive for requesting genetic counseling is the first issue that needs to be addressed. Are they interested in learning whether they might develop the disease so that they can prepare psychologically? Are they thinking of having children and therefore want to know whether they are carrying an aberrant gene that would put their children at risk? Or is there some other reason, perhaps a financial motive, that might be involved?

Another aspect of genetic counseling is an assessment of the psychological impact of test results. Are individuals at high risk of severe emotional upset if the results are distressing? Are there people close to them, such as family members or friends, who would support them if they have inherited the disease gene? Would they be amenable to long-term counseling to help them emotionally if they become significantly upset or depressed?

Finally, genetic counseling helps people consider what they are likely to do with the information and how it may affect their lives. In the past, concerns were raised about bad news leading people to suicide. Experience with the Baltimore Huntington Disease Pre-symptomatic Testing Project at Johns Hopkins suggests that this almost never happens, but suicidal ideation and severe depression are potential risks. Those being counseled are specifically asked to consider how they would anticipate reacting if they are told that they are carrying a gene that puts them at serious risk for developing a very bad disease. Thorough, careful consideration of this question is crucial before genetic testing begins.

Genetic testing of individuals with a family history of dementia is currently most informative for the uncommon families in which a dominant mode of inheritance is present. The population rate of dementia is so high that it is not possible, given the present state of knowledge, to estimate precisely the risk of dementia in most people with a relative who has dementia.

What can be said with certainty for most cases of dementia is that the relatives of people with dementia are at higher risk for developing dementia than the general population and that this risk increases with age. How much greater this risk is cannot be stated with precision except for a few relatively uncommon diseases. One study has suggested that the first-degree relatives (parent, sibling, child) of a person with AD have a 38% chance of developing AD, while another estimate is a 73% risk if persons live to age 90, compared to a 40% chance of developing it if they live into their 90s.

As our understanding of the human genome increases and our ability to link specific genotypes to specific dementia-causing conditions improves, it will be possible to give individuals more precise estimates of their genetic risk. Given the experience of the Baltimore Huntington Disease Presymptomatic Testing Project, we anticipate that this information will be useful to some individuals, but many will not seek testing until effective interventions or preventive treatments are available. Some of these issues will be discussed further in reviewing the genetics of three diseases associated with dementia.

Alzheimer disease

Twin studies have suggested that 60%–70% of the etiology of AD is genetically based. However, the genetics of the disease is complex, because it depends upon several genes that play different roles. For example, AD with onset before age 60 is often of a genetic etiology, transmitted as an autosomal dominant and caused by genetic abnormalities on chromosomes 1, 14, and 21. However, the examination of family pedigrees reveals that many people with age of onset after age 60 also have autosomal dominant inheritance and are likely carriers of aberrant AD-causing genes. The observation that almost 100% of people with Down syndrome develop the pathology of AD by age 40 led to an investigation of chromosome 21 since there is either an extra chromosome 21 or an extra piece of this chromosome in people with Down syndrome. The gene that directs the production of APP (see Chapter 2) is involved in the amyloid plaque found in AD and is found on chromosome 21. Several different mutations in this gene result in the production of an abnormal form of this protein and lead to the development of AD. This overproduction of APP is also likely involved in AD associated with Down syndrome. The presenilin 1 gene on chromosome 14 and the presenilin 2 gene on chromosome 1 produce proteins whose function is not known but that are located in all nerve cell membranes. Carriers of an aberrant form of these genes are destined to develop AD if they live long enough.

A different mode of action is associated with the APOE gene, located on chromosome 19. This gene has three alleles, labeled 2, 3, and 4. Carrying allele 4 (APOE-4) places people at risk for developing AD at a younger age. The gene product does not appear to cause the disease. Individuals who carry two E4 alleles have an earlier age of onset than individuals with one E4 allele, but several people in their 90s have been identified who have two E4 alleles but do not suffer from AD. Other possible genetic abnormalities associated with AD have been proposed but have not been successfully replicated in other studies. For example, it has been reported that an abnormal form of the chromosome 12 gene coding for alpha-2 macroglobulin (alpha-2M) is also a strong risk factor for the onset of AD in later life. As many as 30% of the population carry the mutation. It is still not known precisely how this abnormal gene increases the risk for AD, although it appears that alpha-2M is involved in the clearance of amyloid from brain tissue.

Given the issues reviewed above, we suggest the following. First, it is crucial to conduct a careful evaluation to confirm the diagnosis of AD in affected relatives, if possible, through pathologic investigation of the affected relative. Second, genetic testing of patients and relatives should be considered only when there is a clear genetic pattern in the pedigree, such as autosomal dominant transmission with early-onset disease. In very rare cases, interested relatives, particularly children, may undergo genetic testing to determine whether they possess one of the abnormal genes on chromosomes 1, 14, or 21. At present, genetic testing for APOE-4 and alpha-2M is *not* appropriate for relatives of patients with suspected AD.

In the near future, other genes will be identified that increase or decrease the risk of developing AD. At present, genetic testing is appropriate for only a minority of cases since the majority of AD patients have late-onset disease and most do not have a family history. In the future, combinations of genetic testing, brain imaging, and detailed neuropsychological testing may predict whether individuals are at risk for developing AD and their likelihood of developing symptoms by a specific age.

Huntington disease

From its earliest descriptions, HD has been recognized as a genetic disorder. In affected families it occurs in every generation and afflicts approximately half of each successive generation in an autosomal dominant pattern. In 1984 the disease was linked to a gene on chromosome 4, and in 1993 the aberrant gene was identified. It is now possible to diagnose persons at risk for HD genetically and to determine with nearly 100% certainty whether or not they will develop the disease if they live long enough. This high certainty is possible because HD has a penetrance of 100%.

As discussed in chapter 4, the genetic abnormality causing HD is an increased number of repeat amino acid sequences in a gene that produces a protein called *huntingtin*. By taking a simple blood test and determining the number of CAG triplet repeats in the HD gene, it is possible to determine whether a person will develop the disease with 100% certainty. Thus, genetic counseling is particularly applicable to HD because of the high degree of certainty provided by the testing. Nevertheless, the experience at Johns Hopkins is that less than half of those at risk for HD are interested in finding out whether they carry the aberrant gene.

Vascular dementia

The genetics of vascular dementia are poorly understood. There is evidence that a family history of dementia is more prevalent in patients with vascular dementia than it is in the general population. This suggests a role for genetics in the development of vascular dementia. However, this role remains unclear. One possible explanation involves the observation that many patients diagnosed clinically with vascular dementia turn out to also have AD. Therefore, it may be that this genetic association involves that subcategory of cases with co-morbid AD and vascular dementia.

Another possible explanation is that the genetic association is a linkage of risk factors for stroke. Diabetes, hypertension, and high cholesterol, all conditions with genetic associations, increase the risk for stroke; familial association may be due to the increased risk for diabetes, hypercholesterolemia, and hypertension in relatives of stroke patients. A final possible explanation is that certain types of vascular dementia have specific genetic components.

At this point, it is extremely difficult to disentangle these three possibilities without further evidence. Thus, genetic counseling for patients who have vascular dementia is not currently practical.

APPENDICES

APPENDIX A   Dementia Care Guidelines for Families   279

APPENDIX B   Basic Psychosocial Intervention in Dementia   295

APPENDIX C   Supportive Care Checklists and Calendars   297

277

APPENDIX A

DEMENTIA CARE GUIDELINES
FOR FAMILIES
Third Edition

**Division of Geriatric Psychiatry and Neuropsychiatry
The Johns Hopkins University**

CONTENTS

The Johns Hopkins Model of Care for Dementia	281
What Is Dementia?	282
What Is Alzheimer Disease?	282
Tips for the Caregiver	283
Eating	283
Dressing	284
Bathing	285
Getting to the bathroom	285
Structuring activities	286
Communication	286
Medications	287
Hallucinations	288
Delusions	288
Depression	289
Driving	290
Task Breakdown	290

Prepared by Constantine G. Lyketsos and Peter V. Rabins. May be reproduced and distributed. Forms can also be downloaded from http://www.oup.com/us/pdc.

Taking inventory   291
Catastrophic reactions   291
Rummaging and hoarding   292

The Johns Hopkins Model of Care for Dementia

Most disorders causing dementia such as Alzheimer disease and vascular dementia are progressive and last for many years. This approach to care is grounded in four general areas.

1. Treat the Disease

Currently, the cause of dementia can often be identified with a high degree of certainty through a systematic evaluation. In addition, treatments are now available. So, the first step is to get an evaluation and diagnosis of what is likely causing the dementia and consider treatment.

2. Treat the Symptoms

Dementia is often accompanied by many troublesome symptoms. These include behavior problems such as resisting care, not sleeping at night, pacing and wandering and combativeness and many others. These symptoms can be addressed by a variety of methods including the use of medications to thoughtfully designing a schedule of activities to distract the patient. Different families will find different behaviors more troublesome. It is important to tell your doctor what you find most challenging so that a plan to help can be made.

3. Support the Patient

A person with dementia will need help to stay healthy by monitoring any chronic illnesses and recognizing and gaining prompt treatment for new ones. In most cases, the caregiver must also take responsibility for giving medications. A safe environment must be assured so [that] the patient cannot be harmed in the home. Enjoyable activities are also necessary. Legal protection is addressed by deciding who will make decisions for the patient[s] when they can no longer make them. Identification bracelets can help to identify a patient who has wandered away. Decisions such as when driving is no longer safe must be made.

4. Support the Caregiver

Care for those with dementia is often provided by one person or a small group. It is care that requires vigilance 24 hours per day every day. To help caregivers to do this, the clinical team must support them emotionally, give guidance in decision making, educate them about the disease their loved one has and assist in identifying resources in the community to help.

Prepared by Constantine G. Lyketsos and Peter V. Rabins. May be reproduced and distributed. Forms can also be downloaded from http://www.oup.com/us/pdc.

What Is Dementia?

In the past, terms like "senility," "organic brain syndrome," or "late life confusion" were used to describe the elderly person who had difficulty thinking and remembering. The understanding of what is normal aging and what is abnormal aging has progressed so that new terms are used.

The medical definition of dementia is the following:

> A *global decline* in intellectual abilities of *sufficient severity* to *interfere* with occupational and/or social functioning. This occurs in *clear consciousness*.

What Does This Mean?

- *Global decline* means that more than one aspect of thinking is affected. So, a person who only has memory problems or who only has difficulty in speaking would not be described as demented. Persons who are demented often have difficulty in remembering, communicating, making decisions, and planning.
- *Sufficient severity* to impair functioning means that the problems the patient has are severe enough to produce problems in daily life. Common problems include not remembering to pay bills, not being able to plan, shop, and prepare meals, and getting lost in familiar places.
- *Clear consciousness* means that the person is awake and alert. This is in contrast to a person who is drowsy and not thinking properly due to an illness such as pneumonia and fever or who is impaired by medications, anesthesia, or alcohol.

What Causes Dementia?

Some conditions can mimic dementia and must be identified and treated. These include depression, intoxication from medications, both prescription and over the counter, and thyroid disease, among others.

There are many causes of dementia. Some get worse over time and some do not. Causes include strokes, Parkinson disease, Huntington disease and many others. Alzheimer disease (AD) is the most common cause. It can be diagnosed accurately and a variety of treatments are available.

What is Alzheimer Disease?

Alzheimer disease (AD) is the most common cause of dementia in later life. AD begins gradually and gets worse over a period of years. The common symptoms

Prepared by Constantine G. Lyketsos and Peter V. Rabins. May be reproduced and distributed. Forms can also be downloaded from http://www.oup.com/us/pdc.

of AD begin with the letter *A* and are known as the *4As of AD*. Each of the symptoms causes difficulty in daily life.

- **Amnesia:** *(Memory)* AD causes difficulty in registering new memories and recalling them. Common examples include asking the same question over and over and losing belongings. These problems occur because the part of the brain involved in registering new memories is damaged.
- **Aphasia:** *(Language)* AD affects the ability of the patients to communicate with others. Many patients develop difficulty in finding words and their speech becomes vague and empty. Second, patients will have difficulty in understanding what is being said to them. Language problems are frustrating for both the patient and caregiver.
- **Apraxia:** *(Doing things)* AD damages the parts of the brain that are involved in planning and directing the body to do things. Common problems are putting on clothing backwards and picking up food with the hands instead of using a knife and fork. Tasks must be simplified for the patient who has this symptom. Often, starting a task such as putting food on a fork and handing it to the patient can get a task started.
- **Agnosia:** *(Recognizing the world)* Though patients with AD can see the world, brain disease causes difficulty in recognizing what they see. Common examples of this are the person who stands in front of the refrigerator looking at the milk but being unable to recognize it. Some patients who may be unable to recognize their caregiver become uncooperative or run away.

Tips for the Caregiver

Eating

Many persons with AD develop difficulty with eating and weight loss. There are many causes of decreased eating including not remembering if they have eaten or not, inability to ask for food due to language problems, inability to open complicated packages and to prepare meals, and, lastly, inability to find or recognize food or drinks. Also, any source of pain, such as dental pain, can reduce eating and drinking. The following tips may help:

- Provide meals in a quiet and uncluttered place. TV and other noise can be too distracting for the person with AD.
- Serve one type of food at a time in small amounts. Too many choices can be overwhelming.
- Use simple place settings such as a contrasting plate and placemat and a single utensil.

- Provide meals on a routine schedule and have snacks and fluids readily visible for the person who needs to eat and drink more.
- Provide drinks every 2 hours instead of asking if he is thirsty.
- If the person can no longer cut up food, cut it in the kitchen before serving to preserve dignity.
- If the person chokes on thin liquids, add thickeners available at pharmacies.
- Maintain dental health by regular trips to the dentist or hygienist.
- If the patient eats very little, boost nutrition by adding calories to the regular diet.
- Sometimes, putting something sweet on the tip of the spoon will encourage eating.
- Finger foods will make eating easier for persons who can no longer use utensils.

Dressing

Getting a person with dementia dressed can be a challenge. The process of dressing can break down at many steps including inability to choose clothing, difficulty putting it on correctly, wearing the same clothes over and over and refusing to change clothes. As with other complicated tasks, one must determine where in the process the patient is having trouble and provide the help that is needed. The following tips may help:

- Limit the choices: clear out a closet and place an acceptable outfit in clear view.
- Allow ample time: schedule appointments in late morning or in the afternoon. Rushing can stall the process and upset everyone.
- Remove soiled clothing out of sight when the person is bathing. Replace it with clean clothing.
- Obtain clothing that is easy to put on and to take off. Jogging outfits, elastic waist pants, shoes with Velcro straps and clip on neckties can allow maximum independence.
- Purchasing sets of similar clothing from catalogues can help if the patient insists on wearing the same thing over and over.
- Be prepared for opportunities to change. If the person resists changing, keep spare underwear and clothing in the bathroom so that as he is sitting on the toilet and half undressed, clean clothing can quickly be put on.
- Be flexible: if arguments arise about changing clothes, drop the topic and try again later.
- Sometimes it is better to let people sleep in their clothes and attempt to change the next morning.

Bathing

Problems with bathing are very common in the care of those with dementia. Patients can become uncooperative with bathing for several reasons. They may have forgotten how to bathe, are frightened and cold, or don't recognize their caregiver. Many interpret attempts to bathe them as "someone trying to harm them." The following tips may help:

- Build on past routines. If the person always took showers, he may not resist that as much.
- Get organized: gather soap, towels, washcloths and clean clothes ahead of time.
- Fill the tub ahead of time to decrease frightening noise.
- Plan the bath at the time the patient is rested and most cooperative.
- Give instructions one step at a time.
- Ensure that the person is warm by covering him with a large towel or flannel sheet and washing one body part at a time. Purchase a terry cloth robe to put on as soon as the bath is finished. That will begin the drying process and ensure privacy and warmth.
- Give the person the soap and washcloth so that he can begin the process.
- A handheld showerhead on a flexible cable can allow the caregiver to wash the person easily.
- Obtain a shower or tub bench and install grab bars to avoid slipping. Put a towel on the bench to avoid slipping and to provide comfort.

Getting to the Bathroom

Losing control of the bladder and bowels is not expected in dementia until the late stages. Earlier on, patients can have accidents for many reasons. With good planning, accidents can usually be avoided. Patients can become easily distracted and not realize they need to go until it is too late. They may forget where the bathroom is. Complicated clothing may take too long to undo. They may not recognize the toilet and may use other things like trash cans instead. The following tips may help:

- Establish a routine: Asking the person if she needs to use the bathroom is insufficient to avoid accidents. One must take the person to the bathroom at least every two hours.
- Simplify clothing: eliminate complicated clothing such as panty hose, belts, and zippers. Replace fasteners with Velcro or eliminate them by using elastic waist pants.
- Limit fluids in the evening and avoid caffeine to reduce the risk of nighttime accidents

Prepared by Constantine G. Lyketsos and Peter V. Rabins. May be reproduced and distributed. Forms can also be downloaded from http://www.oup.com/us/pdc.

- Plan ahead: locate family bathrooms in shopping malls and airports. Always take a change of clothes just in case.
- If accidents begin suddenly, take the person to the doctor for a checkup. She may have an infection.
- When traveling, stop at least every two hours and take the person to the bathroom. Placing a sign on the door of the bathroom "Helping ill relative in the bathroom" can enhance privacy.

Structuring Activities

Persons with dementia gradually lose the ability to plan their day. Gradually, things they did in the past such as cooking, yardwork and participating in hobbies become too difficult and can become frustrating. As they lose a sense of time, they may get up during the night and try to go to work. A routine of activities during the day provides security to the patient and promotes rest and sleep at night. Without a routine, many persons with dementia follow their caregiver around all day. The following tips may help:

- Try to get the person up in the morning and in bed at the same times each day. Keeping him up and active during the day helps getting a good night's sleep.
- Write down a schedule allowing ample time to complete tasks such as dressing and bathing. This will be helpful to other caregivers that provide help from time to time.
- Think of activities he liked to do when he was well. Break them down into short, achievable steps and give praise for completing each step.
- Doing the same thing over and over again is reassuring and not boring for many persons with dementia.
- Physical activities and time outside are useful. Even scheduling a walk in the yard or around a shopping mall can be enjoyable.
- Having a schedule also helps in asking for help from others. One can directly say, "Bob goes for a walk at 11 a.m. every day. Can you come over and take him?"
- If the patient becomes tired in the afternoons, allow him to sit and listen to music or look at magazines but avoid naps if possible.
- Planning an activity the person especially enjoys after dinner will encourage him to stay up so that he will sleep all night.

Communication

Communication difficulties are common in dementia and often frustrating for patients and caregivers. Examples of communication problems include: Difficulty

Prepared by Constantine G. Lyketsos and Peter V. Rabins. May be reproduced and distributed. Forms can also be downloaded from http://www.oup.com/us/pdc.

finding words, having words on the "tip of the tongue," losing a train of thought, and not comprehending what is being said. The following tips may help:

- Make sure you have the person's attention before speaking.
- Speak slowly in a calm, low tone of voice.
- Use hand gestures to demonstrate requests ("sit here," patting the seat of the chair).
- Use simple, concrete words.
- Simplify the message into one or two parts.
- Give instructions one step at a time.
- Provide reassurance rather than try to reason or give an explanation. "I'll wait for your return" provides much comfort to someone refusing to attend a day program.
- Respond to repeated questions with simple key words or phrases.
- Try to provide the word the patient is struggling to say.
- Observe facial and body language to better understand what the patient is saying.
- Listen carefully for key words.
- When trying to communicate, eliminate distractions such as radio and TV.

Medications

Taking medications properly is important. Memory loss and difficulty concentrating caused by dementia makes taking medications correctly a challenge. Taking extra doses can be just as harmful as forgetting doses. When dementia patients have more than one doctor prescribing medicine, the chance of mistakes is even greater. Supervision of medications is necessary even early on in the disease process. The following tips may help:

Take inventory:
- List all the medicines, including herbs, vitamins, and supplements, the doses, the frequency and the doctor's name on one card.
- Gather and store all medications in one area.
- Check throughout the house to find medicines (including kitchen cupboards, dressers, purses, coats, bathroom cabinets).
- Take the list of medications to every doctor's visit for review.
- Throw out any expired medicines or those no longer used.

Early in dementia, supervise medicine use:
- Use weekly pill organizers.
- Count the number of pills regularly to check for correct use.
- Make a simple schedule for patients to follow.

When mistakes are noticed:
- Remove all medicine from the person's possession.
- Keep medications stored in a secure place.
- Give the pills immediately when they are to be taken; pills left out may get lost.
- Make sure the person swallows the pill.

If a person with dementia refuses medicine, ask for liquid alternatives or check if the pill can be crushed and added to a favorite food like ice cream or pudding.

Be careful using "over the counter" medicines. Ask your doctor before giving cold and cough medicines or sleep preparations.

Hallucinations

Some people with AD or other dementias will develop hallucinations. These can be distressing symptoms for both the person and the caregiver. When they occur, the doctor should be informed so that treatment can be discussed. These are real experiences for the patient and can be frightening to her.

- Hallucinations are the experience of seeing things or hearing voices when nothing is there.
- Seeing things, animals or people are the most common hallucinations.
- Hallucinations may occur as a result of another illness, an infection, medication side effects or anesthesia.
- When patients hallucinate after surgery, they may be frightened and try to run away from the visions, creating safety risks.

If Hallucinations Develop
- Look for signs of an illness or infection. Examples include sudden onset of incontinence (wetting accidents), a cough, drowsiness, or unsteady walking.
- Let your doctor know this has happened.
- Provide reassurance. For example, you might say: "I don't see those people but I'll keep you safe."
- Provide distraction. Moving the patient to another room or changing the activity can sometimes distract her.
- Stay with the person when she is in the hospital, if possible, to avoid the use of restraints and unnecessary sedation.

Delusions

Many persons with dementia develop delusions. Delusions are fixed false beliefs. Such beliefs are strongly held, and patients cannot be convinced otherwise. Delusions can result in aggression and put patients and their caregivers at risk of harm. *Common delusions* in dementia include believing that:

- Someone is stealing from them.
- People are in the house who are not there.
- Caregivers are not who they say they are.
- Their food or medicines are poisoned.
- Their spouse is unfaithful.

If Delusions Develop

- Avoid arguing or trying to reason. Provide reassurance. Try to find things they say are stolen.
- Inform the doctor of the delusions.
- Try to distract them. For example, if they are looking for their deceased mother, say, "I haven't seen her lately, but let's get a snack and you can tell me about your mother."
- Make sure they are safe and cannot wander out.

Depression

Depression is a common complication of dementia causing needless suffering to patients and their caregivers. Once thought of as a natural consequence of dementia, depression occurs in 20-40% of patients and can be effectively treated. *No one can* "will" away depression by "being stronger." Many patients won't complain of feeling sad or depressed. It is most important to understand that this is a chemical illness much like diabetes and is not a normal reaction to the knowledge of having a dementing illness.

Symptoms of depression in dementia include changes in:

- *Mood*—tearfulness, anxiety, worry, loss of pleasure
- *Behavior*—irritability, uncooperativeness
- *Appetite*—eating less, eating more
- *Thoughts*—low self-esteem, fearfulness, guilt
- *Sleep*—difficulty falling asleep, awakening earlier than usual
- *Energy*—loss of energy, apathy, withdrawal

If Depression Develops

- Have the patient evaluated. Report symptoms to the doctor.
- Encourage small, frequent snacks and meals to ensure adequate nutrition.
- Encourage the patient to get out of bed and change her clothes despite refusals.

- Assist with the change of clothing to promote good hygiene.
- Inform physicians of side effects if taking an antidepressant.
- Offer reassurance and hope, since it may take time for medicine to be effective.

Driving

The issue of whether a patient with AD or other dementia should drive is important. The issue of independence makes driving a sensitive issue. Problems driving occur when something unusual happens, such as a child running into the street or a construction area. Problems in driving include:

- Getting lost
- Using poor judgment
- Driving in the middle of the road or on the wrong side
- Driving too fast or too slow
- Not obeying traffic signals

If There Are Driving Concerns

- If you feel uncomfortable driving with the patient or if you would not allow a grandchild to drive with him, begin steps to stop his driving.
- Enlist the help of your doctor in getting the person to stop driving.
- Disable the car if necessary.
- Provide alternate methods of transportation.
- Relocate or sell the car.
- Obtain a formal driving evaluation if necessary.

Task Breakdown

Task breakdown refers to simplifying the steps of activities in daily life. It can help to overcome frustrating problems like difficulty in remembering the steps of a task, becoming easily distracted, and having difficulty coordinating movements needed to complete a task.

Tips on How to Do Task Breakdown

- Write down all the steps of a task.
- Observe the patient trying to complete a task to identify parts that are difficult.
- Eliminate steps that are frustrating for the patient.
- Give instructions one step at a time.
- Give praise for the completion of each step.

Prepared by Constantine G. Lyketsos and Peter V. Rabins. May be reproduced and distributed. Forms can also be downloaded from http://www.oup.com/us/pdc.

- Begin tasks for patients by getting them started, such as holding a shirt and putting an arm through the armhole.
- Try putting your hand over theirs and guiding it during tasks like holding a fork to eat or brushing teeth. This is called "hand-over-hand" guidance.
- Encourage patients to participate as much as they can without frustration, such as allowing them to stir food when they cannot follow a recipe.
- Re-evaluate task performance regularly. Most patients will have more difficulty over time and will need more help.

Taking Inventory

By the time dementia is recognized, the personal affairs of the patient are often in disarray. Common problems include misplacing checks, forgetting to pay bills, hiding money, and/or repeatedly withdrawing money from the bank. Patients may be reluctant to allow someone to help in these matters. It is important to take inventory of the patient's obligations and assets.

Go Through the House to Find the Following:

- All bills and obligations of the patient.
- The checkbook.
- Account numbers and location of all bank accounts.
- Stock and savings bond certificates.
- Social Security and insurance cards.
- Advance directives.
- Last will and testament.
- Discharge certificates from the armed forces.
- Pensions and other retirement benefits.
- Insurance policies.
- Completed power of attorney to manage finances.
- Jewelry of sentimental or monetary value.
- Costume jewelry to use as substitues for valuable bracelets, rings, necklaces, and earings.

Catastrophic Reactions

A catastrophic reaction is the sudden expression of a negative emotion or behavior such as yelling or running away. Such outbursts are often a reaction to something in the environment or to task failure. This term is useful, as it expresses the idea that the person is reacting to a seemingly minor event as if it were a catastrophe. Catastrophic reactions are associated with brain injury from any cause and are often seen in those who have had head trauma or developmental disabilities.

Prepared by Constantine G. Lyketsos and Peter V. Rabins. May be reproduced and distributed. Forms can also be downloaded from http://www.oup.com/us/pdc.

Example 1: A man with AD struggles to put his pants on and finally puts them on backwards. He then attempts to zip them up the back and can't do it. He then gets so frustrated by this that he takes them off and throws them on the floor, refusing to get dressed.

Example 2: A woman with AD is attending a holiday dinner at her daughter's home. Music is playing; small children are running about; holiday decorations are displayed. Previously, she would have enjoyed such an occasion. When her daughter asks her to carry a plate of food into another room, she suddenly starts crying.

How You Can Help

Know the functional limits of the person and do not expect her to do more than she can to prevent and avoid such reactions.

In *example 1,* simply assisting the man by holding out his pants in the correct presentation can allow him to continue to dress himself.

In *example 2,* limiting the size and complexity of the holiday dinner will help the woman to continue to enjoy it. Also, finding simple things that she can do will reinforce her meaningful contribution to the family.

In general, when you notice someone suddenly getting upset, stop what you are doing with them or move them to a different environment. Catastrophic reactions often stop by themselves. After the person is calm, think about how to avoid further reactions.

Rummaging and Hoarding

Rummaging and hoarding are two common behaviors in persons with more severe dementia. Rummaging is characterized by aimlessly moving objects about, looking through things and touching things. Persons who do this appear to be searching for something and may persist in this behavior for hours, often without accomplishing anything. Examples include going through closets, drawers, purses and briefcases.

Hoarding refers to the collecting of objects. Often the objects being hoarded have little value. They may include scraps of paper, styrofoam cups, and packets of sugar, junk mail or money. Once they are put away, the demented person forgets where they are and the rummaging begins again.

These behaviors can become a problem in several ways. If patients are rummaging in someone else's things, they could be accosted by the owner. If valuable things are being hoarded and lost, this can also be a problem. Examples are hoarding of money, mail, identification cards, and jewelry.

One solution to these problems is to create a small, safe area for rummaging and hoarding. A drawer could be set up with small objects that are not valuable. One closet door could be left unlocked for rummaging.

Another approach is to routinely check the person's room for hoarded items such as food or the possessions of others. This, of course, must be done when the person is not in the room.

Perhaps the most effective way to approach these problems is to provide structured activity programming such as that at a day care center.

Basic Psychosocial Intervention in Dementia

Delivered by: A licensed clinician, such as a primary care or specialist physician, psychologist, nurse or social worker.

Delivered to: The primary caregiver of the person with dementia; it is intended to help both the patient with dementia and the caregiver.

When: After the initial diagnosis is confirmed and at regular intervals thereafter. Follow-ups twice a year are recommended.

This Psychosocial Intervention is targeted at the primary caregiver of a person with dementia and consists of *caregiver counseling, caregiver education, and 24-hour availability for crisis intervention.* It is anchored on in-person visits between the primary caregiver and the clinician. Every effort should be made to have the same person deliver the intervention with the same caregiver.

Procedure*

First Visit (Up to about 30 Minutes)

1. *Explain the purpose of the intervention:*
   - To improve the day-to-day quality of life of Mr./Ms. X (the person with dementia).

Comment: It is recognized that not all caregivers need detailed counseling at every visit and that many refuse to be counseled at specific time points. Such refusals should be honored. All caregivers should be offered the educational materials and information about the clinical team's 24-hour availability. As well, follow up visits may be brief. This too is appropriate. It is left to the clinician to determine the exact length of each counseling session. If caregivers require more support or counseling than can be provided during these sessions, they should be referred to the appropriate resources in the area, as usual care would dictate.

Prepared by Constantine G. Lyketsos, M.D., M.H.S., Cynthia Steele, R.N., M.P.H., and Peter V. Rabins, M.D., M.P.H. May be reproduced and distributed.

- To improve the caregiver's ability to care for the patient.
- To help sustain the caregiver in her or his difficult task.

2. *Provide information in writing* on how to reach the care team on a 24-hour/7-day basis to deal with crises.
3. *Provide and discuss caregiver educational materials:* for example, the book *The 36-hour Day* (Johns Hopkins Press: Baltimore) or the Demential Care Guidelines for Families (Appendix A).
4. *Review systematically* the Supportive Care Checklist (Appendix C) first for the patient and then for the caregiver. Record the elements of the plan on the checklist.
5. *Document* the duration of the intervention and the topics covered, and place the completed checklists in the chart.

Following Visits

1. At each session the clinician will reveiw and update the supportive care plan using the Supportive Care Checklists, provide educational materials as needed, work on caregiving skills, and make any necessary referrals (e.g., P.T., support groups, home health care).
2. Discuss a special topic as follows: Choose a care problem (or issue) to focus on during this visit. Begin by asking: "What is the biggest care problem you are having right now?" You might also focus the discussion on one of the Dementia Care Guidelines for Families, parts of the Supportive Care Checklists, or the recent history that the caregiver provided. Discuss this topic in depth with the caregiver with an eye to teaching caregiving skills and problem-solving strategies. Tailor the discussion to the caregiver's level of sophistication.
3. Document as on a first visit.

Prepared by Constantine G. Lyketsos, M.D., M.H.S., Cynthia Steele, R.N., M.P.H., and Peter V. Rabins, M.D., M.P.H. May be reproduced and distributed.

APPENDIX C

SUPPORTIVE CARE
CHECKLISTS AND CALENDARS

Supportive Care Checklist: Patient

PATIENT   _____
DATE   ___/___/___
CAREGIVER   _____
RELATIONSHIP   _____

Topic	Y/N*	Date Completed	Intervention	Comment
Diagnostic awareness —Patient aware —Patient not aware				
Advanced directives —Health care agent: —Other POA —Will				
Illness education targeted at the patient			Topics covered 1. 2. 3.	
Daily life schedule review			—Sample calendar	—Schedule in place
Safety review				
Driving			—Advised to stop	
Wandering risk			—Driving evaluation	
Level-of-care issues			—Level of care eval.	
Home safety issues			—Home safety eval.	
Fall risk			—PT referral	
Medication administration			—Devise (specify) —Supervision —Administration	
General medical care			PCP: _____ _____ Last seen: _____	
Referrals			—OT —PT —Speech —Home health —Dental —Vision —Hearing	

*Indicate if the area was addressed in a given counseling session.

OT, occupational therapy; PCP, primary care physician; POA, power of attorney; PT, physical therapy.

May be reproduced and distributed.

Supportive Care Checklist: Caregiver

PATIENT _____
DATE ___/___/___
CAREGIVER _____   RELATIONSHIP _____
Who are caregivers?
—Primary (-ies): _____
—Backup plan: _____

Topic	Y/N*	Date Completed	Intervention	Comment
Education			—Verbal (specify) —*The 36 Hour Day* —Dementia Care Family Guidelines —Resource list and telephone numbers —Inventory of important documents	
Resource referrals			—Alzheimer's Association —Eldercare attorney —Office on Aging/ Social Services —Geriatric Case Management	
Caregiver mental health assessment			—Network/activity encouragement —Support group —Counseling referral —Psychiatric referral	
Caregiver physical health assessment			—Primary care	
Caregiver skills counseling			—Activities —Meds/side effects —Supervision —Night time —Behaviors —ADLs —Skills lab referral	
Respite counseling			—Other caregivers —Family/friends —Professional aides —Weekly time off —Monthly time off —Annual vacation	

*Indicate if the area was addressed in a given counseling session.
ADLs, activities of daily living.

May be reproduced and distributed.

Example of a Daily Schedule

Time	Sunday	Monday	Tuesday	Wednesday	Thursday	Friday	Saturday
7:30 A.M.	Awaken	Awaken	Awaken	Awaken	Awaken	Awaken	Awaken
7:30–8:30 A.M.	Morning ADLs	Morning ADLs	Morning ADLs	Morning ADLs	Morning ADLs	Morning ADLs	Morning ADLs
8:30–9:30 A.M.	Breakfast Morning meds	Breakfast Morning meds	Breakfast Morning meds	Breakfast Morning meds	Breakfast Morning meds	Breakfast Morning meds	Breakfast Morning meds
9:30–10:00 A.M.	Exercise*		Exercise*			Exercise*	
10 A.M.–12 P.M.		Out-of-house activity†			Out-of-house activity†		
12–1 P.M.	Lunch Midday meds	Lunch Midday meds	Lunch Midday meds	Lunch Midday meds	Lunch Midday meds	Lunch Midday meds	Lunch Midday meds
1–2 P.M.	Nap/quiet time	Nap/quiet time	Nap/quiet time	Nap/quiet time	Nap/quiet time	Nap/quiet time	Nap/quiet time
2–5 P.M.							Out-of-house activity†
7–8 P.M.	Dinner Evening meds	Dinner Evening meds	Dinner Evening meds	Dinner Evening meds	Dinner Evening meds	Dinner Evening meds	Dinner Evening meds
10–10:30 P.M.	Evening ADLs	Evening ADLs	Evening ADLs	Evening ADLs	Evening ADLs	Evening ADLs	Evening ADLs
10:30 P.M.	Bedtime	Bedtime	Bedtime	Bedtime	Bedtime	Bedtime	Bedtime

*Examples of exercise: mall walk for half an hour, swimming at the local pool.
†Examples of out-of-house activity: out to lunch, adult day care, movie, visit family.
ADLs, activities of daily living.

May be reproduced and distributed.

GLOSSARY

affect   the outward expression of an individual's subjective or emotional state as manifested in his or her behavior. Important elements of affect include range, changeability, and rapidity of change.

aggression   a verbal or physical act that produces harm or carries the potential of harm to the self, another individual, or an object. Examples of aggression in dementia include screaming, the use of profanity, and specific behaviors such as hitting, kicking, spitting, biting, and pushing.

agnosia   a disturbance of perception in which the ability to recognize or interpret primary perceptions is impaired. Agnosia impairs the ability to interpret perceptions in all the senses: vision, hearing, touch, smell, and taste. For example, an individual may be able to see a face and recognize and name the parts of the face but not know that the face belongs to a specific familiar person (prosopagnosia). Another common example is a person whose left side is paralyzed but who is totally unaware of this (anosagnosia) and denies it even when shown the paralyzed limbs.

akathisia   a subjective state of restlessness, sometimes described as the urge to jump out of one's skin. This may be manifested as being in constant motion, pacing, switching weight from one leg to the other when standing, stamping the feet, or crossing and uncrossing the legs when sitting. This is a side effect of antipsychotic medication or a consequence of certain neurologic diseases.

amnesia   a primary disturbance of memory manifested as a loss of memory for previously learned events (retrograde amnesia) or an inability to learn new material (anterograde amnesia.)

amnestic disorder   a cognitive disorder in which memory impairment is the only abnormality. The most common form of amnestic syndrome is Korsakoff's syndrome, which is associated with damage to the thalamus or mammillary bodies.

anosoagnosia (see also agnosia)   lack of awareness of a deficit.

antidepressants   medications from different chemical classes that reduce depressive symptoms in patients with mood disorder. Four classes are distinguished: tricyclic antidepressants, selective serotonin reuptake inhibitors, monoamine oxidase inhibitors, and newer antidepressants.

antidepressants, newer   newer classes of antidepressant medications that appear to have milder side effects. They come from several chemical classes and have been broadly used in dementia, Examples include bupropion (Welbutrin), venlafaxine (Effexor), trazodone (Desyrel), nefazadone (Serzone), and mertazapine (Remeron).

antipsychotic medications   a type of medication typically used to treat delusions, hallucinations, or thought disorder, but also used to treat aggression and other behavioral disturbances in dementia. These medications are called *neuroleptics* because of their neurologic side effects, including parkinsonism, akathisia, dystonia, tardive dyskinesia, and neuroleptic malignant syndrome. Examples include haloperidol (Haldol), risperidone (Risperdal), and thioridazine (Mellaril) (see Chapter 9).

anxiety   a mental symptom characterized by apprehension, tension, uneasiness, and/or worry.

anxiety disorder   a syndrome of sustained anxiety with accompanying physical symptoms (muscle tension, tremor, rapid heartbeat) that may involve panic attacks, obsessions, or compulsions.

apathy   a state of reduced interest and initiative.

aphasia   a disturbance of language manifested as difficulties in communicating. Aphasic individuals may have trouble *understanding* spoken or written language (receptive aphasia, fluent aphasia, Wernicke's aphasia), repeating spoken language (communicating aphasia), or *expressing* themselves in verbal or written language (expressive aphasia, nonfluent aphasia, Broca's aphasia). In *transcortical* aphasia, repetition is intact but there is difficulty with either understanding, expression, or both.

apraxia   the inability to carry out a learned, complex motor task in the absence of paralysis or movement difficulty (such as with Parkinson disease). Common motor tasks affected by apraxia in dementia include dressing, grooming, driving, and eating.

ataxia   a disturbance in gait in which patients have trouble coordinating the movements involved in walking. Ataxic gaits may be broad-based, "magnetic" (the person's feet stick to the ground and are slow to lift and move around), and unstable.

athetosis   a sustained writhing movement of the limbs, trunk, or neck that is involuntary.

atrophy   a loss of tissue in the body. Muscle tissue atrophy occurs after the development of paralysis in the muscles that are no longer used. In dementia, atrophy of the brain is seen when brain tissue is lost.

behavior disorder   an observable activity of an individual that is disruptive or dangerous, or is associated with stress in the patient or those around the patient.

behavioral perspective   the logic of attributing a mental or behavioral disturbance to a disturbance of one of the innate drives (sleep, eating, sexuality) or to the "taking over" of the individual's behavior by a single maladaptive cycle of behavior with a specific goal (e.g., to be seen as sick, to restrict eating, or to abuse alcohol).

benzodiazepines   a class of medications that have activity at a specific receptor site in the brain (the benzodiazepine receptor site) of the GABA system. Typically, these medications have sedating and anxiolytic (anxiety-relieving) properties. Chronic use can lead to addiction. Their use in brain-injured individuals, including patients with dementia, can lead to disinhibition. Examples include diazepam (Valium), chlordiazepoxide (Librium), orazepam (Serax), lorazepam (Ativan), and clonazepam (Clonopin).

catastrophic reaction   a sudden, extreme emotional, physical, or behavioral response to a seemingly minor stimulus as if it were a catastrophe.

catatonia   a clinical syndrome characterized by near immobility of movement and thought, punctuated by shorter periods of excitability and overactivity. Catatonic patients are mute, move very little, and may exhibit "waxy flexibility" (moving their limbs feels to an examiner as if they are being moved through wax).

chorea   a dance-like, rapid, involuntary movement of the limbs, trunk, or neck, seen in Huntington disease.

circumlocutory language (see also aphasia)   a style of language in which an individual appears to use a series of phrases in place of more precise individual words—for example, "hand me the writing instrument while I am preparing to inscribe what I'm trying to say."

cognition   the sum total of human thinking, reasoning, and abstracting capacities.

cognitive disorder, mild   a condition in which there are impairments in two or more areas of cognition, but not severe enough to be a dementia or to affect functioning.

cogwheeling   a neurologic sign elicited by an examiner's moving an individual's limb or muscle group back and forth. It consists of intermittent "catching" followed by relaxation of a muscle, similar to the way the cogs of a wheel catch and release.

compulsion (see also obsession)   an intrusive, repetitive action that cannot be resisted (or leads to discomfort and anxiety if resisted) and that is not perceived as alien by the person (to whom it seems a personal urge). Compulsions may include repetition of trivial acts (checking, counting, tapping) or of complex actions (brushing the teeth in a certain way) or behaviors (washing hands), or may simply be an intrusive repetitive action that distracts the person from other mental activities.

confabulation fabrication of stories in response to questions. It is commonly seen in memory disorders in which patients appear to be filling in gaps in their memory.

cortical dementia a dementia characterized by aphasia, apraxia, agnosia, and amnesia. Cortical dementias typically are due to damage in the temporal, parietal, and posterior lobes of the brain. Alzheimer disease is the most common cause of cortical dementia.

decreased level of consciousness a state of impaired clarity or clouding of awareness of the environment and inability to sustain attention. Terms that describe decreased level of consciousness include *drowsiness, stupor,* and *coma.* It may manifest as hyper- or hypovigilance.

delirium an impairment in the level of consciousness and sensorium. Typically, it has an acute onset and a specific general medical cause and resolves after its primary cause is treated. Delirium is a cognitive disorder with most cognitive functions impaired. Patients may manifest any mental symptom during delirium (including anxiety, depression, delusions, or hallucinations). Patients with delirium can be hypervigilant and active or lethargic and withdrawn.

delusion a fixed, false, idiosyncratic belief.

dementia a global decline in cognitive capacity occurring in clear consciousness.

depression (see also major depression and dysthymia) a subjective state of sadness or low mood ("the blues") that may appear as tearfulness or a sad appearance.

dimensional perspective the logic of causally attributing a mental or behavioral impairment to a mismatch between the person's personality or cognitive vulnerabilities and current circumstances. Dimensional vulnerabilities refer to universal, continuously graded individual attributes (e.g., intelligence, personality dimensions).

disease perspective the logic of causally attributing a mental or behavioral impairment to a process that has broken a part in the brain or the body.

dyskinesia an abnormal involuntary movement that involves a muscle or muscle group. Dyskinesias can affect the oral-facial musculature, the hands, legs, and trunk. Dyskinesias are often a medication side effect. Examples include the dyskinesia associated with L-dopa therapy in Parkinson's disease and those that develop after chronic use of neuroleptic medications. Withdrawal dyskinesias may last for days, weeks, or months after discontinuation of a neuroleptic. Withdrawal dyskinesias that last for more than several months after discontinuation of a neuroleptic are referred to as *tardive dyskinesia,* a chronic disfiguring condition.

dysphoria a state of uncomfortable mood. It may be seen in both major depression and mania.

dysthymia chronic mild depression typically lasting for years. It is not severe enough to qualify as a major depression.

dystonia   a sustained contraction of a muscle or muscle group that usually results in an abnormal position or posture. Examples include tightening of one side of the neck muscles (torticollis), pulling of the eyes up, down, or to the side (occulogyric crisis), or leaning of the trunk to one side (tower of Pisa). Most commonly, dystonia is a side effect of antipsychotic medications (such as haloperidol, risperidone, and others). It also occurs in several brain diseases.

emotional incontinence   a sudden, exaggerated expression of emotion that may or may not occur in response to a stimulus. Examples include pathologic laughing or crying in which an individual unexpectedly cries or laughs but denies the absence of a sad or happy mood. It often occurs when there is damage to subcortical structures, such as in pseudobulbar palsy or Parkinson disease.

euphoria   a state of abnormally elevated mood, usually accompanied by increased confidence in one's abilities. It may be manifested by frequent laughing and giggling or other forms of social disinhibition.

euthymia   a descriptor for normally reactive mood and affect.

executive dysfunction   impairments in the ability to initiate, maintain, or stop a cognitive task or a behavior, abstract, or make sound judgments. It may manifest as slowness in thinking, mental inflexibility, social disinhibition, perseveration, poor judgment, or difficulty changing tasks. It is associated with damage to fronto-subcortical circuits. It may be associated with frontal release signs (reflexes), such as the grab, snout, and glabellar reflexes.

extrapyramidal symptomatology   a set of motor symptoms, including dystonia, akathisia, or parkinsonism, attributed to dysfunction of the extrapyramidal motor systems of the brain and spinal cord. In dementia, these are either side effects of neuroleptic medications or neurologic symptoms of a disease such as disseminated Lewy body disease or Parkinson disease.

festination   a gait disorder initiated by a series of rapid small steps (marche-a-petit-pas) that steadily increases in speed and is difficult for the patient to stop.

frontal-subcortical circuits   neuronal pathways in the brain that join specific areas of the frontal lobes and the basal ganglia in functional units. Damage to frontal-subcortical circuits from any disease is associated with certain types of dementia (subcortical dementia), disturbances of executive function, and disinhibited behavior.

functional impairment   impairment in the ability to carry out routine, everyday activities. Two types are distinguished: impairments of instrumental activities of daily living (IADLs) such as work, household tasks, driving, handling finances, telephone use, and transportation, and impairments in activities of daily living (ADLs) such as dressing, bathing, maintaining continence, feeding, transfering, and mobility.

gait   a medical term for walking.

grasp reflex   a reflex in which patients grab on to things when the underpart of their hand is lightly stroked. This reflex often emerges in advanced dementia and may manifest as grabbing on to clothing, a bedrail, or caregivers. These reflex behaviors may be inappropriately interpreted as uncooperativeness, aggression, or resistance to care.

hallucination   a perception without a stimulus. Hallucinations can occur in all senses: visual—seeing things that are not present; auditory—hearing voices or sounds; gustatory—experiencing taste; olfactory—perceiving odors; and tactile—feeling sensations on the skin.

hydrocephalus   an excess collection of cerebrospinal fluid in the brain that can compress brain tissue and lead to neurologic and mental symptoms.

hypomania   a mild state of mania (see mania) that does not lead to social, interpersonal, or functional impairment.

illusion   a true perception of a physical stimulus, for example, seeing a figure in dark curtains at night.

irritability   a subjective state of becoming easily irritated or of having a short fuse. This may manifest in an individual's easily becoming angry, threatening, or hostile.

judgment   the mental process of choosing among a set of actions, behaviors, or values.

lability   the degree of changeability in a person's mood. Labile moods change rapidly in response to minimal environmental stimuli. Becoming rapidly hostile or angry when unexpected sounds occur and quickly switching from being calm to being depressed or sad are examples.

life story perspective   the logic of explaining an individual's mental or behavioral disturbance as being an understandable psychological reaction to life circumstances—for example, "He is upset because he feels lost" and "He wants to eat because he is unhappy in the nursing home."

major depression   a syndrome consisting of persistent low mood, low vital sense (i.e., fatigability, low energy, insomnia, hypersomnia, anorexia), and low self-attitude (e.g., a sense of being a burden, low self-esteem, limited confidence, and "emotional vulnerability"). Major depression may be secondary to a general medical condition (such as a stroke or hypothyroidism) or may be idiopathic, that is, of unknown cause.

mania   a syndrome characterized by persistent elevation of mood or irritability, elevation in vital sense (i.e., with decreased need for sleep, increased energy, and increased activity), and increased self-attitude (i.e., overconfidence and grandiosity). Mania may also include a flight of ideas, where patients may subjectively feel that their thoughts are moving too fast for them to keep track.

mood   an individual's current pervasive, predominant emotional state. Examples include depression, anxiety, irritability, and euphoria.

mood stabilizers   medications from different chemical classes that have the ability to stabilize swings of mood. These are typically used as treatments for mania, hypomania, and bipolar disorders. Examples include lithium, carbamazepine (Tegretol), divalproex sodium (Depakote), and gabapentin (Neurontin).

myoclonus   a repetitive, intermittent jerking movement of a muscle or muscle group.

neuroleptic malignant syndrome   a syndrome consisting of delirium, stiffness, and fever associated with the use of neuroleptic medications. It can develop with low doses and after short-term use of these medicines. It is life-threatening.

neurotransmitters   chemical substances used by the nervous system for communication between neurons. Many chemical types of neurotransmitters have been described, including peptides and amines. Neurotransmitter systems disturbed in dementia include those that produce acetylcholine, dopamine, norepinephrine, serotonin, and GABA.

obsession (see also compulsion)   an intrusive repetitive urge or thought that an individual tries to resist but ultimately cannot (or that leads to discomfort and anxiety if resisted) and that is not perceived as alien to the person (it seems to be his or her own). Obsessions may drive people to do certain acts (see compulsion) or may be intrusive, repetitive thoughts that distract them from other mental activities.

orthostatic hypotension   a change in blood pressure and pulse that occurs when an individual goes from a lying position to a standing position (after at least 2 minutes). A drop in systolic or diastolic blood pressure of 20 points or more, or an increases in pulse of 20 points or more, constitute, clinically significant orthostatic hypotension. Patients with clinically significant orthostatic hypotension typically complain of dizziness or lightheadedness and are at high risk for falls.

overvalued idea   a strongly held idea or belief that arises out of or is reinforced by an individual's immediate cultural environment. Overvalued ideas are preoccupying in mental life, drive behavior, and lead individuals to act in specific ways. They differ from delusions in that they are not idiosyncratic and are less fixed. Their content is rarely bizarre. Overvalued ideas can be distinguished from ordinary ideas, beliefs, and attitudes in that they typically lead individuals to behave in ways that are outside cultural norms or in some way dangerous to them.

paranoia   a commonly used term referring to suspiciousness or persecutory beliefs. The original Greek term refers to a tendency to misinterpret events and people as being hostile and directed against the person.

paratonia a neurologic sign in which there is increasing muscle tone resistance in response to increasing speed of passive limb movement. Paratonia may manifest itself as resistance to movements by others in advanced dementia and can be misinterpreted as aggression or oppositional behavior.

parkinsonism a motor disturbance in which patients manifest a characteristic tremor (pill rolling), postural disturbance (stooped trunk posture), rigidity or stiffness, mask-like facial expression, slowness in movement (bradykinesia), impaired balance, festination, reduced arm swing, and en-bloc turning.

perseveration the persistence or frequent repetition of a movement or verbal behavior. Examples include repeating a sound or phrase over and over or repeatedly slapping one's thigh. Perseverations are involuntary and may take the form of an intrusion or repetition of an earlier phrase, sound, or behavior into a new conversation. Perseveration has been associated with damage to frontal-subcortical circuits.

personality the pervasive and persistent lifelong set of attributes characteristic of an individual, usually unchanging after early adulthood. In dementia, personality can be changed by brain disease. Personality may also "color" a dementia patient's mental life and behavior during the course of the illness.

praxis the ability to carry out a learned motor intervention in the absence of weakness or movement disorder.

selective serotonin reuptake inhibitors (see also antidepressants) a class of antidepressants whose primary mode of activity is believed to involve inhibition of serotonin reuptake into brain neurons. Examples includes fluoxetine (Prozac), sertraline (Zoloft), paroxetine (Paxil), and fluvoxamine (Luvox).

self-attitude an individual's overall sense of him/herself. Impairments in self-attitude can be positive or negative. Negative self-attitude manifests as reduced confidence, hopelessness, guilt, feeling oneself to be a burden, worthlessness, and low self-esteem. Elevation in self-attitude manifests as overconfidence, grandiosity, and inflated self-esteem.

self-depreciation a symptom of impaired self-attitude in which personal worth is underestimated.

sign an observable abnormality in a patient's behavior, noted on an interview, physical examination, or mental status examination. A sign may be noted by a clinician or a caregiver.

subcortical dementia a dementia characterized by the 4D's: dysmnesia (disturbance in the processing of memory), dysexecutive (executive disturbance), depletion (loss of interest or motivation), and delay (of movement and thought). Subcortical dementias are typically due to disturbances in frontal-subcortical circuits and may be associated with movement disorder and mood. Parkinson disease and Huntington disease are causes of subcortical dementia.

symptom   a complaint reported by a patient, for example, "My head hurts."

syndrome   a characteristic constellation or pattern of signs and symptoms. Dementia is a syndrome characterized by a global decline in intellectual function occurring in clear consciousness.

tardive dyskinesia   see dyskinesia.

tone   the resting "tension" or state of a relaxed muscle or muscle group as felt by an observer. Tone can be diminished (hypotonus), normal, or increased (hypertonus). Examples of abnormal tone are rigidity, cogwheeling, spasticity, and paratonia.

transcortical aphasia   see aphasia.

tremor   a repetitive, stereotyped, regular movement of a muscle or muscle group that has the appearance of "shaking." Tremors occur either at rest or during an action (intention) such as reaching for a glass of water.

tricyclic antidepressants (see also antidepressants)   a class of antidepressants whose basic chemical structure is three rings of carbon molecules. They have activity at several brain neurotransmitter systems. Examples include desipramine (Norpramin and others), imipramine (Tofranil and others), and nortriptyline (Pamelor and others).

vital sense   an individual's subjective sense of pep and energy. Reductions in vital sense manifest as feelings of reduced pep or energy or easy fatigability. Elevations in vital sense manifest as feeling energized, activated, and constantly on the go.

BIBLIOGRAPHY

Textbooks and Other Volumes

American Psychiatric Association. Diagnostic and Statistical Manual, 4th edition. Washington, DC, 1994.

Burns A, Levy R. Dementia. London: Chapman and Hall Medical, 1994.

Cummings JL, Benson DF. Dementia: A Clinical Approach. Boston: Butterworth-Heineman, 1992.

Lishman WA. Organic Psychiatry. Oxford: Blackwell Scientific Publications, 1987.

Chapter 1: Definitions and Overview of the Book

Blessed G, Tomlinson BE, Roth M. The association between quantitative measures of dementia and senile change in the cerebral gray matter of elderly subjects. Br J Psychiatry 1968; 114:797–811.

Erkinjuntti T, Ostbve T, Steenhuis R, Hachinski V. The effect of different diagnostic criteria on the prevalence of dementia. N Engl J Med 1997; 337: 1667–1674.

Hebert LE, Scherr PA, Bienias JL, Bennett DA, Evans D. Alzheimer disease in the population: prevalence estimates using the 2000 census. Arch Neurol 2003; 60:1119–1122

Lyketsos CG, Corazzini K, Steele C. Mania in Alzheimer's disease. J Neuropsychiatry Clin Neurosci 1995; 7:350–352.

Maurer K, Gerbaldo H. Auguste D and Alzheimer's disease. Lancet 1997; 349:1546–1549.

McHugh PR, Slavney PR. The Perspectives of Psychiatry, revised edition. Baltimore: Johns Hopkins University Press, 1998.

Miech RA, Breitner JCS, Zandi PP, Khachaturian AS, Anthony JC, Mayer L for the Cache County Study Group. Incidence of AD may decline in the early 90's for men, later for women. The Cache County Study. Neurology 2002; 58(2):209–218.

Mishima K, Okawa M, Kishikawa Y, Hozumi S, Hori H, Takahashi K. Morning bright light therapy for sleep and behavior disorders in elderly patients with dementia. Acta Psychiatr Scand 1994; 89:1–7.

Chapter 2: The Evaluation and Formulation of Dementia

Alexopoulos GS, Abrams RC, Young RC, Shamoian CA. Cornell scale for depression in dementia. Biol Psychiatry 1988; 23:271–284.

Christensen H, Griffiths K, MacKinnon A, Jacomb P. A quantitative review of cognitive deficits in depression and Alzheimer-type dementia. J Int Neuropsychol Soc 1997; 3:631–651.

Cummings JL, Mega M, Gray K, Rosenberg-Thompson S, Carusi DA, Gornbein J. The Neuropsychiatric Inventory: comprehensive assessment of psychopathology in dementia. Neurology 1994; 44:2308–2314.

Folstein MF, Folstein SE, McHugh PR. "Mini-Mental State": a practical method for grading the cognitive state of patients for the clinician. J Psychiatr Res 1975; 2:189–198.

Iliffe S. Can delays in the recognition of dementia in primary care be avoided? Aging Mental Health 1997; 1(1):7–10.

Loreck DJ, Bylsma FW, Folstein MF. The Dementia Signs and Symptoms Scale: a new scale for comprehensive assessment of psychopathology in Alzheimer's disease. Am J Geriatr Psychiatry 1994; 2:60–74.

Marin RS, Biedrzycki RC, Firinciogullari S. Reliability and validity of the Apathy Evaluation Scale. Psychiatry Res 1991; 38:143–162.

Mayeux R, Saunders AM, Shea S, Mirra S, Evans D, Roses AD, Hyman BT, Crain B, Tange M-X, Phelps CH. Utility of the Apolipoprotein-E genotype in the diagnosis of Alzheimer's disease. N Engl J Med 1998; 338:506–511.

Rabins PV, Steele CS. A scale to measure impairment in severe dementia and similar conditions. Am J Geriatr Psychiatry 1996; 4:247–251.

Sclan SG, Saillon A, Franssen E, Hugonot-Diener L, Saillon A, Reisberg B. The Behavior Pathology in Alzheimer's Disease Rating Scale (Behave-AD): reliability and analysis of symptom category scores. Int J Geriatr Psychiatry 1996; 11:1–12.

Wilkinson IM, Graham-White J. Psychogeriatric Dependency Rating Scales (PGDRS): a method of assessment for use by nurses. Br J Psychiatry 1980; 137: 558–565.

Chapter 3: Diseases Causing a Cortical Pattern of Dementia

Hooten RM, Lyketsos CG. Fronto-temporal dementia: a clinicopathological review of four post-mortem studies. J Neuropsychiatry Clin Neurosci 1996; 8:10–19.

Lyketsos CG. The prion dementias. Maryland Med J 1999; 48:18–22.

McKeith IG, Fairbairn AF, Perry RH, Thompson P. The clinical diagnosis and mis-diagnosis of Senile Dementia of the Lewy Body Type (SDLT). Br J Psychiatry 1994; 165:324–332.

McKeith IG, Perry RH, Fairbairn AF, Perry EK. Operational criteria for SDLT. Psychol Med 1992; 22:911–922.

McKhann G, Drachman D, Folstein MF, et al. Clinical diagnosis of Alzheimer's disease: report of the NINCDS/ADRDA workgroup under the auspices of DHHS task force on Alzheimer's disease. Neurology 1984; 34:939–944.

Terry RD, Katzman R, Bick KL. Alzheimer Disease. New York: Raven Press, 1994.

Chapter 4: Diseases Typically Causing Subcortical or Mixed Pattern Dementia

Alexopoalos GS, Meyers BS, Young RC, Campbell S, Silbersweig D, Charlson M. "Vascular depression" hypothesis. Arch Gen Psych 1997; 54:915–22.

Chabriat H, Vahedi K, Iba-Zizen MT, Joutel A, Nibbio A, Nagy TG, Krebs MO, Julien J, Dubois B, Ducrocq X, Levasseur M, Homeyer P, Mas JL, Lyon-Caen O, Tournier Lasserve E, Bousser MG. Clinical spectrum of CADASIL: a study of 7 families. Lancet 1995; 346:934–938.

Costa PT, Williams TF, Sommerfield M, et al. Recognition and initial assessment of Alzheimer's disease and related dementias. Practice guideline No. 19. AHCPR Publication No. 97–0702. Rockville, MD: U.S. Department of Health and Human Services, Public Health Service, November 1996.

Folstein S. Huntington Disease: A Disorder of Families. Baltimore: Johns Hopkins University Press, 1992.

Huber SJ, Cummings JL. Parkinson's Disease: Neurobehavioral Aspects. New York: Oxford University Press, 1992.

Price RW, Perry SW. HIV, AIDS, and the Brain: Association for Research in Nervous and Mental Disorder ARNMD, Volume 72. New York: Raven Press, 1994.

Rodriguez M, Siva A, Ward J, Stolp-Smith K, O'Brien P, Kurland L. Impairment, disability and handicap in multiple sclerosis. Neurology 1994; 44:28–33.

Romain GC, Tatemichi TK, Erkinjuntti T, et al. Vascular dementia: diagnostic criteria for research studies, report of the NINDS-AIREN international workshop. Neurology 1993; 43:250–259.

Schut LJ. Dementia following stroke. Clin Geriatr Med 1988; 4(4):767–784.

Silver JM, Yudofsky SC, Hales RE (eds). Neuropsychiatry of Traumatic Brain Injury. American Psychiatric Press Institute: Washington, DC: 1994.

Vanneste J, Augustin PA, Dirven C, Tan WF, Goedhart ZD. Shunting normal pressure hydrocephalus: do the benefits outweigh the risks? Neurology 1992; 42:54–59.

Wu J-C, Choo K-B, Chen C-M, Chen T-Z, Huo T, Lee S-D. Genotyping of hepatitis D virus by restriction-fragment length polymorphism and relation to outcome of hepatitis D. Lancet 1995; 356:939–40.

Yatsu FM, Grotta JC, Pettigrew LC. Stroke. London: Edward Arnold, 1995.

Chapter 5: Overview of Dementia Care

Mace N, Rabins PV. The 36-Hour Day, third edition. Baltimore: Johns Hopkins University Press, 1979.

Volicer L, Fabisziewski KJ, Rheuame YL, Lasch KE. Clinical Management of Alzheimer's disease. Rockville, MD: Aspen Publishers, 1988.

Chapter 6: Supportive Care for the Patient with Dementia

Brody J. Guidance in the care of patients with Alzheimer's disease. The New York Times, November 20, 1983.

Zgola JM. Doing Things: A Guide to Programming Activities for Persons with Alzheimer's Disease and Related Disorders. Baltimore: Johns Hopkins University Press, 1987.

Chapter 7: Supporting the Family and the Care Provider

Benbow SM, Marriott A, Morley M, Walsh S. Family therapy and dementia: review and clinical experience. Int J Geriatr Psychiatry 1993; 8:717–725.

Hebert R, Leclerc G, Bravo G, Girouard D, Lefrancois M. Efficacy of a support group programme for caregivers of demented patients in the community: a randomized controlled trial. Arch Gerontol Geriatr 1994; 18:1–14.

Mittleman MS, Ferris SH, Schulman E, et al. A family intervention to delay nursing home placement of patients with Alzheimer disease. JAMA 1996; 276: 1725–1731.

Schulz R, O'Brien AT, Bookwala T, Fleiissner K. Psychiatric and physical morbidity effects of dementia caregiving: prevalence, correlates, and causes. Gerontologist 1995; 35:771–791.

Chapter 8: Noncognitive Behavioral and Psychiatric Disorders

Fitten LJ, Perryman K, Wilkinson C, et al. Alzheimer and vascular dementias and driving. JAMA 1995: 273:1360–1365.

Hall GR. Chronic dementia: challenges in feeding a patient. J Gerontol Nurs 1994; 20:21–30.

Lyketsos CG, Lee HB. Depression and treatment of depression in Alzheimer's disease: a practical update for the clinician. Dementia Geriatri Cogn Disord 2004; 17:55–64.

Robinson A, Spencer B, White L. Understanding difficult behaviors. Ann Arbor: Geriatric Education Center of Michigan, Michigan Department of Mental Hygiene, 1988.

Sloane PD, Rader J, Barrick AL, Hoeffer B, Dwyere S, McKenzie D, Lavelle M, Buckwalter K, Arrington L, Pruitt T. Bathing persons with dementia. Gerontologist 1995; 35:672–678.

Chapter 9: Noncognitive Functional Disorders and Disturbances in Sleeping, Eating, and Sexuality

Burns A, Jacoby R, Levy R. Psychiatric phenomena in Alzheimer's disease. IV: Disorders of behavior. Br J Psychiatry 1990; 157:86–94.

Carlson DL, Fleming KC, Smith GE, Evans JM. Management of dementia-related behavioral disturbances: a non-pharmacologic approach. [Review] Mayo Clin Proc 1995; 70(11):1108–1115.

Devanand DP, Jacobs DM, Tang MX, Del Castillo-Castaneda C, Sano M, Marder K, Bell K, Bylsma FW, Brandt J, Albert M, Stern Y. The course of psychopathologic features in mild to moderate Alzheimer disease. Arch Gen Psychiatry 1997; 54:257–263.

Haddad PM, Benbow SM. Sexual problems associated with dementia: Part 1: Problems and their consequences. Int J Geriatr Psychiatry 1993; 8:547–551.

Kawas C, Resnick S, Morrison A, Brookmeyer R, Corrada M, Zonderman A, Bacal C, Donnell Lingle D, Metter E. A prospective study of estrogen replacement therapy and the risk of developing Alzheimer's disease: the Baltimore Longitudinal Study of Aging. Am Acad Neurol 1997; 48:1517–1521.

Marin RS, Fogel BS, Hawkins J, Duffy J, Krupp B. Apathy: a treatable syndrome. J Neuropsychiatry Clin Neurosci 1995; 7(1):23–30.

Patel V, Hope T. Aggressive behavior in elderly people with dementia: a review. Int J Geriatr Psychiatry 1993; 8:457–472.

Price TR, McAllister TW. Safety and efficacy of ECT in depressed patients with dementia: a review of clinical experience. Convulsive Ther 1989; 5:1–74.

Rao V, Lyketsos CG. Delusions in Alzheimer's disease. J Neuropsychiatry Clin Neurosci 1998; 10:373–382,

Rovner BW, Steele CD, Shmuely Y, Folstein MF. A randomized trial of dementia care in nursing homes. J Am Genet Soc 1996: 44(1):7–13.

Teri L, Wagner A. Alzheimer's disease and depression. J Consult Clin Psychology 1992; 60:379–391.

Wagner AW, Terri L, Orr-Rainey N. Behavior problems of residents with dementia in special care units. Alzheimer Dis Associated Disord 1995; 9: 121–127.

Chapter 10: Pharmacologic and Other Biologic Treatments in Dementia

Burgio LD, Reynolds CF, Janoski JE. A behavioral microanalysis of the effects of haloperidol and oxazepam in demented psychogeriatric inpatients. Int J Geriatr Psychiatry 1992; 7:253–262.

Carlyle W, Ancill RJ, Sheldon L. Aggression in the demented patient: a double-blind study of loxapine versus haloperidol. Int Clin Psychopharmacol 1993: 8:103–108.

Cummings JL, Gorman DG, Shapira J. Physostigmine ameliorates the delusions of Alzheimer disease. Biol Psychiatry 1993; 33:536–541.

Gottlieb GL, McAllister TW, Gus RC. Depot neuroleptic in the treatment of behavioral disorders in patients with Alzheimer disease. J Am Geriatr Soc 1988; 36:642–644.

Kyomen HH, Mobel KW, Wei JY. The use of estrogen to decrease aggressive physical behavior in elderly men with dementia. J Am Geriatr Soc 1991: 39:1110–1112.

Lyketsos CG, DelCampo L, Martin Steinberg M, Miles-Samus Q, Steele CD, Munro C, Baker AS, Sheppard JME, Frangakis C, Brandt J, Rabins PV. Treating depression in Alzheimer's disease: efficacy and safety of sertraline and the benefits of depression reduction: the DIADS Study. Arch Gen Psychiatry 2003; 60:737–746.

Lyketsos CG, Rosenblatt AR, Rabins PV. Forgotten frontal lobe syndrome. Or, executive dysfunction syndrome. Psychosomatics 2004; 45:247–255.

Mellow AM, Solano-Lopez C, Davis S. Sodium valproate in the treatment of behavioral disturbance in dementia. J Geriatr Psychiatry Neurol 1993; 6: 205–209.

Nyth AL, Gottfries CG. The clinical efficacy of citalopram in treatment of emotional disturbances of dementia subjects. Br J Psychiatry 1990; 157: 894–901.

Ott BR. Leuprolide treatment of sexual aggression in a patient with dementia and the Kluver-Bucy syndrome. Clin Neuropharmacol 1995; 18:443–447.

Petracca G, Teson A, et al. A double-blind placebo controlled study of chlomipramine in depressed patients with Alzheimer disease. J Neuropsychiatry Clin Neurosci 1996; 8:270–275.

Reifler BV, Teri L, Raskind M, et al. Double blind trial of imipramine in Alzheimer disease patients with and without depression. Am J Psychiatry 1989; 146:45–49.

Steele C, Lucas M, Tune L. Haloperidol vs. thioridazine in the treatment of behavioral disturbances in patients with Alzheimer disease. J Clin Psychiatry 1986; 47:310–312.

Targano FE, Lyketsos CG, Mangone CA, Allegri RF, Comesaña-Diaz E. Double-blind, randomized, fixed dose trial of fluoxetine versus amitriptyline in the treatment of major depression complicating Alzheimer disease. Psychosomatics 1997; 38:246–252.

Tariot PN, Erb R, Liebovici A, Podgorski CA, Cox C, Asnis J, Kolassa J, Irving C. Carbamazepine treatment of agitation in nursing home patients with dementia: a preliminary study. J Am Geriatr Soc 1994; 42(11):1160–1166.

Chapter 11: Prevention, Early Detection, and Mild Cognitive Impairment

Brandt J. Mild cognitive impairment in the elderly. Am Fam Physician 2001; 63:620–626.

Iliff S, Manthorpe J. The hazards of early recognition of dementia: a risk assessment. Aging Mental Health 2004; 8:99–105.

Morris JC, Storandt M, Miller JP, McKeel DW, Price JL, Rubin E, Berg L. Mild cognitive impairment represents early-stage Alzheimer disease. Arch Neurol 2001; 58:397–405.

Petersen RC, Doody R, Kurtz A, Mohs RC, Morris JC, Rabins PV, Ritchie K, Rossor M, Thal L, Winblad B. Current concepts in mild cognitive impairment. Arch Neurol 2001; 58:1985–1992.

Tuokko H, Freichs RJ. Cognitive impairment with no dementia (CIND): longitudinal studies, the findings, and the issues. Clin Neuropsychol 2000; 14: 504–525.

Chapter 12: Terminal Care

Andrews M, Bell ER, Smith SA, Tischler JF, Veglia JM. Dehydration in terminally ill patients. Postgrad Med 1993; 93:201–208.

Bergstrom N, Braden B, Kemp M, Champagne M, Ruby E. Multi-site study of incidence of pressure ulcers and the relationship between risk level, demographic characteristics, diagnoses, and prescription of preventive interventions. J Am Geriatr Soc 1996; 44:22–30.

Collins C, Ogle K. Patterns of predeath service use by dementia patients with a family caregiver. J Am Geriatr Soc 1994; 42:719–722.

Fabiszewski KJ, Volicer B, Volicer L. Effect of antibiotic treatment on outcome of fevers in institutionalized Alzheimer patients. JAMA 1990; 263:3168–3172.

Hall P, Schroder C, Weaver L. The last 40 hours in long-term care: a focused chart review. J Am Geriatr Soc 2002; 50:501–506.

Hanrahan P, Luchins DJ. Access to hospice programs in end-stage dementia: a national survey of hospice programs. J Am Geriatr Soc 1995; 43:56–59.

Miller SC, Mor V, Wu N, Gozolo P, Lapare K. Does receipt of hospice care in nursing homes improve the management of pain at the end of life? J Am Geriatr Soc 2002; 50:507–512.

Mitchell SL, Kiely DK, Hamel MB. Dying with advanced dementia in the nursing home. Arch Int Med 2004; 164:321–326.

Standards and Accreditation Committee—Medical Guidelines Task Force. Medical Guidelines for Determining Prognosis in Selected Non-Cancer Diseases. Arlington, VA: National Hospice Organization, 1996.

Stern Y, Tang MX, Albert MS, Brandt J, et al. Predicting time to nursing home care and death in individuals with Alzheimer's disease. JAMA 1997; 277:806–813.

Volicer BJ, Hurley A, Fabiszewski KJ, Montgomery P, Volicer L. Predicting short-term survival for patients with advanced Alzheimer's disease. J Am Geriatr Soc 1993; 41:535–540.

Chapter 13: Ethical and Legal Issues

Jonsen A, Siegler M, Winslade WJ. Clinical Ethics. New York: Macmillan, 1982.

Norberg A, Hirschfeld M, Davidson B, Davis A, Lauri S, Lin JY, Phillips L, Pittmen E, Vander Laan R, Ziv L. Ethical reasoning concerning the feeding of severely demented patients: an international perspective. Nursing Ethics 1994; 1:3–13.

Post SG. The Moral Challenge of Alzheimer Disease. Baltimore: Johns Hopkins University Press, 1995.

Chapter 14: Clinical Genetics and Dementia

Connor JM, Ferguson-Smith MA. Essential Medical Genetics. London: Blackwell Scientific Publications, 1984.

Lendon CL, Ashall F, Goate AM. Exploring the etiology of Alzheimer disease using molecular genetics. JAMA 1997; 277:825–831.

Marx J. New gene tied to common form of Alzheimer's. Science 1988; 281: 507–509.

INDEX

Note: Page numbers followed by f and t refer to figures and tables, respectively.

Abilities, identifying, 92–93
Abstraction, in cognitive examination, 35
Accident prevention, household, 101–5
Acetylcholine
  in Alzheimer's disease, 47
  approaches to increase levels of, 209–13.
    See also Cholinesterase inhibitors
  in dementia, 209
  precursors, 209
Activities
  of daily living, 7
  instrumental, 7
  scheduling, 97, 300
  structuring, 286
  task breakdown, 290–91
Acute care hospital, 87–88
Acute psychiatric unit, 88
Adult day care, 85–86
Advance directives, 266–67
Advocacy groups, 129
Affect, in mental status examination, 26–27
Affective disorder, Alzheimer-associated, 155–56
Affective problems, 155–60
  causes, 156–57
  definition, 155–56
  management, 157
Age, dementia and, 10–12, 11f, 12f
Aggression, 143–46
  causes, 144
  definition, 143–44
  management, 145–46
  urinary tract infection and, 202
Agitation, 143–46
  causes, 144
  definition, 143–44
  management, 145–46
Agnosia
  aggression/agitation in, 144
  in Alzheimer's disease, 283
  bathing problems in, 173
  in cortical dementia, 2

dressing problems in, 182
eating problems in, 170
falling and walking/transferring difficulty
  in, 189
sexual problems in, 197
sleep problems in, 185
social withdrawal in, 165
suspiciousness, paranoia, and delusions
  in, 162
uncooperativeness and resistance to care
  in, 139–40, 142
wandering and pacing in, 147
yelling, calling out, and screaming in, 153
AIDS-associated dementia, 65–67
Akathisia
  pacing and, 148
  uncooperativeness and resistance to care
    and, 140
Alcohol abuse, dementia related to, 73–74
Alien hand syndrome, 48
Allele, 270
Alpha-2 macroglobulin gene, in Alzheimer's
  disease, 275
Alzheimer's Association's Safe Return
  program, 101
Alzheimer's disease
  cholinesterase inhibitors for, 211
  clinical picture, 44–45, 45t
  depression in, 155–56, 213–14
  in Down syndrome, 85, 274
  drug therapy, 205–9, 206f
  epidemiology, 46
  four A's of, 282–83
  functional assessment staging system, 7,
    8t–9t, 242, 243t
  genetic counseling and presymptomatic
    testing, 274–75
  noncognitive behavioral and neuro-
    psychiatric symptoms, 44–45,
    213–14
  pathology and etiology, 46–47, 48f, 205,
    206f, 282

Alzheimer's disease (*continued*)
 risk factors, 233
 sleep problems in, 185
 tips for caregiver, 283–93
Amantadine, 227–28
 for disinhibition-induced aggression, 146
 for executive function disorder, 228–29
 for social withdrawal and apathy, 167
Amitriptyline
 for depression in Alzheimer's disease,
  213–14
 side effects, 220t
Amnesia
 in Alzheimer's disease, 283
 bathing problems in, 173
 in cortical dementia, 2
 dressing problems in, 182
 eating problems in, 170
 evaluation. *See* Memory testing
 in fronto-temporal degeneration, 49
 incontinence and toileting problems in, 177
 in mild cognitive impairment, 237
 in Parkinson's disease, 57–58
 sexual problems in, 196
 sleep problems in, 185
 social withdrawal in, 165
 suspiciousness, paranoia, and delusions
  in, 162
 uncooperativeness and resistance to care
  in, 139
 wandering and pacing in, 147
Amyloid hypothesis, 205, 206f
Amyloid precursor protein (APP) gene, in
  Alzheimer's disease, 47, 205, 274
Amyotrophic lateral sclerosis, 49
Anger, in caregivers, 118–19
Anosagnosia, 29, 80
Anti-inflammatory drugs, for Alzheimer's
  disease, 206–7
Anticholinergic side effects
 antidepressants, 219, 220t, 221
 antipsychotic drugs, 216, 218t
Anticipation, genetic, in Huntington disease,
  62
Anticonvulsants
 for aggression/agitation, 145–46
 in end-stage dementia, 248
 for yelling, calling out, and screaming,
  154
Antidepressants, 219–22
 for depressive delusions, 163
 dosage and administration, 221
 indications, 213–14, 219
 selective serotonin reuptake inhibitor
  for aggression/agitation, 145
  for catastrophic reaction, 137

 dosage and administration, 221
 side effects, 220t
 for social withdrawal and apathy, 167
 for yelling, calling out, and screaming,
  154
 side effects, 219–21, 220t
 tricyclic, side effects, 220t, 221–22
Antihistamines, 225
Antioxidant therapy, for Alzheimer's disease,
  207
Antipsychotic drugs, 214–18
 for aggression/agitation, 145–46
 atypical, 214–15, 216, 217–18, 218t
 for catastrophic reaction, 137
 for delirium, 151
 for delusions, 163–64
 dosage and administration, 217–18
 in end-stage dementia, 249
 for hallucinations and illusions, 161
 indications, 215–16
 potency, 216
 side effects, 216–17, 218t
 typical, 214, 218, 218t
 for yelling, calling out, and screaming,
  154
Anxiety, in dementia, 155
Anxiolytics, 224–26
Apathy, 164–68
 causes, 165–66
 definition, 164–65
 incontinence and toileting problems in, 177
 management, 166–68
 in Parkinson's disease, 58
 stimulants for, 229
 versus uncooperativeness and resistance to
  care, 140
Aphasia
 aggression/agitation in, 144
 in Alzheimer's disease, 283
 bathing problems in, 173
 catastrophic reaction in, 134
 in cortical dementia, 2
 fluent (Wernicke), 26
 incontinence and toileting problems in,
  177
 nonfluent (Broca), 26
 receptive, 26
 sexual problems in, 196–97
 social withdrawal in, 165
 suspiciousness, paranoia, and delusions
  in, 162
 uncooperativeness and resistance to care
  in, 139
 wandering and pacing in, 147
 yelling, calling out, and screaming in, 153
Apnea, sleep, versus delirium, 150

Apolipoprotein E gene (APOE)
    in Alzheimer's disease, 47, 275
    test for, 41t
Appearance, in mental status examination,
        24–25
Apraxia
    in Alzheimer's disease, 283
    bathing problems in, 173
    catastrophic reaction in, 134
    in cortical dementia, 2
    dressing problems in, 182
    eating problems in, 170
    evaluation for, 33, 34–35
    falling and walking/transferring difficulty
        in, 189
    incontinence and toileting problems in,
        177
    sexual problems in, 197
    social withdrawal in, 165
    uncooperativeness and resistance to care
        in, 139, 141–42
    wandering and pacing in, 147
Aripiprazole
    for delusions and hallucinations, 215–16
    dosage and administration, 218
    side effects, 218t
Arrhythmia, from antidepressants, 220t,
        221
Arsenic screen, in dementia evaluation, 41t
Artificial feeding
    in end-stage dementia, 244
    ethical issues, 259–61
Asset protection, 101
Assisted living home, 86, 93. See also Place-
        ment
Astrocytosis, in fronto-temporal degenera-
        tion, 50
Asymmetric fronto-temporal degeneration,
        49
Attention, in Mini-Mental State Examina-
        tion, 31–32
Autopsy issues, 250
Autosomal chromosomes, 270
Autosomal dominant inheritance, 271
Autosomal recessive inheritance, 271

Backward training, for incontinence and
        toileting problems, 179
Balance, poor
    in Parkinson's disease, 57
    in progressive supranuclear palsy, 59
Basement effect, in Mini-Mental State
        Examination, 30
Bathing problems, 172–76
    causes, 173–74
    definition, 172–73

management, 174–76
    tips for caregiver, 285
Bed bath, 175–76
Behavior, in mental status examination,
        24–25
Behavior control, ethical issues, 254–55
Behavioral disorders, noncognitive. See
        Noncognitive behavioral and neuro-
        psychiatric symptoms
Benign senescent forgetfulness, 236
Benzodiazepines, 225–26
Beta-amyloid
    in Alzheimer's disease, 46, 205
    test for, 235
    vaccine, 205
Beta blockers, as mood stabilizers, 224
Biological therapy
    brain surgery, 229
    bright light therapy, 229–30
    electroconvulsive therapy, 230
    pharmacologic, 201–29. See also Drug
        therapy
Blood pressure
    in Alzheimer's disease, 207–8
    high, vasculopathy from, 71
    low. See Hypotension
Bovine spongiform encephalitis, 54, 232
Bowel care, 176–81
    in end-stage dementia, 246
    preventive health care, 106–7, 172
    tips for caregiver, 285–86
Bradykinesia
    in Parkinson's disease, 57
    in progressive supranuclear palsy, 59
Brain
    infarction, vascular dementia from, 69,
        71
    infection, AIDS-associated dementia from,
        65–67
    lymphoma, AIDS-associated dementia
        from, 65, 67
    surgery, in dementia patient, 229
    traumatic injury, dementia after, 71–73
    vascular disease. See Cerebrovascular
        disease
Bright light therapy, for sleep problems, 188,
        229–30
Broca aphasia, 26
Bromocriptine, 228
    for executive function disorder, 228–29
Bupropion
    dosage and administration, 221
    for executive function disorder, 228–29
    side effects, 220t
    for social withdrawal and apathy, 167
Buspirone, 224, 226

Caffeine, wandering and pacing from, 148
CAG repeat
  in dementia evaluation, 41t
  in Huntington disease, 61–62, 276
Calendar, 300
Calling out. *See* Yelling, calling out, and
    screaming
Capacity
  determination, 261–65, 264t
  ethical issues, 257–58
  testamentary, 265
Carbamazepine, 222–23
Carbidopa, 227
Cardiac arrhythmia, from antidepressants,
    220t, 221
Cardiopulmonary resuscitation (CPR), in
    terminal phase, 244
Caregiver(s), 10
  anger in, 118–19
  communication among, 81
  demoralization in, 112–13
  dependency on, rating scales, 36
  emotional problems, 110–15
  family, 109–15
  fatigue in, 114
  grief in, 111–12
  guilt in, 113–14
  nonfamily, 115
  supportive care for, 115–29. *See also*
      Caregiving interventions
  tips for, 283–93
Caregiver factors
  in affective and mood problems, 157
  in aggression/agitation, 144
  in bathing problems, 174
  in catastrophic reaction, 135
  in delirium, 151
  in dressing problems, 183
  in driving problems, 194
  in eating problems, 171
  in falling and walking/transferring diffi-
      culty, 190
  in hallucinations and illusions, 160
  in incontinence and toileting problems,
      178
  in sexual problems, 197
  in sleep problems, 186
  in social withdrawal and apathy, 166
  in suspiciousness, paranoia, and delu-
      sions, 163
  in uncooperativeness and resistance to
      care, 141
  in wandering and pacing, 148
  in yelling, calling out, and screaming,
      153

Caregiving interventions, 119–29, 120t
  addressing personal needs, 123–24
  advocacy groups, 129
  checklist, 299
  coaching on how to approach patient,
      121
  education, 120–21
    on genetics, 129
    on myths and misunderstandings, 117
  emotional support, 124–26
  general approaches, 117–19
  long-range planning, 122
  placement, 127–28
  problem-solving, 121
  psychosocial, 295–96
  resolving family conflicts, 126–27
  respite, 122–23
  substitute decision making, 123
  support groups, 124–26
  tips, 283–93
Carotid endarterectomy, in dementia
    patient, 229
Catastrophic reaction, 27, 133–37
  aggression/agitation in, 145
  causes, 134–35
  definition, 133–34
  documentation, 137
  management, 135–37
  tips for caregiver, 291–92
  warning signs, 134
Caudate nucleus, atrophy, in Huntington
    disease, 62
Ceiling effect, in Mini-Mental State Exami-
    nation, 30
Cerebral spinal fluid pressure waves, in nor-
    mal pressure hydrocephalus, 63–64
Cerebrovascular disease
  in Alzheimer's disease, 207–8
  atypical antipsychotic drugs and, 216
  in dementia, 69–71, 70t
  preventive interventions, 232–33
Ceruloplasmin, arylsulfatase electrophoresis,
    in dementia evaluation, 41t
Checklist(s)
  dementia symptoms, 22, 23t
  supportive care, 298, 299
Chloral hydrate, 225
  side effects, 225
  for sleep problems, 188
Cholesterol, monitoring, in Alzheimer's
    disease, 208
Cholinergic dysfunction
  in Alzheimer's disease, 47
  in Lewy Body dementia, 52–53
Cholinergic receptors, stimulation, 209

Cholinesterase inhibitors, 204, 210–13, 212f
    dosage and administration, 211
    indications, 211
    for mild cognitive impairment, 238
    side effects, 213
Chromosomes, 270
Citalopram
    for depression in Alzheimer's disease, 213
    dosage and administration, 221
    side effects, 220t
Clonazepam, 226
Closed head injury, dementia after, 71
Clothing
    dressing problems. *See* Dressing problems
    tugging at or removing, 182–83
    underwear, with hip pads, 191
Clozapine
    for delusions and hallucinations, 215–16
    side effects, 218t
Co-morbid medical illnesses, 7, 10
Coaching, on how to approach dementia
        patient, 121
Cognitive examination, 29–36
    expanded, 33–36
    Mini-Mental State Examination, 30–33
    patient refusal, 251–52
    rating scales, 36
Cognitive impairment
    affective and mood problems in, 156–57
    aggression/agitation in, 144
    in Alzheimer's disease, 44, 282–83
    apathy in, 165
    bathing problems in, 173
    catastrophic reaction in, 134–35
    in definition of dementia, 2–3, 3t
    delirium in, 150
    depression-induced, 67–69
    dressing problems in, 182
    driving problems in, 193
    drug therapy, 209–13, 212f
    eating problems in, 170
    evaluation for. *See* Cognitive examination
    falling and walking/transferring difficulty
        in, 189
    in fronto-temporal degeneration, 48
    hallucinations and illusions in, 159
    incontinence and toileting problems in,
        177
    in Lewy Body dementia, 51
    mild, 236–38
    versus noncognitive neuropsychiatric
        symptoms, 4–5
    in Parkinson's disease, 57
    sexual problems in, 196–97
    sleep problems in, 185

    social withdrawal in, 165
    suspiciousness, paranoia, and delusions
        in, 162
    uncooperativeness and resistance to care
        in, 139–40
    wandering and pacing in, 147
    yelling, calling out, and screaming in,
        153
Cognitive impairment, not dementia
        (CIND), 236–38
Cognitive slowness, in progressive supra-
        nuclear palsy, 60
Communication
    among caregivers, 81
    with dementia patient, 90–92, 93t,
        286–87
    of diagnosis and treatment options, 79–80
    nonverbal, 92
Competence, determination, 261–65, 264t
Compulsions, in mental status examination,
        28
Computed tomography, in dementia evalua-
        tion, 41
Concentration, in Mini-Mental State
        Examination, 31–32
Consciousness, level of
    in definition of dementia, 3
    evaluation, 34
Consensus building, 268
Constipation
    delirium from, 150
    prevention, 246
Cornell Scale for Depression in Dementia
        (CSDD), 36
Cortical dementia, 43–55
    in Alzheimer's disease, 44–47, 45t
    definition, 2
    in disseminated Lewy Body disease,
        51–53, 53t
    in fronto-temporal degeneration, 47–51,
        50t
    in prion disease, 53–55
    versus subcortical dementia, 3, 4t
Cortico-basalganglionic degeneration, 49,
        50
Costs of dementia, 12
Counseling
    for dementia patient, 98
    genetic. *See* Genetic counseling and
        presymptomatic testing
Coup/countercoup injury, dementia after, 73
Creutzfeld-Jakob disease, 53–55
    variant, 54, 232
Crisis preparation in dementia care, 83–84
Cultural issues, in dementia care, 84–85

Daily living
    activities of, 7
    dementia care in, 92–100
Day program, 85–86
Death
    of dementia patient
        family reactions, 249–50
        predictors, 242, 243t
    thoughts of, in mental status examination,
        27
Decision making
    substitute, caregiver support, 123
    in terminal phase of dementia, 242–44
Decision-making capacity, determination,
    261–65, 264t
Deconditioning, falling due to, 189, 190
Decubitus ulcers, prevention, 246
Dehydration
    delirium from, 150
    in end-stage dementia, 248
    pain question, 260
Delay, in subcortical dementia, 2–3
Delirium, 149–52
    causes, 150–51
    definition, 149–50
    in dementia, 3–4
    versus dementia, 3
    management, 151–52
    postoperative, 108
Delusions, 161–64
    in Alzheimer's disease, 44
    antipsychotic drugs for, 215–16
    causes, 162–63
    definition, 161–62
    depressive, 162
        management, 163
        uncooperativeness and resistance to
            care in, 140
    dressing problems in, 182
    eating problems in, 170
    versus hallucinations, 159
    in Lewy Body dementia, 51
    management, 163–64
    in mental status examination, 28
    in Parkinson's disease, 58
    tips for caregiver, 288–89
    yelling, calling out, and screaming in, 153
Dementia
    classification, 2–3, 4t, 39–40
    co-morbidity, 7, 10
    cognitive symptoms. See Cognitive im-
        pairment
    cortical pattern. See Cortical dementia
    definition, 1–4, 3t, 282
    diseases causing, 4, 5t

early diagnosis, benefits, 16, 235–36
evaluation. See Dementia evaluation
impairment and disability, 7, 8t–9t
mixed, 3
    after traumatic brain injury, 71–73
    in substance abuse, 73–74
noncognitive functional symptoms. See
    Noncognitive functional symptoms
noncognitive neuropsychiatric symptoms.
    See Noncognitive behavioral and
    neuropsychiatric symptoms
psychosocial intervention, 295–96
scope of problem, 10–12, 11f, 12f
subcortical pattern. See Subcortical
    dementia
terminal phase, 241–44
toxic, 73–74
vascular. See Vascular dementia
Dementia care, 75–108
    in adult with mental retardation, 85
    complexities, 12–13
    cultural and ethnic issues, 84–85
    in day-to-day living, 92–100
    goals, 75–77
    good clinical practices, 82–84, 83t
    guidelines for families, 279–93
    health maintenance, 105–8
    Johns Hopkins model, 281
    principles, 75, 76t
    safety-proofing, 101–4
    setting, 81–82, 85–88, 93–94
        acute care hospital, 87–88
        acute psychiatric unit, 88
        day program, 85–86
        emergency department, 87
        group and assisted living home, 86, 93
        home, 93
        hospice, 88
        nursing home, 86–87, 93
    supervision, 104–5, 105t
    supportive, 89–108. See also Supportive
        care, for dementia patient
    team approach, 81
    in terminal phase, 241–50. See also
        Terminal care
    treatment plan
        attributes, 77–79, 78t
        implementing, 79–82
    in young, 84
Dementia caregiver. See Caregiver(s)
Dementia evaluation
    differential diagnosis and workup, 5t,
        37–42, 39f
    family assessment, 37, 38t
    formulation, 38–39

indications, 15–16, 17t
laboratory tests, 40–41, 40t, 41t
neuropsychiatric assessment, 20–37
 history, 20–22, 22f, 23t
 mental status examination, 22–36, 25t.
  See also Mental status examination
 in mild cognitive impairment, 237–38
 patient refusal, 251–52
 purposes, 17–18
 settings, 18
 stages, 18–19, 19t
 supplemental scales, 36–37
 symptom checklist, 22, 23t
Demoralization, in caregivers, 112–13
Demyelination, in multiple sclerosis, 64
Dental health
 in end-stage dementia, 247
 maintenance, 106
Denture care, 106
Dependency on caregivers, rating scales, 36
Depletion, in subcortical dementia, 2–3
Depression
 after traumatic brain injury, 72
 in Alzheimer's disease, 45
 delusions in, 162
  management, 163
  uncooperativeness and resistance to
   care in, 140
 in dementia, 67–69, 155–56, 158, 209
 dressing problems in, 182
 drug therapy, 213–14. *See also* Antidepressants
 eating problems in, 170
 electroconvulsive therapy, 230
 in Huntington disease, 61
 in multiple sclerosis, 64
 in Parkinson's disease, 58
 rating scales, 36
 sleep problems in, 188
 social withdrawal and apathy in, 165
 suspiciousness and paranoia in, 162
 tips for caregiver, 289–90
 uncooperativeness and resistance to care
  in, 140
 vascular, 68–69, 70, 213
 wandering and pacing in, 147
 yelling, calling out, and screaming in, 153
Depression-induced cognitive impairment,
 67–69
Desipramine, side effects, 220t
Dexadrine, for social withdrawal and
 apathy, 167
Dignity, patient, in end-stage dementia,
 247–48
Diphenhydramine, 225

Disabilities, in dementia, 7
Disinhibition, 146
Disrobing, 182–83
Distraction
 for affective and mood problems, 158
 for catastrophic reaction, 136
 for hallucinations and illusions, 160
Diuretics, wandering and pacing from, 148
Divalproex sodium, 222
DNA testing, 271–72
Donepezil, for Alzheimer's disease, 210–13,
 212f
L-Dopa, 227
 for disinhibition-induced aggression, 146
 for executive function disorder, 228–29
Dopamine agonists, 227–28
 aggression/agitation from, 144
Dopamine loss, in Parkinson's disease,
 58–59
Down syndrome, Alzheimer's disease in, 85,
 274
Dressing problems, 181–84
 causes, 182–83
 definition, 181
 management, 183–84
 tips for caregiver, 284
Drinking apraxia, 170
Driving concerns, 192–96
 causes, 193–94
 definition, 192–93
 ethical issues, 253–54
 management, 194–96
 tips for caregiver, 290
Drug(s)
 aggression/agitation from, 144
 delirium from, 150
 delusions from, 162
 hallucinations from, 160
 pacing from, 148
 sexual problems from, 197
 sleep problems from, 185, 186
 social withdrawal and apathy from, 166
Drug therapy, 201–29. *See also specific
  drugs, e.g.,* Antipsychotic drugs
 administration of medications, 107,
  287–88
 for aggression/agitation, 145
 for Alzheimer's dementia, 205–9, 206f
 for behavior control, ethical issues,
  254–55
 for catastrophic reaction, 137
 for cognitive symptomatology, 209–13,
  212f
 for delirium, 151
 indications, 203

Drug therapy (*continued*)
   for noncognitive neuropsychiatric
      symptoms, 213–29
   principles, 201–3
   resistance to taking medications, 142
   for social withdrawal and apathy, 167
   for uncooperativeness and resistance to
      care, 143
   for underlying disease, 203–9
   for yelling, calling out, and screaming,
      154
Durable power of attorney, 242, 266
Dyskinesia
   drug therapy, 227–28
   tardive, from antipsychotic drugs, 217
Dysmnesia, in subcortical dementia, 2–3
Dysthymia, in dementia, 155

Early diagnosis of dementia, benefits, 16,
   235–36
Eating problems, 169–72
   causes, 170–71
   definition, 169–70
   in end-stage dementia, 245
   ethical issues, 259–61
   management, 171–72
   tips for caregiver, 283–84
Education, caregiver, 120–21
   on genetics of dementia, 129
   on myths and misunderstandings about
      dementia, 117
Electroconvulsive therapy
   for aggression/agitation, 146
   for depression, 230
Electroencephalography
   in dementia evaluation, 41t
   in prion dementia, 54
Electrophoresis, 41t
Elimination patterns, 176–81
   in end-stage dementia, 246
   preventive health care, 106–7, 172
   tips for caregiver, 285–86
Elopement, 146–47
Embolic stroke, 71
Emergency department, dementia care in, 87
Emotional incontinence, 27
Emotional problems
   in caregivers, 110–15
   in end-stage dementia, 249
Emotional support
   for caregivers, 124–26
   for dementia patient, 98
Encephalitis, bovine spongiform, 54, 232
Encephalopathy, spongiform, in prion
      dementia, 55

Environmental factors
   in affective and mood problems, 157
   in aggression/agitation, 144
   in bathing problems, 174
   in catastrophic reaction, 135
   in delirium, 151
   in dressing problems, 183
   in driving problems, 194
   in eating problems, 171
   in falling and walking/transferring diffi-
      culty, 190, 191
   in hallucinations and illusions, 160, 161
   in incontinence and toileting problems,
      178
   in sexual problems, 197
   in sleep problems, 186
   in social withdrawal and apathy, 166
   in suspiciousness, paranoia, and delu-
      sions, 163
   in uncooperativeness and resistance to
      care, 140–41
   in wandering and pacing, 148
   in yelling, calling out, and screaming, 153
Environmental stimulation, for social
      withdrawal and apathy, 166–67
Epidemiology of dementia, 10–12, 11f, 12f
Escitalopram, side effects, 220t
Estrogen-replacement therapy, for Alz-
      heimer's disease, 206
Ethical issues, 251–61
   driving problems, 253–54
   general principles, 267–68
   health decisions for incapacitated patient,
      257–58
   living alone, 252–53
   lying to dementia patient, 255–57
   medications and restraints to control
      behavior, 254–55
   refusal of evaluation by memory impaired
      patient, 251–52
   refusal to eat, 259–61
Ethnic issues, in dementia care, 84–85
Euphoria, in dementia, 155
Euthymia, in dementia, 155
Eutonia, in dementia of multiple sclerosis,
      64–65
Executive function, in cognitive examina-
      tion, 35–36
Executive function disorder
   aggression/agitation in, 144
   apathy in, 165
   drug therapy, 222, 228–29
   eating problems in, 170
   in fronto-temporal degeneration, 48
   sexual problems in, 197

in subcortical dementia, 2–3
suspiciousness, paranoia, and delusions in, 162
yelling, calling out, and screaming in, 153
Extrapyramidal side effects, antipsychotic drugs, 216, 218t
Eye movement disorder, in progressive supranuclear palsy, 59–60

Falls, 188–92
causes, 189–90
in Lewy Body dementia, 51
prevention, 190–92
risk factors, 188–89
Family
assessment, in dementia evaluation, 37, 38t
dementia care guidelines, 279–93
Family caregivers, 109–15. See also Caregiver(s)
Family conference, 79, 118
Family conflicts, resolving, 126–27
Family history, in neuropsychiatric assessment, 20, 22f
Family pedigree, 20, 22f
FAST (Functional Assessment Staging of Alzheimer's Disease) system, 7, 8t–9t, 242, 243t
Fatigue, in caregivers, 114
Feeding problems, 169–72
causes, 170–71
definition, 169–70
in end-stage dementia, 245
ethical issues, 259–61
management, 171–72
Feeding tube
in end-stage dementia, 244
ethical issues, 259–61
Fever, in end-stage dementia, 244
Fluent aphasia, 26
Fluid(s)
intake
in end-stage dementia, 248
maintenance, 94–95, 172
loss. See Dehydration
Fluoxetine
dosage and administration, 221
side effects, 220t
Fluphenazine, side effects, 218t
Foot care, preventive, 106
Formulation, in dementia evaluation, 38–39
Frontal lobe fronto-temporal degeneration, 49
Frontal lobe injury
catastrophic reaction in, 134–35
yelling, calling out, and screaming in, 153

Frontal-subcortical dementia, apathy in, 165
Fronto-temporal degeneration, 47–51, 50t
clinical picture, 48–49, 50t
epidemiology, 49–50
pathology, 50–51
subtypes, 49
Function
executive, in expanded cognitive examination, 35–36
maximizing, 92–93
visuospatial
in expanded cognitive examination, 34–35
in Mini-Mental State Examination, 33
Functional Assessment Staging of Alzheimer's Disease (FAST) system, 7, 8t–9t, 242, 243t
Functional impairment, 169–200
bathing problems, 172–76
dressing problems, 181–84
driving problems, 192–96
eating problems and weight loss, 169–72
executive. See Executive function disorder
falls and walking/transferring difficulty, 188–92
incontinence and toileting problems, 176–81
rating scales, 36
sexual problems, 196–200
sleep problems, 184–88
staging system, 7, 8t–9t, 242, 243t
types, 7
visuospatial, in Parkinson's disease, 58

Gait ataxia, in normal pressure hydrocephalus, 62–63
Gait disorders, falling in, 189
Galantamine, for Alzheimer's disease, 210–13, 212f
Gastrostomy tube
in end-stage dementia, 244
ethical issues, 259–61
Genetic anticipation, in Huntington disease, 62
Genetic counseling and presymptomatic testing
in Alzheimer's disease, 274–75
in dementia evaluation, 41t
in Huntington disease, 275–76
issues, 272–74
types of tests, 271–72
in vascular dementia, 276
Genetics, 269–76
of Alzheimer's disease, 47
caregiver education on, 129

Genetics (*continued*)
  of fronto-temporal degeneration, 50
  of Huntington disease, 61–62
  primer, 270–72
Genogram, 20, 22f
Gerstman-Straussler-Scheinker syndrome,
  53–55
Ginkgo biloba, for Alzheimer's disease, 207
Glossary of terms, 301–9
Glucose, monitoring, in Alzheimer's disease,
  208
Go–No Go Test, 36
Grasp reflex, uncooperativeness due to, 140,
  142
Grief
  in caregivers, 111–12
  in dementia patient, 155, 156–57
Group home, 86, 93. *See also* Placement
Guilt, in caregivers, 113–14
Guns, safety considerations, 101

Hallucinations, 159–61
  in Alzheimer's disease, 44
  antipsychotic drugs for, 215–16
  causes, 159–60
  definition, 159
  versus delusions, 159
  versus illusions, 159
  in Lewy Body dementia, 51
  management, 160–61
  in mental status examination, 28
  in progressive supranuclear palsy, 60
  tips for caregiver, 288
  uncooperativeness and resistance to care
    in, 140
  yelling, calling out, and screaming in, 153
Haloperidol
  dosage and administration, 218
  side effects, 218t
Head injury, traumatic, dementia after, 71–73
Health care
  coordination, 105–6
  preventive, 106–7
Health decisions for incapacitated patient,
  ethical issues, 257–58
Health maintenance, in dementia care, 105–8
Heavy metal exposure, dementia related to,
  41t, 74
Hemorrhagic stroke, 71
Hepatitis, from atypical antipsychotic drugs,
  217
Hip pads, underwear with, 191
Hippocampal sclerosis, 49
History, 20–22
  family, 20, 22f

medical, 20–21
  past neuropsychiatric, 21–22
  personal, 20
  premorbid personality, 21
  present illness, 22, 23t
  substance abuse, 20
HIV (human immunodeficiency virus)
  AIDS-associated dementia from, 65–67
  test for, in dementia evaluation, 41t
Hoarding, tips for caregiver, 292–93
Home
  dementia care in, 93
  leaving patient alone in, 104–5, 105t
  safety-proofing, 101–3
Homicidal thoughts, in mental status
    examination, 27
Homocysteine, monitoring, in Alzheimer's
    disease, 208
Hope, caregiver need for, 117
Hospice care, 88
  certification formula, 242, 243t
  in end-stage dementia, 243–44, 249
Hospitalization
  for aggression/agitation, 145
  for pneumonia or sepsis, 245
Human immunodeficiency virus (HIV)
  AIDS-associated dementia from, 65–67
  test for, in dementia evaluation, 41t
Huntingtin protein, 62, 276
Huntington disease
  clinical picture, 60–61
  epidemiology, 61
  genetic counseling and presymptomatic
    testing, 275–76
  pathology and etiology, 61–62
Huperzine-A, for Alzheimer's disease, 210
Hydration. *See also* Dehydration
  in end-stage dementia, 248
  maintenance, 94–95, 172
Hydrocephalus, normal pressure, 62–64
Hydroxyprogesterone, for sexual problems,
  199
Hydroxyzine, 225
Hygiene
  basic, 106–7
  sleep, 95–96, 186–87
Hyperorality, 170
Hypertension therapy, in Alzheimer's
    disease, 207–8
Hypertensive vasculopathy, 71
Hypomania, in dementia, 156
Hypotension, orthostatic, 190
  from antidepressants, 220t
  from antipsychotic drugs, 216, 218t
Hypothyroidism, dementia and, 235

Identification items, wearing, 102
Illusions, 159–61
  causes, 159–60
  definition, 159
  management, 160–61
  in mental status examination, 28
Imipramine, side effects, 220t
Immunotherapy, for Alzheimer's disease, 205
Implicit learning, 96
Incidence of dementia, 11–12, 12f
Incontinence, 176–81
  causes, 177–78
  definition, 176–77
  emotional, 27
  in end-stage dementia, 246
  management, 178–81
  in normal pressure hydrocephalus, 62
Infection
  brain, AIDS-associated dementia from, 65–67
  delirium from, 150
  urinary tract
    aggression from, 202
    delirium from, 150
    incontinence and toileting problems from, 177–78
Information resources, 79
Inhalant abuse, dementia related to, 73–74
Inheritance patterns, 271
Insight
  lack of, in dementia, 80
  in mental status examination, 29
Institutional settings, safety-proofing, 103–4
Instrumental activities of daily living (IADLs), 7
Inventory, taking, 291
Irritability, in dementia, 155

Johns Hopkins model of care for dementia, 281
Judgment, in mental status examination, 29

Karyotyping, 271
Knowledge assessment, in cognitive examination, 35

Labile mood, in dementia, 155
Laboratory tests, in dementia evaluation, 40–41, 40t, 41t
Language assessment, 32–33. See also Talk (speech)
Late-life depression, treatment, 209
Lead exposure, dementia related to, 41t, 74
Learning, implicit, 96

Leaving alone, versus supervision of dementia patient, 104–5, 105t
Leg, restless, 187
Legal issues, 261–67
  advance directives, 266–67
  determination of capacity or competence, 261–65, 264t
  driving concerns, 194–95
  durable power of attorney, 266
  testamentary capacity, 265
Leukoareosis, vascular dementia from, 69
Leuprolide, for sexual problems, 146, 199
Level of consciousness
  in definition of dementia, 3
  evaluation, 34
Lewy bodies, in Parkinson's disease, 59
Lewy Body dementia
  cholinesterase inhibitors for, 211
  clinical picture, 51–52, 53t
  epidemiology, 52
  pathology, 52–53
Limbic circuit injury, catastrophic reaction in, 135
Lithium carbonate, 223–24
Living alone, 93–94, 252–53
Living will, 266
Local resources, 82, 118
Lorazepam, 226
  in end-stage dementia, 249
Lou Gehrig's disease, 49
Lumbar puncture, in dementia evaluation, 41t
Luria Hand-Sequencing Test, 36
Lying, ethical issues, 255–57
Lyme disease titer, in dementia evaluation, 41t
Lymphoma, brain, AIDS-associated dementia from, 65, 67

Mad cow disease, 54, 232
Magnetic resonance imaging, in dementia evaluation, 41
Malnutrition, delirium from, 150
Mania
  after traumatic brain injury, 72
  in dementia, 156
  dressing problems in, 182
  eating problems in, 170
  mood stabilizers for, 222–24
  uncooperativeness and resistance to care in, 140
Mass action principle
  in traumatic brain injury, 73
  in vascular dementia, 71
Massage, in end-stage dementia, 246

Masturbation, public, 198
Medical disorders
  affective and mood problems in, 157
  aggression/agitation in, 144
  bathing problems in, 173
  catastrophic reaction in, 135
  co-morbid, 7, 10
  delirium in, 150
  dressing problems in, 182–83
  driving problems in, 193
  eating problems in, 170–71
  falling and walking/transferring difficulty
    in, 189–90
  hallucinations in, 159–60
  incontinence and toileting problems in,
    177–78
  sexual problems in, 197
  sleep problems in, 185–86
  social withdrawal and apathy in, 165–66
  suspiciousness, paranoia, and delusions
    in, 162
  uncooperativeness and resistance to care
    in, 140
  wandering and pacing in, 147–48
  yelling, calling out, and screaming in,
    153
Medical history, in neuropsychiatric assess-
    ment, 20–21
Medical interventions, in end-stage demen-
    tia, benefits and burdens, 244–45
Medications. See Drug(s); Drug therapy
Memantine, for Alzheimer's disease, 208–9
Memory disorder. See Amnesia
Memory testing
  in expanded cognitive examination, 34
  in Mini-Mental State Examination,
    30–31, 32
  patient refusal, 251–52
Mental status examination, 22–36, 25t
  appearance and behavior in, 24–25
  cognition in, 29–36
  insight and judgment in, 29
  mood and affect in, 26–27
  perception in, 28
  resistance to, 22–24, 251–52
  self-attitude in, 27
  talk (speech) in, 25–26
  thought content in, 28–29
  thoughts of death, suicide, or homicide in,
    27
  vital sense in, 27
Mentally retarded adult, dementia care, 85
Mercury screen, in dementia evaluation,
    41t
Metals, heavy, dementia related to, 41t, 74

Methylphenidate
  for executive function disorder, 229
  for social withdrawal and apathy, 167
Microtubule-associated proteins
  in fronto-temporal degeneration, 50–51
  in progressive supranuclear palsy, 60
Mild cognitive impairment (MCI), 236–38
Mini-Mental State Examination, 30–33
  dementia evaluation need based on, 16
  limitations, 30
  Modified, 33
  strengths, 30
Mirtazapine
  dosage and administration, 221
  side effects, 220t
Misunderstandings, about dementia, 117
Mixed dementia, 3
  after traumatic brain injury, 71–73
  in substance abuse, 73–74
Modafenil, for social withdrawal and
    apathy, 167
Modified Mini-Mental State Examination, 33
Monoamine oxidase inhibitors, side effects,
    220t
Mood, in mental status examination, 26–27
Mood disorders, 155–60. See also Depres-
    sion; Mania
  after traumatic brain injury, 72
  causes, 156–57
  definition, 155–56
  dementia in, 67–69
  management, 157
  in multiple sclerosis, 64–65
Mood stabilizers, 222–24
  for catastrophic reaction, 137
  indications, 222
Mood states, 155
Mood syndromes, 155–56
Motor disorders
  in AIDS-associated dementia, 66
  in depression-induced cognitive impair-
    ment, 67–69
  drug therapy, 227–28
  in Huntington disease, 60–61
  in normal pressure hydrocephalus, 62–63
Motor neuron fronto-temporal degenera-
    tion, 49
Motor slowness
  in Parkinson's disease, 57
  in progressive supranuclear palsy, 59
Motor vehicle bureau, notification of
    driving problems, 194–95, 254
Mouth care
  in end-stage dementia, 247
  maintenance, 106

Multi-infarct dementia, 69–71, 70t
Multifactorial inheritance, 271
Multiple sclerosis, 64–65
Muscle weakness, falling due to, 189, 190
Myths, about dementia, 117

Naming, in Mini-Mental State Examination,
    32
Negative predictive value, screening test,
    234–35
Neuritic plaques
    in Alzheimer's disease, 46
    in Lewy Body dementia, 52
Neurofibrillary tangles, in Alzheimer's
    disease, 46
Neuroleptic malignant syndrome, from
    atypical antipsychotic drugs, 217
Neurologic symptoms, in Alzheimer's
    disease, 45
Neuronal loss
    in Alzheimer's disease, 46
    in fronto-temporal degeneration, 50
    in Lewy Body dementia, 53
    in Parkinson's disease, 58–59
    in progressive supranuclear palsy, 60
Neuropsychiatric assessment, 20–37
    history, 20–22, 22f, 23t
    mental status examination, 22–36, 25t.
        See also Mental status examination
    in mild cognitive impairment, 237–38
Neuropsychiatric disorders. See Psychiatric
    disorders
Neuropsychiatric history, past, 21–22
Neuropsychiatric Inventory (NPI), 36–37
Neuropsychiatric symptoms
    cognitive. See Cognitive impairment
    noncognitive. See Noncognitive behav-
        ioral and neuropsychiatric symptoms
Neuropsychological testing, in dementia
    evaluation, 38–39
Neurosyphilis, preventive interventions,
    231–32
NMDA receptor antagonists, for Alzheimer's
    disease, 208–9
Noncognitive behavioral and neuropsychi-
    atric symptoms, 4–7, 6t, 131–68. See
    also Psychiatric disorders
    affective and mood problems, 155–60
    after traumatic brain injury, 72
    aggression/agitation, 143–46
    in AIDS-associated dementia, 66
    in Alzheimer's disease, 44–45, 213–14
    catastrophic reactions, 133–37
    delirium, 149–52
    drug therapy, 213–29

etiology and pathogenesis, 6
4D approach, 131–33, 132t
    in fronto-temporal degeneration, 48
    hallucinations and illusions, 159–61
    in Huntington disease, 61
    in Lewy Body dementia, 51
    morbidity, 6–7
    prevalence, 6
    rating scales, 36–37
    social withdrawal and apathy, 164–68
    suspiciousness, paranoia, and delusions,
        161–64
    uncooperativeness and resistance to care,
        138–43
    in vascular dementia, 69–70
    wandering and pacing, 146–49
    yelling, calling out, and screaming,
        152–55
Noncognitive functional symptoms,
    169–200
    bathing problems, 172–76
    dressing problems, 181–84
    driving problems, 192–96
    eating problems and weight loss,
        169–72
    falls and walking/transferring diffi-
        culty, 188–92
    incontinence and toileting problems,
        176–81
    rating scales, 36
    sexual problems, 196–200
    sleep problems, 184–88
    staging system, 7, 8t–9t, 242, 243t
    types, 7
    visuospatial, in Parkinson's disease,
        58
Nonfluent aphasia, 26
Nonsteroidal anti-inflammatory drugs, for
    Alzheimer's disease, 206–7
Nonverbal communication, 92
Normal pressure hydrocephalus
    clinical picture, 62–63
    epidemiology, 63
    pathology and etiology, 63–64
Nortriptyline
    dosage and administration, 221
    side effects, 220t
    for vascular depression, 213
Nursing home. See also Placement
    dementia care in, 86–87, 93
    safety-proofing, 103–4
Nutrition. See also Feeding problems
    maintenance, 94–95
    poor, delirium from, 150
Nutritional supplements, 172

Obsessions, in mental status examination, 28
Occupational therapist, 93–94
Olanzapine
  dosage and administration, 218
  side effects, 218t
Opioids, in end-stage dementia, 249
Opisthotonos, in progressive supranuclear palsy, 60
Opportunistic brain infection, AIDS-associated dementia from, 65, 67
Oral health
  in end-stage dementia, 247
  maintenance, 106
Orientation, in Mini-Mental State Examination, 30
Orthostatic hypotension, 190
  from antidepressants, 220t
  from antipsychotic drugs, 216, 218t
Out-of-home placement. See Placement
Oxygen supplementation, in end-stage dementia, 248

Pacing, 146–49
  causes, 147–48
  definition, 146–47
  management, 148–49
Pain
  catastrophic reaction and, 135
  dehydration and, 260
  in end-stage dementia, 249
  uncooperativeness and resistance to care and, 140
  wandering and pacing and, 147–48
  yelling, calling out, and screaming and, 153, 154
Pallilalic speech, 26
Palsy, progressive supranuclear, 49, 50, 59–60
Panic attack, 156
Panic disorder
  in dementia, 156
  in multiple sclerosis, 64
Paranoia, 161–64
  causes, 162–63
  definition, 161–62
  management, 163–64
Paraphasic speech, 26
Parkinsonism
  causes, 59
  drug therapy, 227–28
  in Lewy Body dementia, 51
Parkinson's disease
  clinical picture, 57–58
  epidemiology, 58
  pathology and etiology, 58–59

Paroxetine
  dosage and administration, 221
  side effects, 220t
Pellagra, preventive interventions, 232
Penetrating head injury, dementia after, 71–72
Perception, in mental status examination, 28
Perphenazine
  dosage and administration, 218
  side effects, 218t
Personal affairs, taking inventory, 291
Personal history, in neuropsychiatric assessment, 20
Personal needs, caregiver, 123–24
Personality change
  after traumatic brain injury, 72
  in fronto-temporal degeneration, 48, 49
  in vascular dementia, 70
Phobias, in mental status examination, 28
Physical restraints
  in end-stage dementia, 248–49
  ethical issues, 254–55
  for prevention of falling, 191
Pick's disease, 50
Place orientation, in Mini-Mental State Examination, 30
Placement, 99–100
  caregiver support, 127–28
  reasons for, 100t
Planning
  ability, assessment, 34–35
  long-range, caregiver, 122
Pneumonia, in end-stage dementia, 245
Polymorphism
  definition, 270
  restriction fragment length, 272
Positive predictive value, screening test, 234
Positron emission tomography, in dementia evaluation, 41
Postconcussion syndrome, after traumatic brain injury, 72
Power of attorney, durable, 242, 266
Praxis. See also Apraxia
  in expanded cognitive examination, 34–35
  in Mini-Mental State Examination, 33
Prednisone, for Alzheimer's disease, 206–7
Premorbid personality, in neuropsychiatric assessment, 21
Presenillin-1 gene
  in Alzheimer's disease, 47, 274
  test for, in dementia evaluation, 41t
Presenillin-2 gene, in Alzheimer's disease, 47, 274–75

Present illness, in neuropsychiatric assessment, 22, 23t
Prevalence of dementia, 10–11, 11f
Prevention, accident, household, 101–5
Preventive health care, 106–7
Preventive interventions for dementia, 231–35
    approaches, 233
    examples, 231–33
    recommendations, 238–39
    screening test characteristics, 234–35
    target groups, 234
Primary prevention, 231
Prion dementia
    clinical picture, 53–54
    epidemiology, 54–55
    pathology, 54–55
Prion (proteinous infectious particle) protein, 55
Problem solving
    skill development, 121
    trial-and-error, 83
Procedures, surgical, for dementia patient, 107–8
Progesterone, for sexual aggression, 146
Progressive supranuclear palsy, 49, 50, 59–60
Prosody, in communication with dementia patient, 90
Pseudodementia, 68
Psychiatric disorders
    aggression/agitation in, 144
    bathing problems in, 173
    delirium in, 150
    depression in, 157
    dressing problems in, 182
    driving problems in, 193
    falling and walking/transferring difficulty in, 189
    hallucinations and illusions in, 159
    incontinence and toileting problems in, 177
    sexual problems in, 197
    sleep problems in, 185
    social withdrawal and apathy in, 165
    suspiciousness, paranoia, and delusions in, 162
    uncooperativeness and resistance to care in, 140
    wandering and pacing in, 147
    yelling, calling out, and screaming in, 153
Psychiatric units, acute, dementia care in, 88
Psychogeriatric Dependency Rating Scale, 36

Psychological symptoms, noncognitive. See Noncognitive behavioral and neuropsychiatric symptoms
Psychosocial intervention, 295–96
Psychotherapy, for dementia patient, 98

Quetiapine
    for delusions and hallucinations, 215–16
    dosage and administration, 217
    side effects, 218t

Raphe nuclei, serotonin cell loss in, in progressive supranuclear palsy, 60
Rash, from atypical antipsychotic drugs, 217
Rating scales, in dementia evaluation, 36–37
Receptive aphasia, 26
Refusal
    to eat, 259–61
    of evaluation by memory impaired patient, 251–52
Registration, in Mini-Mental State Examination, 30–31
Relationship with dementia patient
    communication in, 90–92, 93t
    establishing, 89–90
Repetition, in Mini-Mental State Examination, 32–33
Resistance
    to care, 138–43
        causes, 139–41
        definition, 138–39
        management, 141–43
    to mental status examination, 22–24, 251–52
Resources
    information, 79
    local, 82, 118
Respite, for caregivers, 122–23
Restless leg syndrome, 187
Restraints
    in end-stage dementia, 248–49
    ethical issues, 254–55
    for prevention of falling, 191
Restriction fragment length polymorphism (RFLP) studies, 272
Rigidity
    in Parkinson's disease, 57
    in progressive supranuclear palsy, 59
Risperidone
    dosage and administration, 218
    side effects, 218t
Rivastigmine, for Alzheimer's disease, 210–13, 212f
Routines, establishing, 96–97
Rummaging, tips for caregiver, 292–93

Safety-proofing, 101–4
  in home, 101–3
  in institutional settings, 103–4
  living alone and, 94
Sclerosis
  amyotrophic lateral, 49
  hippocampal, 49
  multiple, 64–65
Screaming. *See* Yelling, calling out, and
    screaming
Screening tests, characteristics, 234–35
Secondary prevention, 231
Sedation
  from antidepressants, 220t, 221
  from antipsychotic drugs, 216, 218t
Sedative-hypnotics, 224–26
  indications, 224–25
  side effects, 225
  for sleep problems, 187–88
  for yelling, calling out, and screaming,
    154
Seizures
  from atypical antipsychotic drugs, 217
  in end-stage dementia, 248
Selective serotonin reuptake inhibitors
  for aggression/agitation, 145
  for catastrophic reaction, 137
  dosage and administration, 221
  side effects, 220t
  for social withdrawal and apathy, 167
  for yelling, calling out, and screaming,
    154
Self-attitude, in mental status examination,
    27
Senile plaques
  in Alzheimer's disease, 46
  in Lewy Body dementia, 52
Sensitivity, screening test, 234
Sepsis, in end-stage dementia, 245
Serial sevens, in Mini-Mental State Exami-
    nation, 31
Serotonergic side effects, antidepressants,
    219, 220t
Serotonin cell loss, in progressive supra-
    nuclear palsy, 60
Serotonin reuptake inhibitors
  for aggression/agitation, 145
  for catastrophic reaction, 137
  dosage and administration, 221
  side effects, 220t
  for social withdrawal and apathy, 167
  for yelling, calling out, and screaming, 154
Serotonin syndrome, 219
Sertraline
  for depression in Alzheimer's disease, 213

  dosage and administration, 221
  side effects, 220t
Severe Impairment Rating Scale (SIRS), 36
Sex chromosomes, 270
Sex-linked inheritance, 271
Sexual aggression, management, 146
Sexual problems, 196–200
  causes, 196–97
  definition, 196
  management, 198–200
Shunt surgery
  in dementia patient, 229
  for normal pressure hydrocephalus, 63
Signs and symptoms
  checklist, 22, 23t
  as indication for dementia evaluation, 16,
    17t
Single photon emission computed tomog-
    raphy, in dementia evaluation, 41
Skin care
  in end-stage dementia, 246
  preventive, 106
Skin rash, from atypical antipsychotic drugs,
    217
Sleep apnea, versus delirium, 150
Sleep hygiene, 95–96, 186–87
Sleep problems, 184–88
  bright light therapy, 229–30
  causes, 185–86
  definition, 184–85
  drug therapy, 224–26
  management, 186–88
Slit lamp examination, in dementia evalua-
    tion, 41t
Slowness
  cognitive, in progressive supranuclear
    palsy, 60
  motor
    in Parkinson's disease, 57
    in progressive supranuclear palsy, 59
Smoking, safety considerations, 101
Social withdrawal, 164–68
  causes, 165–66
  definition, 164–65
  management, 166–68
  stimulants for, 229
Specialist input, in dementia assessment, 18
Specificity, screening test, 234
Speech
  in mental status examination, 25–26
  pragmatics, in communication with
    dementia patient, 90
Spongiform encephalitis, bovine, 54, 232
Spongiform encephalopathy, in prion
    dementia, 55

Steroids, aggression/agitation from, 144
Stiffness, in Parkinson's disease, 57
Stimulants
    for disinhibition-induced aggression, 146
    for executive function disorder, 229
    for social withdrawal and apathy, 167
Stimulus-bound behavior, eating problems
        in, 170
Stroke-related dementia, 69–71, 70t
Subcortical dementia, 57–74
    in cerebrovascular disease, 69–71, 70t
    definition, 2–3
    in HIV-AIDS, 65–67
    in Huntington disease, 60–62
    in mood disorders, 67–69
    in multiple sclerosis, 64–65
    in normal pressure hydrocephalus, 62–64
    in Parkinson's disease, 57–59
    in progressive supranuclear palsy, 59–60
Substance abuse
    dementia related to, 73–74
    history, in neuropsychiatric assessment, 20
Substantia nigra, dopamine loss in, in
        Parkinson's disease, 58–59
Substitute decision making, caregiver
        support, 123
Suicidal thoughts, in mental status examina-
        tion, 27
Supervision, in dementia care, 104–5, 105t
Support groups, caregiver, 124–26
Supported living situation. See Placement
Supportive care
    for caregivers, 115–29. See also Care-
        giving interventions
        checklist, 299
        general approaches, 117–19
        interventions, 119–29, 120t
        psychosocial, 295–96
    for dementia patient, 89–108
        accident prevention, 100–105
        approach to patient, 89–92, 93t
        checklist, 298
        communication, 90–92, 93t
        in day-to-day living, 92–100
        emotional support, 98
        establishing daily routine, 96–97
        establishing relationship, 89–90
        health care coordination, 105–6
        health maintenance, 105–8
        hygiene and preventive health care,
            106–7
        maximizing function and identifying
            abilities, 92–93
        medication administration, 107
        nutrition and hydration, 94–95

        placement, 99–100, 100t
        procedures/surgery, 107–8
        safety-proofing, 101–4
        sleep hygiene, 95–96, 186–87
        successful activities, 97
        supervision, 104–5, 105t
        travel, 98–99
    for family, in end-stage dementia, 249, 250
Surgery, for dementia patient, 107–8
Suspiciousness, 161–64
    causes, 162–63
    definition, 161–62
    eating problems in, 170
    management, 163–64

Tacrine, 210
Talk (speech)
    in mental status examination, 25–26
    pragmatics, in communication with
        dementia patient, 90
Tardive dyskinesia, from antipsychotic
        drugs, 217
Task breakdown, 290–91
Tau protein
    in fronto-temporal degeneration, 49, 50
    test for, 235
Team approach
    to dementia care, 81
    to evaluation of dementia, 18
Temporal lobe injury, catastrophic reaction
        in, 135
Terminal care, 241–50
    autopsy issues, 250
    bowel care, 246
    dehydration, 248
    emotional upheaval, 249
    family and patient wishes, 242–44
    family reactions to death, 249–50
    family supportive care, 249, 250
    feeding problems, 245
    hospice care, 243–44, 249
    maintaining patient dignity, 247–48
    medical interventions, benefits and
        burdens, 244–45
    oral health, 247
    predictors of death, 242, 243t
    restraints, 248–49
    seizures, 248
    skin care, 246
Tertiary prevention, 231
Testamentary capacity, 265
Thalamostriatal fronto-temporal degenera-
        tion, 49
Thermoregulation, impaired, from anti-
        psychotic drugs, 216

Thiothixine, side effects, 218t
Thought content, in mental status examination, 28–29
Thoughts of death, suicide, or homicide, in mental status examination, 27
Three-step command, in Mini-Mental State Examination, 33
Thrombotic stroke, 71
Time orientation, in Mini-Mental State Examination, 30
Toileting problems, 176–81
    in end-stage dementia, 246
    preventive health care, 106–7, 172
    tips for caregiver, 285–86
Tolcapone, 228
Toxic dementia, 73–74
Trail Making Test, verbal form, 35–36
Transferring difficulty, 188–92
Tranylcypromine, side effects, 220t
Traumatic brain injury, dementia after, 71–73
Travel, with dementia patient, 98–99
Trazodone
    indications, 219
    side effects, 220t
    for sleep problems, 187–88
    for yelling, calling out, and screaming, 154
Treatment plan
    attributes, 77–79, 78t
    implementing, 79–82
Tremor, in Parkinson's disease, 57
Tricyclic antidepressants
    cardiotoxicity, 221–22
    side effects, 220t
Truth-telling, ethical issues, 255–57
Tube feeding
    in end-stage dementia, 244
    ethical issues, 259–61

Ulcers, decubitus, prevention, 246
Uncooperativeness, 138–43
    causes, 139–41
    definition, 138–39
    management, 141–43
Underwear, with hip pads, 191
Urinary incontinence, 176–81
    causes, 177–78
    definition, 176–77
    in end-stage dementia, 246
    management, 178–81
    in normal pressure hydrocephalus, 62
Urinary tract infection
    aggression from, 202

delirium from, 150
incontinence and toileting problems from, 177–78

Vaccine, beta-amyloid, 205
Vacuolization, in fronto-temporal degeneration, 50
Vascular dementia, 69–71, 70t
    cholinesterase inhibitors for, 211
    genetic counseling and presymptomatic testing, 276
    preventive interventions, 232–33
Vascular depression, 68–69, 70, 213
Vasculopathy, hypertensive, 71
Venlafaxine
    dosage and administration, 221
    side effects, 220t
Visuospatial function
    in expanded cognitive examination, 34–35
    in Mini-Mental State Examination, 33
    in Parkinson's disease, 58
Vital sense, in mental status examination, 27
Vitamin B_{12}, dementia and, 235
Vitamin C, for Alzheimer's disease, 207
Vitamin E, for Alzheimer's disease, 207
Vocalizations. See Yelling, calling out, and screaming

Walking problems, 188–92
Wandering, 146–49
    causes, 147–48
    definition, 146–47
    management, 148–49
Wandering garden, 149
Weakness, falling due to, 189, 190
Weight loss, 169–72, 259–61
Wernicke aphasia, 26
Wernicke-Korsakoff syndrome, 74
White matter loss, vascular dementia from, 69
Will, living, 266

Yelling, calling out, and screaming, 152–55
    causes, 152–53
    definition, 152
    management, 153–55
Young person, dementia care for, 84

Zalepelon, 226
    for sleep problems, 188
Zolpidem, 226
    side effects, 225
    for sleep problems, 188